LIBRARY

Direct Line: 020 7290 2940 Direct Fax: 020 7290 2939
Direct Line: 0171 290 2940 Direct Fax: 0171 290 2939

DIFFICULT HYPERTENSION PRACTICAL MANAGEMENT AND DECISION MAKING

Martin J Kendall MD FRCP
Reader in Clinical Pharmacology
Clinical Pharmacology Section
Department of Medicine
University of Birmingham
Queen Elizabeth Hospital
Birmingham, UK

Norman M Kaplan MD
Professor of Internal Medicine
Department of Internal Medicine
University of Texas Southwestern Medical School
Dallas TX, USA

Richard C Horton BSc MB
North American Editor
The Lancet
New York NY, USA

MARTIN DUNITZ

1995

© Martin Dunitz Ltd 1995

First published in the United Kingdom in 1995 by
Martin Dunitz Ltd
The Livery House
7–9 Pratt Street
London NW1 0AE

A CIP catalogue record for this book is available
from the British Library

ISBN 1-85317-214-6

Composition by Scribe Design, Gillingham, Kent
Printed and bound in Great Britain

CONTENTS

List of Contributors

Dr Dwomoa Adu MA MB MD BChir FRCP
Consultant Physician and Nephrologist, Queen Elizabeth Hospital, Birmingham B15 2TH, UK.

Professor Anthony H Barnett BSc MD FRCP
Professor of Diabetic Medicine, the University of Birmingham, and Honorary Consultant Physician, Department of Medicine, Birmingham Heartlands Hospital, Birmingham B9 5SS, UK.

Professor Christopher Bulpitt
Professor of Geriatric Medicine, Royal Postgraduate Medical School, Hammersmith Hospital, London W12 0HS, UK.

Dr Ian G Chadwick MB ChB MRCP
Sheffield Hypertension Clinic, University Department of Medicine & Pharmacology, Royal Hallamshire Hospital, Sheffield S10 2JF, UK.

Dr Michael de Swiet MD FRCP FRCOG
Academic Sub-Dean to the Institute of Obstetrics and Gynaecology, Royal Postgraduate Medical School, and Honorary Consultant Physician Queen Charlotte's and Chelsea Hospital, Hammersmith Hospital, Northwick Park Hospital and University College Hospital, London, UK.

Dr Jane E Deal MRCP DCH
Consultant Paediatrician and Paediatric Nephrologist, Department of Paediatrics, St Mary's Hospital, London W2 1NY, UK.

Dr Astrid Fletcher
Senior Lecturer in Epidemiology, Department of Epidemiology and Population Sciences, London School of Hygiene and Tropical Medicine, London, UK.

Dr Neil J L Gittoes BSc MB ChB MRCP
Registrar in Endocrinology, Department of Medicine, University of Birmingham, Queen Elizabeth Hospital, Birmingham B15 2TH, UK.

Dr Iftikhar Ul Haq MB ChB MRCP
Sheffield Hypertension Clinic, University Department of Medicine & Pharmacology, University of Sheffield, Royal Hallamshire Hospital, Sheffield S10 2JF, UK.

Professor Peter Hutton PhD FFA RCS
Hickman Professor of Anaesthesia, Department of Anaesthesia and Intensive Care, University of Birmingham, Queen Elizabeth Hospital, Birmingham B15 2TH, UK.

Dr Peter R Jackson PhD MB ChB
Senior Lecturer, University of Sheffield, Department of Medicine & Pharmacology, Section of Pharmacology & Therapeutics, Royal Hallamshire Hospital, Sheffield S10 2JF, UK.

Dr Ulf Lindblad MD PhD
Skaraborg Institute, S-541 45 Skövde, Sweden.

Dr Simon R J Maxwell BSc MB ChB MRCP
Lecturer in Clinical Pharmacology, Department of Medicine, University of Birmingham, Queen Elizabeth Hospital, Birmingham B15 2TH, UK.

Dr Anthony F Nash MB BCh MRCP
Medical Adviser, Cardiovascular Group, Medical Research Department, ZENECA Pharmaceuticals, Mereside, Alderley Park, Nr Macclesfield, Cheshire, SK10 4TG, UK.

Dr Barnabas Panayiotou BM BS MRCP
Senior Registrar in General and Geriatric Medicine, Department of Clinical Pharmacology, City General Hospital, Stoke-on-Trent ST4 6QG, UK.

Dr Iris Rajman
Medical Research Fellow, Department of Clinical Pharmacology, Queen Elizabeth Hospital, Birmingham B15 2TH, UK.

Professor Lawrence E Ramsay MB ChB FRCP FFPM RCP
Professor of Clinical Pharmacology & Therapeutics, University of Sheffield, Department of Medicine & Pharmacology, Section of Pharmacology & Therapeutics, and Consultant Physician, Royal Hallamshire Hospital, Sheffield S10 2JF, UK.

Dr Lennart Råstam MD PhD
Associate Professor of Family Medicine, Division of Epidemiology, School of Public Health, University of Minnesota, Minneapolis MN 55454-1015, USA, and Department of Community Health Sciences, Lund University, S-21401 Malmö, Sweden.

Dr Ali Raza BSc MB BS
Director of Clinical and Medical Affairs, Clinical and Medical Affairs Group, ZENECA Pharma Inc, Mississuaga ON, L5N 5R7, Canada.

Dr Scott H Russell FRCA
Senior Registrar and Honorary Lecturer in Anaesthesia, Department of Anaesthesia and Intensive Care, University of Birmingham, Queen Elizabeth Hospital, Birmingham B15 2TH, UK.

Professor Lars Rydén MD PhD
Professor of Cardiology, Department of Cardiology, Karolinska Hospital, S-171 76 Stockholm, Sweden.

Professor Michael C Sheppard PhD MB ChB FRCP
Professor of Endocrinology, University of Birmingham, and Honorary Consultant Physician, Queen Elizabeth Hospital, Birmingham B15 2TH, UK.

Dr Roger Shinton MSc MA MB BChir MRCP
Consultant Physician, Department of Medicine for the Elderly, Birmingham Heartlands NHS Trust, Yardley Green Hospital, Birmingham B9 5PX, UK.

Dr Donald Stribling MA PhD
International Product Development Manager, International Development Department, ZENECA Pharmaceuticals, Mereside, Alderley Park, Nr Macclesfield, Cheshire, SK10 4TG, UK.

Dr Wai Y Tse
Registrar in Renal Medicine, Department of Nephrology, Queen Elizabeth Hospital, Birmingham B15 2TH, UK.

Dr Wilfred W Yeo MB ChB MRCP
Lecturer, University of Sheffield,
Department of Medicine & Pharmacology,
Section of Pharmacology & Therapeutics,
Royal Hallamshire Hospital, Sheffield
S10 2JF, UK.

Acknowledgements

Charles Darwin wrote that 'a naturalist's life would be a happy one if he had only to observe, and never to write'. The writing of any book involves the toil of people well beyond a small circle of authors. We owe especially warm thanks to Debbie Eaton in Birmingham, UK, for coordinating the efficent assembling of our contributors' (and our own) manuscripts. And, of course, at moments of profound doubt and self searching, one relies on the irrepressible optimism and good cheer of one's editor. All three of us have many reasons to thank Alan Burgess of Martin Dunitz Ltd. His unusual blend of indefatigable trust, patience, and diplomacy in handling our occasionally divergent enthusiasms has allowed us to produce a book for which the epithet 'difficult' deservedly applies to the subject and not, thankfully, to the project.

MJK
NMK
RCH

To Andrew, Mark and Adam
MJK

To my wife Audrey
NMK

To Ingrid Wolfe
RCH

Introduction

Hypertension is common. For instance, in the USA, about 50 million people have a mean blood pressure consistently greater than 140/90 mm.[1] If left untreated, the consequences are severe. Patients with hypertension are at markedly increased risk of suffering and dying from the effects of coronary, cerebrovascular, renal, and peripheral vascular disease. The key aim of treatment is therefore to lower the blood pressure and thereby to reduce the risks and prolong the patient's life while not worsening the quality of that life.

Treatment of moderate and severe hypertension can be profoundly beneficial.[2,3] Successful control of blood pressure is associated with a diminution in the incidence of stroke.[4] The beneficial effects on coronary artery disease are less clear[5] but control of blood pressure has probably contributed substantially to the steady decline in mortality from ischaemic heart disease since the early 1970s. Furthermore, the incidence of congestive heart failure and hypertensive renal damage have been favorably influenced by treatment. The evidence about the treatment of mild hypertension and hypertension in the elderly is open to several interpretations because of the difficulty in balancing risk and benefit; however, the trend is towards benefit, and recent studies in older subjects have shown that the detection and treatment of elderly hypertensives with a simple and inexpensive regimen will have a major impact upon strokes, heart failure and coronary disease. There remains concern about the relatively lesser protection from coronary disease seen in the clinical trials involving both younger and older patients. Vascular diseases, particularly coronary events and strokes, remain the most frequent cause of death in the developed world, and it is therefore abundantly clear that the battle to reduce risk must go on.

Since hypertension is largely a mechanical problem and there are drugs available that can reduce the pressure in the vascular tree, the management of hypertension should, in theory, be relatively easy. However, hypertension is not a single entity and patients come in different sizes and from different ethnic groups, and they present at any age and under varying circumstances, from childhood, through pregnancy, and into old age. Furthermore, they may suffer from co-existing diseases that require competing therapies, and they may first present with extensive atheromatous disease of the coronary or cerebral arteries (i.e. when the diseases we are trying to prevent are already well advanced). Finally, the drug treatments available to correct hypertension all have their merits and defects. Determining the optimal therapeutic strategy may therefore be quite difficult, a fact that makes the treatment of hypertension interesting and challenging.

Many books on therapeutics or clinical pharmacology are available which cover the theoretical aspects of drugs. In this book, we attempt to mimic clinical practice and to address the problems posed when the doctor faces patients of different ages, ethnic backgrounds, coexisting conditions, and concomitant diseases.

Therefore, a discussion of hypertension in children, pregnancy, the elderly, and ethnic groups makes up Part I of this book. As the patient will present with a particular type of high blood pressure, in Part II we have focused on secondary, accelerated, unresponsive, and isolated systolic hypertension as the especially relevant and 'difficult' areas for physicians. Because the patient with a particular type of hypertension will present in various settings, in Part III we have included discussions of hypertension in diabetes mellitus and renal disease, after myocardial infarction, in stroke, under general anaesthesia, and with other concomitant diseases. Finally, whenever one is deciding about management, one must have a firm grasp of how to interpret published evidence on treatment and how to relate that evidence to a patient's quality of life. These topics are to be found in Part IV.

A greater impact on the complications of hypertension will result from more effective therapy producing better blood pressure control. To achieve the greatest benefit with the least costs, the therapeutic plan must be based on a better understanding of the disease, the particular problems of different patient groups, and the drugs available to treat hypertension. Patients who have hypertension but are undetected and untreated need to be found and offered appropriate therapy. This raises important concerns about the scale of the task, the feasibility with which it can be overcome, and the cost, both medical and economic. A pragmatic, patient-centered approach offers one means of achieving our goals.

Martin J Kendall
Norman M Kaplan
Richard C Horton

References

1 National High Blood Pressure Education Program Working Group. *Ann Intern Med* 1993; **153**:186–208.

2 Kaplan NM. *Clinical Hypertension*. Baltimore: Williams and Wilkins, 1994.

3 Swales JD. Pharmacological treatment of hypertension. *Lancet* 1994; **344**:380–5.

4 Garraway WM, Whisnant JP. The changing pattern of hypertension and the declining incidence of stroke. *JAMA* 1987; **258**:214–17.

5 Kendall MJ, Horton RC. *Preventing Coronary Artery Disease*. London: Martin Dunitz, 1994.

SECTION I

THE PATIENT

1

Treatment of children with hypertension

Jane E Deal

The management of hypertension in children has many principles and practices in common with the management of hypertension in adults, but it also presents its own unique problems:

- The initial recognition of what is a significantly raised blood pressure for a child;
- the spectrum of causes and underlying diseases that may be involved;
- the natural history of the underlying cause of the hypertension in relation to growth and maturation;
- the problems of deciding which therapeutic approach will be most effective;
- which drugs are the most appropriate and what dose to use;
- the issues of compliance and the long-term effects of therapy.

Normal standards exist for blood pressure in children, and these are expressed either relative to the child's age, or more usefully, to the child's height.[1,2] Using these standards, hypertension is defined as a blood pressure value that is consistently above the 95th centile for sex and age or sex and height.

The majority of children who have sustained significant hypertension will be found to have secondary hypertension; however a small percentage will have essential hypertension, the prevalence of primary hypertension increasing through childhood and approaching adult levels in late adolescence. Of those children found to have secondary hypertension the majority will

have underlying renal disease, most commonly coarse renal scarring secondary to reflux or obstructive nephropathy or glomerular disease. Coarctation of the aorta is the commonest non-renal cause of hypertension in children (see Table 1.1).[3–7]

Because of the high prevalence of secondary causes of hypertension in children investigation of the hypertensive child usually needs to be extensive. Investigation is aimed not only at elucidating the underlying cause of the hypertension, in the hope that a potentially curable cause will be found, but also at detecting any evidence of end-organ effect from the hypertension (e.g. retinopathy, left ventricular hypertrophy, or renal damage) which will influence the decision as to whether the blood pressure requires treatment or not. For children with blood pressures consistently just above the 95th centile for age or height but without evidence of end-organ effect, it is difficult to decide the best therapeutic approach, and many paediatricians will begin with non-pharmacological measures and follow these children carefully and closely.

Management of hypertensive emergencies

Between 6 and 27% of children with significant hypertension present as a hypertensive emergency, i.e. with a blood pressure above

	Aderele et al, 1974[3]	Gill et al, 1976[4]	Deal et al, 1992[5]	Wyszynska et al, 1992[6]	Arar et al, 1994[7]
Coarse renal scars					
Reflux nephropathy	1.5	14	18	11	20
Obstructive uropathy	0.7	6	16	5	2
Glomerular disease	89	35	27.5	6	28
Renovascular disease	2.2	6	8	4	5
Haemolytic uraemic syndrome	0.7	6	7	1.3	—
Polycystic kidney disease	—	4	5	2	8
Renal dysplasia	—	5	3	—	—
Wilms' tumour	0.7	1	2	—	1
Coarctation of the aorta	—	15	1.5	29	2
Phaeochromocytoma	—	—	1	0.7	—
Renal vein thrombosis	—	—	1	—	—
Idiopathic (essential)	4.4	2	4	33	23
Miscellaneous	0.7	6	6	8	11

Table 1.1
Prevalence of different causes of hypertension in children, expressed as a percentage.

the 99th centile for sex and age or sex and height, and with associated neurological signs and symptoms.[3–5,8] It is important that the blood pressure in these children is controlled as soon as is possible to prevent the development of further hypertensive complications. However, care must be taken not to lower the blood pressure too quickly as relative hypotension could occur with catastrophic consequences for the child.[5] Initial assessment is aimed at estimating the duration of symptoms and the possible underlying aetiology, and there must be a careful examination looking for signs of end-organ damage and neurological abnormalities. Cardiac function and the child's fluid status must also be assessed. These children should ideally be managed in units skilled at the management of severely ill children where close and frequent monitoring can occur.

As a general rule of thumb, if the hypertension is of short duration (i.e. hours or a few days at most), then the blood pressure can be brought down relatively quickly. If there is any possibility that the hypertension is of long standing, then the blood pressure must be brought down to the desired level slowly over a period of at least 3 days. Ideally, blood pressure reduction should always be controlled and incremental, thereby avoiding sudden hypotensive or hypertensive swings.

Drugs in hypertensive emergencies

The choice of drugs for use in a hypertensive emergency should be governed by the need for an agent with rapid onset of action, short duration of effect, and easy administration. Angiotensin converting enzyme (ACE) inhibitors should not be used as first line drugs in hypertensive emergencies in children because of the possibility of an underlying renal artery stenosis and the well-recognized association of renal failure with ACE inhibitor use in this situation. Beta-blocking agents must be avoided or used with caution in any child with a history of asthma or with features of cardiac failure. Unless it is clear that the child is fluid overloaded (e.g. as in acute glomerulonephritis), diuretics should be avoided because, in many cases of hypertension in children, the hypertension is due to a chronic excess of plasma renin activity and the child will therefore be relatively salt and water depleted. In this situation the use of a diuretic may result in a profound and exaggerated hypotensive response.[9]

Routes of drug administration

The best and safest route of drug administration is the intravenous route. This will also allow venous access if hypotensive complications occur and the blood pressure needs to be raised again by the infusion of normal saline. Bolus therapy by whatever route, but particularly oral or intramuscular administration, should be avoided as unpredictable and sustained drops in pressure can occur.[6,11]

In an emergency, drugs may be administered by the oral or sublingual route, but in some children this may be either impractical because of altered levels of consciousness or unsuitable because of the unpredictable rate of absorption of the drug from the gastrointestinal tract. Successful administration of nifedipine via the rectal route has been reported in children with acute, severe hypertension, and this may overcome some of the difficulties of drug administration in this situation, though care must be taken as with any other bolus therapy.[10] Intramuscular injections can be used but are unpleasant for children and are best avoided. Furthermore, the rate of absorption of the drug via this route in a severely ill child is unpredictable.

Therefore, on admission, any child deemed to require emergency treatment for hypertension should have an intravenous line inserted. During the treatment of any hypertensive emergency the child must be closely monitored. This not only includes frequent blood pressure measurements but also looking for signs of hypotensive complications, which can be assessed by testing pupillary responses, monitoring the level of consciousness, and measuring urine output.

After initial examination and assessment, treatment with one of the suggested first line drugs should be commenced. Goals for the control of the hypertension should be set by assessing what the ideal blood pressure for the sex, age and height of the child is and then aiming to reduce the blood pressure by only a third of the eventual desired fall in the first 24 hours after the start of treatment, a third in the subsequent 24 hours, with the final reduction of blood pressure during the third day (Table 1.2).

Treatment should be commenced using the lowest recommended dose, which should be increased if the desired reduction in blood pressure is not achieved. If on reaching the maximum recommended dose an adequate effect on blood pressure has not been seen then a second agent should be added. Drugs used in the treatment of hypertensive emergencies are shown in Table 1.3. Drugs of choice include labetalol, sodium nitroprusside, nifedipine, or diazoxide.

A 7-year-old girl, height 125 cm, weight 24 kg, is admitted with a blood pressure of 220/165 mmHg.

"Ideal" BP for child 87–120 mmHg systolic	(104 mmHg 50th centile)
Therefore total BP reduction to be achieved	100 mmHg systolic
Lowest desired BP at end of 1st 24 hours	185 mmHg systolic
Lowest desired BP at end of 2nd 24 hours	150 mmHg systolic
Lowest desired BP at end of 3rd 24 hours	120 mmHg systolic

Initial sliding scale prescription for intravenous infusion:

Make up 100 mg labetalol to 50 ml with 5% dextrose (1 ml = 2 mg)

If systolic BP > 230 mmHg call doctor

If systolic BP 210–230 mmHg run labetalol at 12 ml/hr
    (= 1 mg/kg/hr)

If systolic BP 190–210 mmHg run labetalol at 6 ml/hr
    (= 0.5 mg/kg/hr)

If systolic BP 180–190 mmHg run 5% dextrose at 5 ml/hr

If systolic BP < 180 mmHg run in 50 ml N saline and call doctor

Changes in the infusion rate should only be made after 2 consistent BP readings 5 minutes apart.

Table 1.2

Example of an emergency treatment programme for a hypertensive child admitted to hospital. This programme would be attached to the patient's drug chart or nursing orders.

Surgical treatment of hypertension in children

A number of children with significant, sustained hypertension will have a potentially surgically remediable underlying cause. Treatment in this situation is aimed at not only curing the hypertension or reducing the need for antihypertensive medication but also at the preservation of functioning renal tissue. Techniques used in the surgical management of hypertensive children are shown in Table 1.4.

Before any surgical procedure or invasive investigation is carried out, it is important that the blood pressure is adequately controlled medically and that the fluid status of the child is satisfactory. In the past, high mortality rates were reported for children with phaeochromocytomata in the perioperative period because of inadequate catecholamine blockade resulting in either catastrophic hypotension or hypertension.[12]

Tumours causing hypertension

The hypertension associated with tumours of the adrenal or renal cortex may not only be associated with excess secretion of catecholamines or renin but have also been reported to be associated with stenosis of renal arteries.[13,14] This can be anticipated by thorough preoperative investigation. In addition, tumours of the autonomic nervous system are more likely to be multiple and extra-adrenal in site in children than in

Drug	Dose	Mode of action	Onset of action	Half life	Comments
First line drugs					
Labetalol	1–3 mg/kg/hr iv infusion	alpha- and beta-receptor blocker	minutes	4–6 hours	contraindicated in asthma or cardiac failure
Sodium nitroprusside	0.5–8.0 µg/kg/min iv infusion	vasodilator	immediate	minutes	risk of cyanide and thiocyanate toxicity if used for prolonged time
Diazoxide	2–5 mg/kg iv	vasodilator	immediate	20–36 hours	risk of hyperglycaemia
Nifedipine	0.25–0.5 mg/kg, sublingual, oral, or rectal	calcium channel blocker	10–30 minutes	2–6 hours	
Second line drugs					
Hydralazine	0.2–0.4 mg/kg iv	vasodilator	10–20 minutes	3 hours	
Minoxidil	0.1–0.2 mg/kg oral	vasodilator	1–2 hours	1–4 hours	
Captopril	0.05–2 mg/kg oral	ACE inhibitor	15–30 minutes	1–2 hours	avoid if suspected renovascular disease
Frusemide	1–5 mg/kg iv	diuretic	minutes	2–3 hours	use only if fluid overload exists

Table 1.3
Drugs used in the treatment of hypertensive emergencies in children.

adults;[15] hence a careful search must be made before any surgery to detect the sites of all the tumours that may be present. With these precautions, operative mortality should be low.

Renovascular disease
Success rates varying between 36% and 86% have been reported for the surgical treatment of renal artery stenoses in children.[16–21] This is in part due to the more widespread nature of renovascular disease in children than in adults, with bilateral disease reported in 15–70% and small vessel intrarenal disease in 36–76% of children.[16,18,19,22] With improvement in surgical vascular reconstructive techniques fewer children are undergoing nephrectomy or heminephrectomy, and smaller children and smaller vessels are being tackled. Success has also been reported recently using selective embolization in children with small vessel

Repair of coarctation of the aorta
Removal of renal tumours and tumours of the sympathetic nervous system and adrenal cortex
Renovascular disease
• nephrectomy or partial nephrectomy
• reconstructive vascular surgery
  (aortorenal anastomosis, splenorenal
  anastomosis, iliorenal anastomosis,
  saphenous vein bypass grafts,
  autotransplantation)
• percutaneous transluminal angioplasty
• segmental renal artery embolization
Renal parenchymal disease
• nephrectomy
• partial nephrectomy

Table 1.4
Indications for surgical treatment of hypertension.

intrarenal disease to cure renovascular hypertension.[23]

Percutaneous transluminal angioplasty (PTA) is being increasingly used in the management of renovascular disease in children. Success rates vary between 38% and 90%, depending upon the site and cause of the stenosis, the appropriate selection of patients for treatment and the extent of their disease.[17,24,25] Even if cure of the hypertension is not achieved by PTA, improvement in hypertension and a decrease in the need for antihypertensive medication may be seen and functioning renal tissue preserved by the procedure. PTA has also been reported to be of use in the long term management of children with widespread vascular disease, by the use of repeat angioplasty when restenosis or progression of the stenosis is seen in a growing child.[26]

Renal scarring

Children with hypertension caused by renal scarring that is secondary to either reflux nephropathy or urological problems may be helped by the removal of renal tissue by complete or partial nephrectomy. Before this is undertaken, the child should be carefully assessed, and this preoperative assessment should include renin sampling from the renal veins, inferior vena cava, and the segmental renal veins to document the extent of disease involvement. If possible, surgical intervention should be delayed until there is no further risk of damage to the renal parenchyma (from continuing urinary tract infections, vesicoureteric reflux, or obstruction), and maximum renal growth has occurred.

Medical treatment of significant hypertension in children

Children with sustained, significant hypertension should be treated with antihypertensive agents because the mortality and morbidity of untreated hypertension is high in this group.[27] Treatment may need to be long term. The choice of the most appropriate agent to use is guided by a knowledge of the underlying cause,

Drug	Dose	Number of doses per day	Preparations available
Beta-blockers			
Atenolol	1–2 mg/kg/day	1–2	tablets, syrup
Propranolol	1–10 mg/kg/day	3–4	tablets, syrup
Metoprolol	1–2 mg/kg/day	2–4	tablets
Vasodilators			
Hydralazine	1–8 mg/kg/day	2–3	tablets
Minoxidil	0.1–2.0 mg/kg/day	1–2	tablets
Calcium channel blockers			
Nifedipine	0.25–2 mg/kg/day	3	capsules
		2	slow release tablets
ACE inhibitors			
Enalapril	0.1–0.5 mg/kg/day	1	tablets
Captopril	0.3–5.0 mg/kg/day	3	tablets
Diuretics			
Hydrochlorothiazide	1–4 mg/kg/day	1–2	tablets
Frusemide	0.5–15 mg/kg/day	2–3	tablets, syrup
Metolazone	0.1–5 mg/kg/day	1–2	tablets
Spironolactone	1–3 mg/kg/day	1–3	tablets, syrup
Triamterene	1–3 mg/kg/day	1–2	capsules
Amiloride	0.2–1 mg/kg/day	1–2	tablets
Alpha-blockers			
Prazosin	0.05–0.4 mg/kg/day	2–3	tablets
Phenoxybenzamine	1–4 mg/kg/day	1–2	capsules
Centrally acting agents			
Methyldopa	5–10 mg/kg/day	2	tablets, syrup
Clonidine	0.002–0.1 mg/kg/day	2	tablets, capsules

Table 1.5
Oral drugs used in the treatment of hypertension in children.

the age and size of the child, and the medical unit's experience with the various agents that are available. In addition, it is recommended that as few drugs as is possible are used and that they are given as infrequently as possible in order to improve compliance. For very young children, liquid preparations are often necessary, and these may need to be prepared by a paediatric pharmacist. Even so, quite young children can often manage tablets, either swallowed whole or crushed. A child who needs to take crushed tablets will not be able to use the currently available slow-release preparations.

Many drugs used in the treatment of hypertension have not been specifically licensed for use in children, though most of the commoner antihypertensive drugs have been safely used for many years and numerous reports are to be found in the literature regarding their use in children.

When prescribing drugs for children, dosages are worked out on a per kilogram weight basis. Tablet sizes that are available are not always suitable for very small children and a specialist paediatric pharmacy may be needed to ensure that suitable doses are available. Drugs that have been used in the medical management of hypertension are shown in Table 1.5.

First-line therapy
As in adult practice, a step-wise approach to the introduction of oral drugs is used in children (Figure 1.1).[1,9] Recommendations for first-line therapy have in the past advised the use of beta-blockers and/or diuretics as initial therapy,[9,28] and many paediatricians have successfully used the combination of a beta-blocker with a vasodilator in their initial management of the hypertensive child. Nowadays, because of concerns regarding these drugs and their long-term effects on serum lipid levels, recommendations are changing to the more frequent use of calcium channel blockers and ACE inhibitors as first line therapy.[29] No studies have yet been reported in children regarding the use of the various antihypertensive drugs and their long-term effects on cardiovascular and cerebrovascular morbidity and mortality or on their relationship to risk factors such as lipid levels and insulin sensitivity.

ACE inhibitors are attractive for use in children with hypertension, given the high incidence of secondary renal causes of hypertension. However, care must be taken with use of ACE inhibitors in children in whom renal artery stenosis has not been excluded and in children who have other forms of renin dependent hypertension. It is recommended that lower doses are used in infants, particularly those under the age of 6 months, as this younger age-group has a more active renin–angiotensin system.[30]

Although largely superceded by the newer antihypertensive agents drugs such as prazosin, minoxidil, methyldopa, and clonidine still have a place as second-line therapy for children with resistant hypertension or for those who suffer unacceptable side effects; they are often highly effective in these situations.

Treatment of mild hypertension in children

Although there is good evidence that tracking of blood pressure occurs during childhood, the predictive value of a high blood pressure reading for the future development of hypertension is not as useful in children as it is in adults.[31] As a consequence, the potential benefits of early pharmacological treatment of mild hypertension versus the risks of long term drug therapy for the growing and developing child are unknown. When faced with a child who has mild hypertension, as defined by the accepted criteria, but who has no evidence of retinopathy, left ventricular hypertrophy, or proteinuria and in whom there is no known, progressive, underlying, secondary cause of hypertension, most paediatricians will opt for careful follow-up and the initial use of non-pharmacological strategies for lowering the blood pressure.

Hypertension and diet
Good correlations exist between the presence of obesity and hypertension in children and adolescents,[32–35] the relationship between body size and blood pressure being present by the age of 6 years.[36] Studies in children have shown

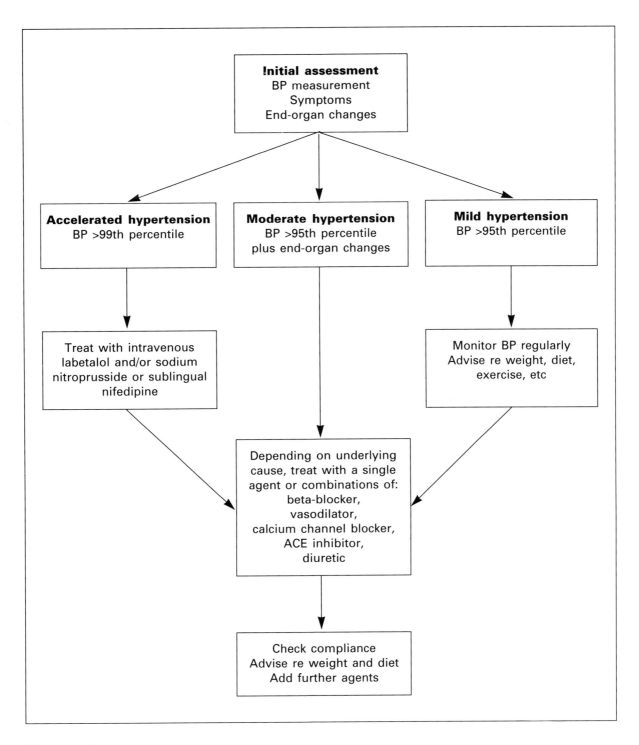

Figure 1.1
Scheme for the management of hypertension in children

an improvement in both systolic and diastolic blood pressure with weight loss.[34,37,38] In addition, weight loss is associated with an improvement in other cardiovascular risk factors (such as serum lipid levels), and so it should be encouraged in children with mild hypertension.

The role of salt restriction in the management of the child with mild hypertension is controversial. Although clinical studies have demonstrated an effect of salt restriction on blood pressure in children the results are confounded in some studies by the associated effects on other dietary components such as potassium supplementation, calorie restriction, and changes in levels of fitness.[1,39–43] Nevertheless, most paediatricians would recommend a reduction in salt intake in the hypertensive child, although this is often difficult to achieve because of the high salt content of the sorts of food that are popular with children. Compliance with a diet, unless the child and his or her family are well motivated, is often poor.

Other dietary approaches, such as potassium supplementation, calcium supplementation, and the use of high-fibre and vegetarian diets, have been proposed. Although they are associated with a fall in blood pressure in the short term, the evidence for their long-term efficacy in children with mild hypertension is not available.[40,44–46]

A low-level correlation has been reported between blood pressure and the intake of dietary protein, fat, and carbohydrate in children in the USA.[47] However, it is not clear if reductions in serum cholesterol and lipid on their own will result in a lowering of blood pressure in the hypertensive child. Nevertheless, dietary restriction of lipids are seen to be an important part of the general advice given to patients as part of a cardiovascular disease prevention programme.[29]

Hypertension and exercise

Studies have shown that improvement in physical fitness by a programme of regular exercise has lowered blood pressure in children and adolescents.[48,49] It is not known whether exercise will have long-term benefits for children with mild hypertension, and some studies have shown an acute rise in blood pressure in association with exercise in children who are hypertensive.[50,51] Therefore, advice regarding exercise and participation in sports must be cautious for the child who has established hypertension, particularly if it is severe.

Compliance

Compliance with antihypertensive treatment can be a problem in children. Compliance is usually best in young children whose drugs are supervised by their parents. It is also improved by the use of as few agents as possible and once- or twice-a-day doses at most. Compliance usually worsens in adolescence and it is important that children, as they grow older, receive adequate explanation as to their underlying disease and therapy so that they feel supported and involved in their care. Non-pharmacological therapy is particularly difficult for some children who are not suitably motivated, and this particularly applies to compliance with dietary restrictions. With constructive support, compliance of 80–90% has been reported in adolescents.[29]

References

1 Report of the Second Task Force on Blood Pressure Control in Children. *Pediatrics* 1987; **79:**1–25.

2 de Man SA, Andre J-L, Bachmann H et al. Blood pressure in childhood: pooled findings of six European studies. *J Hypertens* 1991; **9:** 109–14.

3 Aderele WI, Seriki O. Hypertension in Nigerian children. *Arch Dis Child* 1974; **49:**313–17.

4 Gill DG, Mendes da Costa B, Cameron JS, Joseph MC, Ogg CS, Chantler C. Analysis of 100 children with severe and persistent hypertension. *Arch Dis Child* 1976; **51:**951–6.

5 Deal J, Barratt TM, Dillon MJ. Management of hypertensive emergencies. *Arch Dis Child* 1992; **67:**1089–92.

6 Wyszynska T, Cichocka E, Wieteska-Klimczak A, Jobs K, Januszewicz P. A single pediatric center experience with 1025 children with hypertension. *Acta Paediatr* 1992; **81:**244–6.

7 Arar MY, Hogg RJ, Arant BS Jr, Seikaly MG. Etiology of sustained hypertension in children in the southwestern United States. *Pediatr Nephrol* 1994; **8:**186–9.

8 Still JL, Cottom D. Severe hypertension in childhood. *Arch Dis Child* 1967; **42:**34–9.

9 Dillon MJ. Investigation and management of hypertension in children. A personal perspective. *Pediatr Nephrol* 1987; **1:**59-68.

10 Uchiyama M, Sakai K. Rectal administration of perforated nifedipine capsules in acute severe hypertension in children. *Br J Clin Pract* 1992; **46:**100–1.

11 Wachter RM. Symptomatic hypotension induced by nifedipine in the acute treatment of severe hypertension. *Arch Intern Med* 1987; **147:**556–8.

12 Ellis D, Gartner JC. The intraoperative medical management of childhood phaeochromocytoma. *J Pediatr Surg* 1980; **15:**655–9.

13 Robinson MJ, Kent M, Stocks J. Phaeochromocytoma in childhood. *Arch Dis Child* 1973; **48:**137–142.

14 Rosenheim ML, Ross EJ, Wrong OM, Hodson CJ, Davis DR, Smith JF. Unilateral renal ischaemia due to compression of a renal artery by a phaeochromocytoma. *Ann J Med* 1963; **34:**735–48.

15 Stackpole RH, Melicow MM, Uson AC. Pheochromocytoma in children. *J Pediatr* 1963; **63:**315–30.

16 Daniels SR, Loggie JMH, McEnery PT, Towbin RB. Clinical spectrum of intrinsic renovascular hypertension in children. *Pediatr* 1987; **80:**698–704.

17 Guzzetta PC, Potter BM, Ruley EJ, Majd M, Bock GH. Renovascular hypertension in children: current concepts in evaluation and treatment. *J Pediatr Surg* 1989; **24:**1236–40.

18 Wise KL, McCann RL, Dunnick NR, Paulson DF. Renovascular hypertension. *J Urol* 1988; **140:**911–24.

19 Deal JE, Snell MF, Barratt TM, Dillon MJ. Renovascular disease in childhood. *J Pediatr* 1992; **121:**378–84.

20 Merguerian PA, McLorie GA, Balfe JW, Khoury AE, Churchill BM. Renal autotransplantation in children: a successful treatment for renovascular hypertension. *J Urol* 1990; **144:**1443–5.

21 Berkowitz HD, O'Neill JA Jr. Renovascular hypertension in children. Surgical repair with special reference to the use of reinforced vein grafts. *J Vasc Surg* 1989; **9:**46–55.

22 Stanley JC, Fry WJ. Pediatric renal artery occlusive disease and renovascular hypertension. Etiology, diagnosis and operative treatment. *Arch Surg* 1981; **116:**669–76.

23 Teigen CL, Mitchell SE, Venbrux AC, Christenson MJ, McLean RH. Segmental renal artery embolization for treatment of pediatric renovascular hypertension. *J Vasc Interv Radiol* 1992; **3:**111–17.

24 Chevalier RL, Tegtmeyer CJ, Gomez RA. Percutaneous transluminal angioplasty for renovascular hypertension in children. *Pediatr Nephrol* 1987; **1:**89–98.

25 Cicuto KP, McLean GK, Oleaga JA, Freiman DB, Grossman RA, Ring EJ. Renal artery stenosis: anatomic classification for percutaneous

transluminal angioplasty. *AJR Am J Roentgenol* 1981; **137**:599–601.

26 Simunic S, Winter-Fuduric I, Radanovic B et al. Percutaneous transluminal angioplasty (PTRA) as a method of therapy for renovascular hypertension in children. *Eur J Radiol* 1990; **10**:143–6.

27 Uhari M, Saukkonen AL, Koskimies O. Central nervous system involvement in severe arterial hypertension in childhood. *Eur J Pediatr* 1979; **132**:141–6.

28 Scharer K. Hypertension in children and adolescents – 1986. *Pediatr Nephrol* 1987; **1**:50–8.

29 Sinaiko AR. General considerations and clinical approach to the management of hypertension. In: Loggie JM, ed. *Pediatric and Adolescent Hypertension*. Boston: Blackwell Scientific, 1992: 119–26.

30 Dillon MJ, Ryness JM. Plasma renin activity and aldosterone concentration in children. *Br Med J* 1975: **4**:316–19.

31 Lauer RM, Mahoney LT, Clarke WR. Tracking of blood pressure during childhood: the Muscatine Study. *Clin Exp Hypertens* 1986; **A8**(4, 5):515–37.

32 Lauer RM, Clarke WR. Childhood risk factors for high adult blood pressure: the Muscatine Study. *Pediatrics* 1989; **84**:633–41.

33 Voors AW, Webber LS, Fredrichs RR, Berenson GS. Body height and body mass as determinants of basal blood pressure in children. The Bogalusa Heart Study. *Am J Epidemiol* 1977; **106**:101–8.

34 Rocchini AP. Adolescent obesity and hypertension. *Pediatr Clin North Am* 1993; **40**:81–92.

35 Londe S. Causes of hypertension in the young. *Pediatr Clin North Am* 1978; **25**:55–65.

36 Prineas RJ, Gillum RF, Gomez-Marin O. The determinants of blood pressure levels in children: the Minneapolis children's blood pressure study. In: Loggie JMH, Horan MJ, Gruskin AB, Hohn AR, Dunbar JB, Havlik RJ, eds. *NHLBI Workshop on Juvenile Hypertension*. New York: Biomedical Information, 1984: 21–35.

37 Brownell KD, Kelman JH, Stunkard AJ. Treatment of obese children with and without their mothers: changes in weight and blood pressure. *Pediatrics* 1983; **71**:515–23.

38 Reisin E, Abel R, Modan M, Silverberg DS, Eliahou HE, Modan B. Effect of weight loss without salt restriction on the reduction of blood pressure in overweight hypertensive patients. *N Engl J Med* 1978; **298**:1–6.

39 Gillum RF, Elmer PJ, Prineas RJ. Changing sodium intake in children: the Minneapolis Children's Blood Pressure Study. Hypertension 1981; **3**:698–703.

40 Miller JZ, Weinberger MH. Blood pressure response to sodium restriction and potassium supplementation in healthy normotensive children. *Clin Exp Hypertens* 1986: **A8**:823–7.

41 Howe PRC, Cobiac L, Smith RM. Lack of effect of short-term changes in sodium intake on blood pressure in adolescent school children. *J Hypertens* 1991; **9**:181–6.

42 Whitten CF, Stewart RA. The effect of dietary sodium in infancy on blood pressure and related factors: studies of infants fed salted and unsalted diets for five months at eight months and eight years of age. *Acta Paediatr Scand Suppl* 1980; **279**:2–17.

43 Lauer RM, Filer LJ, Reiter MA, Clarke WR. Blood pressure, salt preference, salt threshold and relative weight. *Am J Dis Child* 1976; **130**:493–7.

44 Grobbee DE, Hofman A. Effect of calcium supplementation on diastolic blood pressure in young people with mild hypertension. *Lancet* 1986; **ii**:703–6.

45 Jenner DA, English DR, Vandongen R et al. Diet and blood pressure in 9 year old Australian children. *Am J Clin Nutr* 1988; **47**:1052–9.

46 Margetts BM, Beilin LJ, Vandongen R, Armstrong BK. Vegetarian diet in mild hypertension: a randomised controlled trial. *Br Med J* 1986; **293**:1468–71.

47 Frank GC, Berenson GS, Webber F. Dietary studies and the relationship of diet to cardiovascular disease risk factor variables in 10 year old children: The Bogalusa Heart Study. *Am J Clin Nutr* 1978; **31**:328–40.

48 Hofman A, Walter HJ, Connelly PA, Vaughan RD. Blood pressure and physical fitness in children. *Hypertension* 1987; **9**:188–91.

49 Fripp RR, Hodgson JL, Kwiterovich PO, Werner JC, Schuler HG, Whitman V. Aerobic capacity, obesity, and atherosclerotic risk factors in male adolescents. *Pediatrics* 1985; **75**:813–18.

50 Dlin R. Blood pressure response to dynamic exercise in healthy and hypertensive youth. *Pediatrician* 1986; **13:**34–43.

51 Chaix RL, Dimitriu VM, Wagniart PR, Safer ME. A simple exercise test in borderline and sustained essential hypertension. *Int J Cardiol* 1982; **1:**371–82.

2

Hypertension in pregnancy
Michael de Swiet

Hypertension in pregnancy can have many different causes but by far the most important is pre-eclampsia. It is pre-eclampsia that makes hypertension the leading cause of maternal mortality in the United Kingdom and a major cause of maternal mortality in all countries.[1] Some of the points to be considered in the management of hypertension in pregnancy and of pre-eclampsia in particular are shown in Table 2.1.

Pre-eclampsia is responsible for about half of induced preterm delivery; and the need to detect pre-eclampsia as early as possible is a major rationale for antenatal care. Although pre-eclampsia was formally diagnosed on the basis of oedema, albuminuria, and raised blood pressure, it is now realized that the condition is caused by an unknown placental factor that affects the endothelium of blood vessels.[2] Since every organ has a blood supply, pre-eclampsia has the potential to be a multi-system disease (see Table 2.2). Therefore the management of pre-eclampsia involves far more than the treatment of hypertension alone.

The precise cause of pre-eclampsia is still unknown, and largely because of this there is no specific marker that distinguishes patients who have pre-eclampsia from those who do not. There is no blood test that precisely diagnoses pre-eclampsia, and even renal biopsy, formerly thought to be specific[3] has now been shown to yield false positive and

Blood Pressure Measurement
Management

   Management of Pre-eclampsia (usually presenting after 30 week's gestation)

      Antihypertensive therapy for severe pre-eclampsia
         Hydralazine
         Labetalol
         Nifedipine
      Anticonvulsant drugs for severe pre-eclampsia and their interactions with antihypertensives

   Hypertension presenting before 30 weeks' gestation
      Differential diagnosis
         Essential hypertension
         Pre-eclampsia
         Phaeochromocytoma
         Coarctation
         Renal failure
      Antihypertensive therapy
         Methyldopa
         Beta-blocking drugs
         Hydralazine
         Labetalol
         Nifedipine

   Prevention of pre-eclampsia

   Management of hypertension before pregnancy

Table 2.1
Points to consider in the management of hypertension in pregnancy

- **Central nevous system**
  Eclamptic convulsions
  Cerebral haemorrhage (intraventricular or subarachnoid)
  Cerebral infarction (microinfarction or macroinfarction, e.g.
    cortical blindness due to infarction of occipital cortex)

- **Eyes**
  Retinal detachment
  Retinal oedema

- **Liver**
  Rupture
  Infarction
  Jaundice
  Decreased synthesis of soluble clotting substances
  HELLP syndrome
  (Haemolysis, Elevated Liver Enzymes, Low Platelets)

- **Kidney**
  Acute tubular necrosis
  Acute cortical necrosis
  Unspecified renal failure

- **Respiratory system**
  Laryngeal oedema
  Pulmonary oedema
  Adult respiratory distress syndrome

- **Coagulation system**
  Thrombocytopenia
  Microhaemangiopathic haemolysis
  HELLP syndrome
  Disseminated intravascular coagulation

Table 2.2
Clinical features of pre-eclampsia

false negative results.[4] However, it is generally accepted that

- pre-eclampsia is a condition most common in primigravidae, in whom the blood pressures rises in the second half of pregnancy in association with proteinuria;

- pre-eclampsia can result in eclamptic grand mal convulsions; and
- pre-eclampsia entirely remits after delivery.

Of course, patients may have hypertension before they are pregnant and these patients may or may not develop superadded pre-eclampsia.

- The maternal syndrome
    Hyperuricaemia (elevated serum urate
        or uric acid)*
    Proteinuria*
    Hypocalcaemia*
    Raised Von Willebrand factor in plasma
    Raised fibronectin in plasma
    Reduced Antithrombin III
    Thrombocytopenia*
    Increased haematocrit*
    Abnormal liver function tests*

- The fetal syndrome
    Intrauterine growth retardation (growth
        scan)*
    Intrauterine hypoxia
        (cardiotochography)*

* Commonly used tests in the clinical practice

Table 2.3
Features of pre-eclampsia found on investigation

In normal patients, the blood pressure tends to fall in the first half of pregnancy, rising to pre-pregnancy levels or higher from about 30 weeks' gestation.[5] Any definition of pre-eclampsia based on blood pressure criteria must take account of these trends. The Redman and Jeffries[6] definition is: 'a diastolic blood pressure below 90 mmHg before 20 weeks, a rise in diastolic blood pressure after 20 weeks gestation to above 90 mmHg and by at least 25 mmHg above the first blood pressure recorded in pregnancy.' This definition has a high probability of predicting the subsequent association with proteinuria in primigravidae but, for the reasons given above, it is not infallible. Some patients meeting these criteria will

not have other features of pre-eclampsia and other patients will appear to have pre-eclampsia without meeting these blood pressure criteria; because we do not have a specific marker for pre-eclampsia no definition based on blood pressure alone will be precise.

Pre-eclampsia is therefore recognized in patients who have the clinical features listed in Table 2.2 and who also have abnormalities that may be found on investigation (Table 2.3).

Blood pressure measurement

All the well-known problems of conventional sphygmomanometry, such as cuff size, observer error and bias, and blood pressure variability, apply to blood pressure measurement in pregnancy. But in addition the blood pressure will be lower in the second half of pregnancy in patients lying supine. This is because the gravid uterus obstructs the venous return from the lower limbs. Therefore blood pressure should be measured in the left lateral position with patients either lying or sitting. Because of difficulties in maintaining the sphygmomanometer cuff at the level of the heart in the left lateral position, sitting is the preferred patient position.[7] Much has been written about the audibility of Korotkoff sounds in pregnancy at very low pressures, caused by the vasodilation of pregnancy. In practice, this is rarely a problem; K5 is usually nearer to intra-arterial pressure than K4, but the difference between them is only a few mmHg, and this is unlikely to affect clinical decisions. 'White coat hypertension', where the blood pressure is excessively elevated because of arousal due to the clinical environment, is as much of a problem of pregnancy as in other situations, if not more. Its significance is being assessed by devices that allow blood pressure to be measured frequently and outside the hospital, such as 24-hour ambulatory monitoring.[8]

Management

First, pre-eclampsia will be considered, followed by other causes of hypertension in pregnancy.

There are two important differences between the management of hypertension due to pre-eclampsia and the management of hypertension outside pregnancy. Most cases of non-pregnant hypertension are idiopathic or 'essential', and the major aim of their treatment is to prevent the long-term complications of stroke and myocardial infarction. Some patients present outside pregnancy with hypertensive encephalopathy but these are now very uncommon. It is realized that acute lowering of blood pressure has major risks. Pregnancy and pre-eclampsia do not last for long enough to justify or need treatment of hypertension because of a long-term risk – the long term risks do not exist. But there are major acute risks of eclampsia and cerebral haemorrhage; the latter is the dominant cause of the increase in maternal mortality seen in pre-eclampsia.[1] In contrast with the situation outside pregnancy, this is the most important reason for treatment.

Secondly, hypertension is only one aspect of pre-eclampsia; other features must be looked for (see Table 2.2) and managed appropriately. The presence of these features is variable, and different aspects of the pre-eclamptic process may progress at different speeds. Progression is, however, relentless and no intervention except delivery has been shown to stop this progression.

Management of pre-eclampsia (usually presenting after 30 weeks)

Patients who have a rise in blood pressure that is only suggestive of pre-eclampsia, who are asymptomatic and whose blood pressure remains less than 150 mmHg systolic and less than 100 mmHg diastolic do not need to be admitted to hospital, particularly if there are day-care facilities available.

All other patients should be managed in hospital, not because hospital admission affects the progression of pre-eclampsia,[9] but because it allows more intensive monitoring of mother and fetus, both of whom are at risk. Since the only intervention that affects the progression of pre-eclampsia is delivery, the purpose of such monitoring is to detect a deterioration in maternal or fetal condition that demands delivery.

Other ancillary measures that may help are glucocortcoids that cross the placenta (dexamethasone, betamethasone), which will aid fetal lung maturation; and treatment of maternal hypertension to allow the pregnancy to continue for long enough to allow the glucocorticoids to take effect. In general, once pre-eclampsia has caused the blood pressure to rise to the level that demands antihypertensive treatment (greater than 170 systolic or greater than 110 diastolic) it is unlikely that the pregnancy will be able to continue for more than a few days: one of the fetal or maternal features noted in Table 2.1 will necessitate delivery.

Antihypertensive therapy

The reason for using antihypertensive drugs is to reduce the risk of the cerebral complications of pre-eclampsia. It is generally believed that blood pressures in excess of 170 systolic or 110 diastolic due to pre-eclampsia, carry a distinct risk of cerebral haemorrhage and eclampsia (though the latter may certainly occur at lower blood pressures). For this reason, clinicians feel that antihypertensive therapy is mandatory once the blood pressure reaches these levels. The target blood pressure should be about 140/90.

Blood pressures reduced to below this put the fetus and maternal brain at risk owing to impaired perfusion. This has never been subjected to clinical trial and almost certainly never will be, for obvious reasons. However, a blood pressure of 170/110 is just below the level of mean blood pressure (180–190/120–130 mmHg) at which cerebral regulation fails.[10]

By contrast, there is no evidence that treatment of lower degrees of hypertension (where there is no acute maternal risk) improves the fetal outcome once the gestation has exceeded 32 weeks. At gestations less than 32 weeks and in pregnancies complicated by pre-existing hypertension, this situation is not so clear and long-term antihypertensive therapy probably has a place.

Antihypertensive drugs

Hydralazine

Hydralazine is the drug most frequently used for blood pressure control in acute severe hypertension. Intravenous boluses will lower the blood pressure to a safe level in most acute episodes of pre-eclampsia.[11] The drug may also be given intramuscularly and by intravenous infusion. The patient should be managed in an intensive care environment. As indicated above, once the blood pressure has risen to levels greater than 170/110 because of pre-eclampsia, the patient is likely to require delivery soon, so blood pressure control for more than a few weeks is not very relevant.

Labetalol

Labetalol is a combined alpha-adrenergic and beta-adrenergic blocking agent. It too may be given by intravenous infusion for acute blood pressure control.[12] Patients with a history of asthma should not be given labetalol because of its beta-blocking component. No formal comparisons of labetalol and hydralazine have

been made for blood pressure control. Clinicians tend to use the drug that they are most familiar with in this emergency situation.

Nifedipine

The calcium antagonist Nifedipine is also used and is effective for oral control of acute severe hypertension[13] even though it has not been licensed for this purpose in the United Kingdom. It should not be given in conjunction with magnesium (for seizure control), as this will dangerously potentiate its hypotensive effect.[14]

Anticonvulsant drugs

If a patient has an eclamptic fit, most obstetricians in the United Kingdom would use intravenous diazepam to control the seizure.[15,16] Once the patient's condition is stable with regard to blood pressure and other acute problems such as thrombocytopenia (see Table 2.3) have been controlled, she would be delivered if the fit occurred antenatally. In the United States of America, parenteral magnesium sulphate would be used to control the seizure as well as diazepam, and magnesium sulphate would certainly be used for seizure prophylaxis, both in the woman who has had a fit and in the woman with severe pre-eclampsia.[17]

In the United Kingdom, further anticonvulsant treatment would be given to all women who have had an eclamptic seizure – either more diazepam or phenytoin or magnesium sulphate; but there is dispute as to whether anticonvulsant prophylaxis reduces the risk of eclampsia in patients who have severe pre-eclampsia and who already have good blood pressure control.[18]

The controversy arises because the eclampsia rate is similar (about 3%) in series of women who have and who have not had anticonvulsant prophylaxis in addition to meticulous blood pressure control; and because of the well-documented occurrence of eclamptic seizures in women who have had phenytoin blood levels that are considered within the therapeutic range in the non-pregnant state. Furthermore, anticonvulsant prophylaxis has serious potential side effects – diazepam causes sedation and depressed respiration in mothers and neonates, who may also be 'floppy' and hypothermic;[19] phenytoin causes dystonic reactions and pain at the injection site; magnesium in overdose causes neuromuscular paralysis and respiratory arrest.[20] But if anticonvulsants are to be withheld, blood pressure control must be meticulous, and this is difficult to achieve. It also requires a sufficient number of well trained and well-motivated staff.[18]

Other features of the management of fulminating pre-eclampsia, such as fluid balance, the correction of coagulopathy, and the timing and route of delivery, are beyond the scope of this chapter.

Hypertension presenting before 30 weeks

Pre-eclampsia can occur at gestations between 20 and 30 weeks and if it does, it is very severe. In the average obstetric service no more than 5 women in 1000 have pre-eclampsia presenting before 30 weeks. The earlier that hypertension presents before 30 weeks, the more likely is it that non-toxaemic hypertension is the cause or is a major contributing factor.

The reason for choosing a 'watershed' of 30 weeks is that there are clinical trial data to support improved fetal survival from long-term antihypertensive therapy, particularly with methyldopa, when compared with placebo in patients presenting before 30 weeks' gestation.[21,22] In Redman's trial of methyldopa

compared to placebo, there was a significant reduction in the perinatal loss rate from 6% to 1% in 106 women treated with methyldopa, compared to 107 women treated with placebo.[21] Entry criteria were blood pressures consistently greater than 95 mmHg diastolic before 30 weeks' gestation but not so high as to demand antihypertensive therapy. What is uncertain is why the methyldopa group did better, since the improvement could not be correlated with the antihypertensive effect. In the Redman trial, it was not clear to what extent there was any improvement in women who had pre-eclampsia as opposed to non-toxaemic hypertension.[21]

Management of non-toxaemic hypertension and of hypertension presenting before 30 weeks

As indicated above, the earlier in pregnancy that hypertension presents, the more likely is it to be due to non-toxaemic hypertension. As in the non-pregnant state, most cases of non-toxaemic hypertension in pregnancy have no obvious cause (essential hypertension) – in fewer than 5% of cases can a cause be found. However, some forms of secondary hypertension have specific problems in pregnancy, which must be considered.

Phaeochromocytoma

Nearly every maternal mortality report has a death from phaeochromocytoma. The condition which can mimic all features of pre-eclampsia[23] has a mortality of 50% when undiagnosed.[24] As in the non-pregnant state, most cases lack the typical features of phaeochromocytoma, so all patients with severe hypertension in pregnancy should be screened for phaeochromocytoma by whatever method is used locally. Since methyldopa interferes with many biochemical screens for phaeochromocytoma, and since methyldopa is the preferred long-term treatment for hypertension in pregnancy (see below), the necessity to screen for phaeochromocytoma must be considered before instigating treatment. If the patient screens positive, treatment should be started immediately with alpha-adrenergic and beta-adrenergic blockade. The author prefers phenoxybenzamine and propanolol, not withstanding any concern about the use of beta-blocking agents in pregnancy (see below). Once effective alpha- and beta-blockade have been instigated, the maternal risk is effectively eliminated.[25]

The tumour may well be localized antenatally by ultrasound or MRI, which is generally considered safe in pregnancy. If the tumour has been localized with confidence, it may be removed by a combined approach at the time of delivery[25] or subsequently.[26] If the tumour has not been localized before delivery, which is more likely with lesions outside the adrenal glands, delivery is safe under combined alpha- and beta-adrenergic blockade. The tumour can be localized and removed after delivery.

Coarctation of the aorta

Most patients with significant coarctation have the lesion repaired before pregnancy. If this has not been done, there is a risk of dissection of the aorta because of the increased cardiac output of pregnancy.[27] Patients who have any degree of coarctation should have their blood pressure scrupulously controlled by beta-adrenergic blockade, notwithstanding any possible risks to the fetus (see below). Beta-blockade is preferred because it reduces the cardiac contractility and therefore the shear stress on the aorta.

Renal disease

Renovascular hypertension causes no particular problems in pregnancy but renal parenchymal disease does: hypertension and renal impairment interact in a way that is not understood to increase the risks of superadded pre-eclampsia and acute and chronic fetal distress. For example, in renal disease the presence of hypertension increases the incidences of intrauterine growth retardation from 2% to 16% and the risk of preterm delivery from 11% to 20%.[28]

Essential hypertension

This will be the diagnosis in the majority of women presenting early in pregnancy. It is now realized that essential hypertension *per se* does not put the fetus at risk: and that the risk to the fetus is the risk of developing superadded pre-eclampsia (up to 20%) compared to the risk in a normotensive woman (up to 10%, depending on gravidity and other factors in the obstetric history). The management of patients with essential hypertension early in pregnancy therefore depends on treatment that might stop them developing pre-eclampsia or stop them developing life-threatening hypertension.

Occasionally, there is concern about very severe hypertension early in pregnancy and about whether such a pregnancy should be terminated, i.e. that continuing the pregnancy will put the mother's life at extra risk. In practice this does not happen: women with very severe hypertension do not often get pregnant; the blood pressure can usually be controlled more easily in early pregnancy; and if it cannot, the pregnancy usually terminates itself.

Antihypertensive therapy

Methyldopa

There are no good data to indicate that treatment with antihypertensive drugs reduces the risk of pre-eclampsia but, as indicated above, the Redman trial did show that fetal outcome was improved with methyldopa compared to placebo.[21] There are also long-term follow-up data at seven years, which show no detriment to the offspring in the methyldopa treated group.[29]

It is for these reasons that methyldopa is the drug most frequently used for long-term control of blood pressure in pregnancy. It may be given in divided doses of 2–3 g per day, though at high doses the sedative effects are marked. It should not be used if there is a significant risk of maternal depression, and for this reason the author changes therapy in all patients to a beta-blocking agent, calcium antagonist, or ACE inhibitor after delivery.

Although there is almost uniform agreement about methyldopa as the first drug for long-term treatment of hypertension, there is no consensus about alternative or additional medication, largely because of a lack of adequate clinical trials.

Beta-blocking drugs

Oxprenolol has been compared to methyldopa using the same entry criteria as in the methyldopa versus placebo trial.[21] Initial reports that the use of oxprenolol was associated with larger babies[30] were not supported in a subsequent study.[31] Atenolol has been compared to placebo; although there was no difference in fetal outcome, the authors found less proteinuric pre-eclampsia (a remarkable outcome) and fewer hospital admissions, hardly surprising since the blood pressures were lower.[32]

But worryingly, the same authors,[33] in another placebo-controlled trial of atenolol in early pregnancy, found a very high incidence of subsequent severe growth retardation in the atenolol group. For this reason, atenolol should not be used in the first half of pregnancy. It is not clear whether the risk of growth retardation is specific to atenolol or general to all beta-blocking drugs. Since atenolol does not have intrinsic sympathomimetic activity (unlike oxprenolol) the drug's, pharamacological profile may be important.

However, until the situation is clearer, the author does not use beta-blocking drugs for blood pressure control in the first half of pregnancy unless there is some specific reason to do so, e.g. coarctation of the aorta (see above). Nevertheless, beta-blocking drugs do not need to be stopped before conception, and neither does any other antihypertensive drug (see below).

Hydralazine

Hydralazine can be used as an adjuvant to methyldopa. The side effects of tachycardia and headache are usually not a problem if methyldopa is being taken as well. Treatment in pregnancy does not last long enough for the development of lupus to be a problem. Tachyphylaxis limits the use of hydralazine to late pregnancy.

Labetalol

Like hydralazine, labetalol has been used for long-term as well as acute blood pressure control. Comparative trials between labetalol and methyldopa have not been large enough to exclude important differences in outcome. There has been a trend towards an increased risk of growth retardation with labetalol.

Nifedipine

Nifedipine is the only calcium antagonist for which there is any extensive experience in pregnancy, and this is anecdotal rather than in the context of a clinical trial.[13,34] This is at least in part because of the lack of a product license for its use in hypertension in pregnancy in the United Kingdom. The most extensive report of its long-term use[34] showed a poor fetal outcome, but the study was conducted in a particularly high-risk group of pregnancies. At present, nifedipine is the author's preferred additional or alternative drug for long-term use in pregnancy when methyldopa is either inadequate or contra-indicated.

Diuretics

Diuretics were formally extensively used for the 'treatment' or prevention of pre-eclampsia. Meta-analysis has shown that they reduce oedema but have no impact on perinatal survival.[35] Diuretics are theoretically contraindicated since in severe pre-eclampsia the circulating blood volume is already contracted and any further reduction might impair placental perfusion. Diuretics also raise the level of serum urate, which is used to monitor the progress of pre-eclampsia (see Table 2.3). In pre-eclampsia the serum urate is disproportionately elevated when compared to tests of renal function. For these reasons, and because they do not appear to be very effective as hypotensive agents, diuretics are not used to control blood pressure in pregnancy.

Angiotensin converting enzyme inhibitors

These drugs should not be used after the first trimester unless there is no other way of controlling blood pressure. They cause renal failure in the fetus, which is shown before delivery as oligohydramnios and after delivery as oliguria and anuria.[36] The condition has been fatal; both captopril and enalapril have been implicated.

Prevention of pre-eclampsia

Because of the importance of pre-eclampsia and because no treatment will cure the condition except delivery, the possibility of prevention of pre-eclampsia is particularly important. There are two main groups at risk: those who have had it before and those who have some underlying condition such as hypertension or renal disease that has been shown to predispose patients to the condition. Early trials with antiplatelet agents, in particular low-dose aspirin 60–150 mg per day were encouraging, and there were suggestions of a 70% reduction in risk.[37,38] However, the most recent and largest trial, CLASP[39] showed no overall reduction in risk, and meta-analysis indicates no more than a 12% reduction of risk. Even so, secondary analysis of the CLASP data did suggest that early-onset pre-eclampsia might be reduced by as much as 50%,[39] and early-onset pre-eclampsia (occurring before 34 weeks' gestation) is the most severe form of the disease.

If a patient has early-onset pre-eclampsia occurring in the second trimester, the risk of recurrence of some form of pre-eclampsia is 40% with a 10% recurrence risk of early-onset pre-eclampsia.[40] Other risk factors for early-onset pre-eclampsia are pre-existing renal disease[41] and pre-existing hypertension,[40] though how severe the hypertension has to be is uncertain.

The author's criteria are to advise aspirin 75 mg per day from 12 weeks' gestation for the following patients:

- women who have had a fetal loss because of pre-eclampsia or unexplained intrauterine growth retardation (similar placental pathologies);
- women who have had pre-eclampsia before 34 weeks;
- women who have documented impaired renal function; and
- women who have been treated with antihypertensive drugs before pregnancy.

The CLASP trial showed that aspirin given in this way is safe for mother and child.[39]

Management of hypertension before pregnancy and in early pregnancy

Patients should be investigated for hypertension in the usual way and treatment should be instigated and optimized with regard to blood pressure control. There are no mandatory levels of blood pressure above which pregnancy cannot be countenanced. Patients should be counselled about the risks of pre-eclampsia and the possible benefits of antiplatelet therapy.

No antihypertensive drug has been shown to teratogenic. None are likely to be harmful in the first weeks of pregnancy. Therefore, the choice of drugs to be used before pregnancy may be made, irrespective of any consideration of a possible future pregnancy. Once the patient becomes pregnant, her blood pressure is likely to fall because of the marked vasodilation that occurs in early pregnancy. (Indeed if this does not occur it is an ominous sign for the success of the pregnancy). As soon as the patient knows she is pregnant, it should be possible to withdraw antihypertensive drugs, or to substitute methyldopa, depending on the amount of antihypertensive therapy necessary before pregnancy.

References

1 Department of Health, Welsh Office, Scottish Office and Health Department, Department of Health and Social Security, Northern Ireland. Report on confidential enquiries into maternal deaths in the United Kingdom 1988–1990. HMSO 1994.

2 Roberts JM, Taylor RN, Musci TJ et al. Preeclampsia: an endothelial cell disorder. *Am J Obstet Gynecol* 1989; **161**:1200–4.

3 Spargo B, McCartney CP, Winemiller R. Glomerular capillary endotheliosis in toxemia of pregnancy. *Arch Path* 1959; **68**:593–9.

4 Fisher ER, Pardo V, Paul R, Hayrashi TT. Ultrastructural studies in hypertension. IV. Toxemia in pregnancy, *Am J Path* 1969; **55**:109–31.

5 MacGillivray I, Rose GA, Rowe B. Blood pressure survey in pregnancy, *Clin Sci* 1969; **37**:395–407.

6 Redman CWG, Jeffries M. Revised definition of pre-eclampsia, *Lancet* 1988; **ii**:809–12.

7 National High Blood Pressure Education Programme. National High Blood Pressure Education Programme Working Group Report on High Blood Pressure in Pregnancy, *Am J Obstet Gynecol* 1990; **163**:1691–712.

8 Shennan AH, Kissane J, de Swiet M. Validation of the Spacelabs 90207. *Br J Obstet Gynaecol* 1993; **100**:904–8.

9 Matthews DD. A randomised controlled trial of bed rest and sedation or normal activity and non-sedation in the management of non-albuminuric hypertension in late pregnancy. *Br J Obstet Gynaecol* 1977; **84**:108–14.

10 Redman CWG. Hypertension in pregnancy. In: *Medical Disorders in Obstetric Practice*. de Swiet M (ed). Blackwell Scientific Publications: Oxford, 1995:200.

11 Patterson-Brown S, Robson SC, Redfern N et al. Hydralazine boluses for the treatment of severe hypertension. *Br J Obstet Gynaecol* 1994; **101**:409–13.

12 Garden A, Davey DA, Dommisse J. Intravenous labetalol and intravenous dihydralazine in severe hypertension in pregnancy. *Clin Exp Hypertens* 1982; **1**:371–83.

13 Walters BNJ, Redman CWG. Treatment of severe pregnancy-associated hypertension with the calcium antagonist nifedipine, *Br J Obstet Gynaecol* 1984; **91**:330–6.

14 Waisman CD, Mayorga LM, Camera MI et al. Magnesium plus nifedipine: potentiation of hypotensive effect in preeclampsia? *Am J Obstet Gynecol* 1988; **159**:308–9.

15 Chamberlain GVP, Lewis PJ, de Swiet M et al. How obstetricians manage hypertension in pregnancy. *Br Med J* 1978; **i**:626–7.

16 Hutton JD, James DK, Stirrat GM et al. Managment of severe pre-eclampsia and eclampsia by UK consultants. *Br J Obstet Gynaecol* 1992; **99**:554–6.

17 Pritchard JA, Cunningham FG, Pritchard SA. The Parkland Memorial Hospital protocol for treatment of eclampsia: evaluation of 245 cases. *Am J Obstet Gynecol* 1984; **148**:951–63.

18 Chua S, Redman CWG. Are prophylactic anticonvulsants required in severe pre-eclampsia? *Lancet* 1991; **337**:250–1.

19 Cree JE, Meyer J, Hailey DM. Diazepam in labour: its metabolism and effect on the clinical condition and thermogenesis of the newborn. *Br Med J* 1973; **iv**:251–5.

20 Hibbard BM, Rosen M. The managment of severe pre-eclampsia, *Br J Anaesth* 1977; **49**:3–9.

21 Redman CWG, Beilin LJ, Bonnar J et al. Fetal outcome in trial of antihypertensive treatment in pregnancy, *Lancet* 1976; **ii**:753–6.

22 Leather HM, Humphreys DM, Baker P. A controlled trial of hypotensive agents in hypertension in pregnancy. *Lancet* 1968; 488–90.

23 Lamming GD, Symonds EM, Rubin PC. Phaeochromocytoma in pregnancy: still a cause of maternal death. *Clin Exp Hypertens* 1990; **9**:57–68.

24 Blair RG. Phaeochromocytoma and pregnancy. *J Obstet Gynaecol Br Commonw* 1963; **70**:110–19.

25 Harper MA, Murnaghan GA, Kennedy L et al. Phaeochromocytoma in pregnancy. Five cases and a review of the literature. *Br J Obstet Gynaecol* 1989; **96**:594–606.

26 Schenker JG, Chowers I. Phaeochromocytoma and pregnancy. *Obstet Gynecol Surv* 1971; **26**:739–47.

27 Deal K, Wooley CF. Coarctation of the aorta and pregnancy. *Ann Intern Med* 1973; **78**:706–10.

28 Surian M, Ibascia E et al. Glomerular disease and pregnancy: A study of 123 pregnancies in patients with primary and secondary glomerular disease. *Nephron* 1984; **36**:101–5.

29 Redman CWG, Ounsted MK. Safety for the child of drug treatment for hypertension in pregnancy. *Lancet* 1982; **i**:1237.

30 Gallery EDM, Saunders DM, Hunyor SN et al. Randomised comparison of methyldopa and oxprenolol for treatment of hypertension in pregnancy. *Br Med J* 1979; **i**:1591–4.

31 Fidler J, Smith V, de Swiet M. Randomised controlled comparative study of methyldopa and oxprenolol for the treatment of hypertension in pregnancy. *Br Med J* 1983; **286**:1927–30.

32 Rubin PC, Butters L et al. Placebo-controlled trial of atenolol treatment of pregnancy-associated hypertension. *Lancet* 1983; **i**:431–4.

33 Butters L, Kennedy S, Rubin PC. Atenolol in essential hypertension during pregnancy. *Br Med J* 1990; **301**:587–9.

34 Constantine G, Beevers DG, Reynolds AC. Nifedipine as a second line antihypertensive drug in pregnancy. *Br J Obstet Gynaecol* 1987; **94**:1136–42.

35 Collins R, Yusuf S, Peto R. Overview of randomised trials of diuretics in pregnancy. *Br Med J* 1985; **290**:17–23.

36 Rosa FW, Bosco LA, Graham CF. Neonatal anuria with maternal angiotensin-converting enzyme inhibition. *Obstet Gynecol* 1989; **74**:371–4.

37 Beaufils M, Uzan S, Donsimoni R et al. Prevention of eclampsia by early platelet therapy. *Lancet* 1985; **i**:840–2.

38 Wallenburg HCS, Dekker GA, Makovitz JW et al. Low-dose aspirin prevents pregnancy-induced hypertension and pre-eclampsia in angiotensin-sensitive primigravidae. *Lancet* 1986; **i**:1–3.

39 CLASP (Collaborative Low-dose Aspirin Study in Pregnancy) Collaborative Group. CLASP: a randomised trial of low-dose aspirin for the prevention and treatment of pre-eclampsia among 9364 pregnant women. *Lancet* 1994; **343**:619–29.

40 Sibai BM, Mercer B, Sarinoglu C. Severe pre-eclampsia in the second trimester: recurrent risk and long-term prognosis, *Am J Obstet Gynacol* 1991; **165**:1408–512.

41 Ihle BU, Long P, Oats J. Early onset pre-eclampsia: recognition of underlying renal disease. *Br Med J* 1987; **294**:79–81.

3

Treatment of the elderly hypertensive

Martin J Kendall

Until recently most doctors were reluctant to treat hypertensive patients over 70 years old. It seemed illogical to offer treatment designed to reduce the risk of long-term cardiovascular complications to patients with a limited life expectancy. It seemed inappropriate to lower blood pressure when it was known that blood pressure tends to rise as people grow older and when moderate hypertension might be considered normal in the old. Furthermore, antihypertensive drugs might not only lower blood pressure but also thereby reduce cerebral perfusion and so predispose to cerebrovascular events, confusion, and other adverse effects on higher mental function. These views are not acceptable today.

Investigation of hypertension in the elderly

Several studies[1-5] have shown beyond reasonable doubt that the treatment of hypertension in elderly people reduces morbidity and prolongs life. Furthermore, very thorough investigation has shown that blood pressure reduction in the elderly does not affect cognitive and behavioural function,[6] and several trials have failed to produce good evidence that older people tolerate antihypertensives particularly badly,[7] even though they assessed the effects of antihypertensive drugs on the quality of life of elderly hypertensives.[8] However, this does not mean that all elderly hypertensives should be treated

or that all antihypertensive drugs are equally safe and effective in this group of patients. These trials have evaluated the efficacy and safety of a limited number of antihypertensive drugs in a highly selected group of elderly hypertensives. The prescribing doctor now needs to:

- consider the clinical trial data currently available on the treatment of elderly hypertensive patients;
- remember the problems associated with treating older patients;
- decide which elderly hypertensives should be offered treatment; and
- review the different drug groups currently available to treat hypertension and decide which might be most appropriate for treating the older patient.

Clinical trials

There have been five major trials[1-5] and some smaller trials on the treatment of elderly hypertensives; it is the former, particularly the more recent trials,[3-5] which have provoked a re-evaluation of our views on this subject.[9,10]

EWPHE trial

The European Working Party on Hypertension in the Elderly (EWPHE)[1] enrolled 840 patients over 60 years old (mean age 72±8 years) from 18 centres. It was a double-blind randomized comparative group study in which patients with a systolic pressure of 160–239 mmHg and a diastolic pressure of 90–120 mmHg were initially given a diuretic combination (25 mg hydrochlorthiazide plus 50 mg triamterene) or a placebo. Further treatment could be added.

This study showed that diuretic therapy producing a reduction in blood pressure could also reduce cardiac mortality and non-fatal cerebrovascular events. In this study, cardiac mortality included a number of deaths from heart failure, and non-fatal myocardial infarcts were slightly commoner in the actively treated group.

Coope and Warrender's trial
The open trial in 13 general practices in England and Wales reported by Coope and Warrender[2] received much less attention than the EWPHE trial, but it was a major landmark study. In it, 884 patients, aged 60–79 years, with a systolic pressure of 170–280 mmHg and a diastolic pressure of 105–120 mmHg were randomized into a treated or an untreated group. The former were treated with atenolol 100 mg daily to which bendrofluazide 5 mg daily was added if necessary to lower blood pressure. Active therapy effectively lowered the blood pressure over a mean follow period of 4.4 years. Fatal stroke was reduced by 70% (p=0.025) and cardiac mortality reduced by 26% (NS), though coronary events and sudden deaths were slightly commoner in the treated group.

The conclusions of the above trials were supported in general terms by the data on the older patients in the Australian trial[11] and the HDFP study.[12] However, the results from all the clinical trials conducted before 1990 failed to persuade most prescribers of the potential benefits of treating elderly hypertensives.

SHEP trial
In 1991, the results of the study the SHEP trial (Systolic Hypertension in the Elderly Programme) were reported.[3] As the name implies, this study was directed specifically towards answering the questions: is isolated systolic hypertension dangerous, and does blood pressure reduction help? Patients (4376, of whom 57% were female) who were over 60 years old (mean age 72, 14% over 80 years) with a systolic pressure of 160–219 mmHg and a diastolic pressure under 90 mmHg were randomized double blind to either a diuretic-based regimen (starting with chlorthalidone 12.5 mg a day) or placebo. The mean follow-up period was 4.5 years.

During this time, diuretic therapy dramatically reduced the incidence of strokes: 96 non-fatal cerebrovascular events in the treated group versus 149 in the placebo group; and 10 fatal cerebrovascular events in the treated group versus 14 in the placebo group (Table 3.1 and Figs 3.1, 3.2). The stroke rates were

	Cerebrovascular disease		Myocardial infarction	
	Active	Placebo	Active	Placebo
SHEP[3]	96	149	50	74
STOP-H[4]*	26	41	19	22
MRC-Elderly[5]	64	92	43	49
*Primary end-point data				

Table 3.1
Impact of antihypertensive therapy on the number of non-fatal events in recent trials.[3–5]

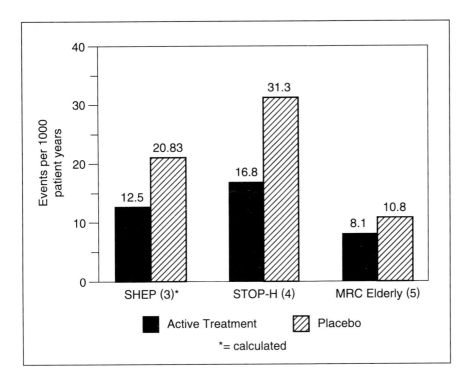

Figure 3.1
Total number of cerebrovascular events (per 1000 patient years) on active treatment and placebo from recent trial reports.[3–5]

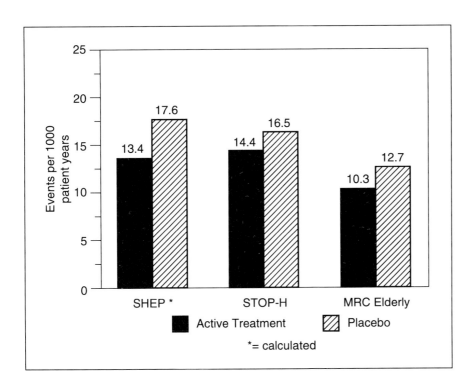

Figure 3.2
Total number of coronary events (per 1000 patient years) on active treatment and placebo from recent trial reports.[3–5]

reported as 5.2 versus 8.2 per 500 patient years. This means that treating 1000 patients for 5 years with a relatively inexpensive drug prevented 30 strokes.

The impact on coronary events was less dramatic though there was a reduction in the number of myocardial infarcts but not sudden deaths (see Tables 3.1, 3.2 and Fig 3.2).

STOP-Hypertension trial
The Swedish trial in Old Patients with Hypertension, the so-called STOP-Hypertension trial, was also reported in 1991.[4] This prospective randomized double-blind trial compared active therapy (beta-blocker or diuretic therapy) with placebo in hypertensive males and females aged 70–84 years. The inclusion criteria were a systolic pressure of 180–230 mmHg with a diastolic pressure over 90 mmHg, or a diastolic pressure of 105–120 mmHg. The 812 patients on active therapy and the 815 patients on

placebo were followed for an average of 25 months and no patients were lost to follow up. The active regimen effectively lowered blood pressure by a mean of 19.5/8.1 mmHg more than placebo. This was associated with a significant reduction in total mortality – 36 vs 63 (p=0.0079). The other results are presented in Tables 3.1 and 3.2 and Figs 3.1 and 3.2.

MRC Elderly trial
The MRC (Elderly) trial (The Medical Research Council Trial of treatment of hypertension in older adults) was published in February 1992.[5] This trial was designed to determine whether treatment with a diuretic or a beta-blocker would reduce the risk of stroke, coronary events, and death in older hypertensive patients. This single-blind study, performed in a general practice setting in the United Kingdom, included 4396 patients of whom 58% were females aged 65–74 years.

Trial (Numbers in each group)	Totals		Cerebrovascular		Myocardial infarcts		Sudden death	
	Active	Placebo	Active	Placebo	Active	Placebo	Active	Placebo
SHEP[3] (Active – 2362, Placebo – 2371)	213	242	10	14	15	26	44	47
STOP-H[4] (Active – 812, Placebo – 815)	36	63	3	12	6	6	4	12
MRC-Elderly[5]	301	315	37	42	85	110	—	—

*Primary end point data

Table 3.2
Impact of antihypertensive therapy on the numbers of deaths in recent trials.[3–5]

The entry blood pressures were 160–209 mmHg systolic and a diastolic pressure of less than 115 mmHg. The patients were allocated randomly to one of three groups: atenolol 50 mg daily; hydrochlorothiazide 25 mg daily plus amiloride 2.5 mg daily; or placebo. The doses were increased as necessary to meet target pressures. The mean follow up time was 5.8 years.

As in the other trials, active therapy reduced the blood pressures and reduced the incidence of strokes (101 vs 134; p=0.04). Myocardial infarct rates were also reduced but, whereas the 2 drug regimens had comparable effects on stroke rates, the reduction in coronary events was greater on diuretics (see Table 3.1 and Fig. 3.1). Unfortunately, up to 25% of patients were lost to follow-up in this trial.

Treating the elderly

Whatever the condition to be treated, the fact that the patient is elderly may have a major impact on the response to treatment. Furthermore, older patients are more likely than young patients to suffer from other disorders and to be taking other drugs. These coexisting diseases and the concomitant medications may have a greater effect on the patient's response to therapy than the well-known functional deteriorations that accompany advancing age. The impact of diseases and current drug therapy on the decision whether to treat and how to treat will be considered below. First, let us consider briefly compliance and drug handling (pharmacokinetic factors) in the old.

Compliance

Doctors tend to assume that patients will take the tablets that are prescribed for them. It would be more reasonable to anticipate that when drugs are prescribed for elderly hypertensives they will not be taken properly. Good compliance usually requires that

- the regimen is simple;
- the therapy is effective;
- the reasons for taking the treatment are clear; and
- there are few unwanted effects.

Oral contraceptive fulfil these criteria and compliance is usually good. By comparison, the elderly hypertensive

- may already be taking other drugs, and any additional tablets tend to make it difficult to remember what to take and when;
- may have difficulty appreciating the long-term benefits, particularly if he or she is already concerned about other short-term problems like diabetic control, dyspnoea, pain, or urinary retention;
- may experience difficulty because of trouble hearing the instructions, remembering what he or she has been told, reading the labels on the bottles, or unscrewing the tops of the bottles;
- may be more prone to suffer adverse effects such as postural hypotension or confusion.

These considerations should not prevent doctors prescribing for the old, but they emphasize the need for careful patient selection, clear instructions, well-tolerated therapy, and a simple regimen.

Advancing age also influences drug handling in the body. In the past, reviewers of this subject made the subject unnecessarily complicated and suggested that with the passing of the years all body functions deteriorate. In clinical practice two organs merit concern in this context: the kidneys and the brain. Renal function deteriorates with age, and drugs should be prescribed in lower doses and their effects – both therapeutic and adverse – should be monitored. The impact of ageing on the brain is much more variable but the tendency is for the elderly to tolerate rapid falls in pressure and metabolic changes badly.

Patient selection

All trials have inclusion and exclusion criteria. As a result the patient population, particularly in studies on the elderly, is highly selected and generally includes predominantly relatively fit people who do not suffer from other serious disorders and who are not taking drugs considered likely to modify the response to the antihypertensive agent under

investigation. This selection process is important for both the smooth running and scientific validity of the trial, but it results in the exclusion of relatively large numbers of patients (often over 90%).[3] Considerable care is therefore needed in applying the results of the trials described[1-5] to the whole population of elderly hypertensives.[9,10]

When considering guidelines for treating elderly hypertensives, it may be helped to divide (somewhat arbitrarily) the potential patient population into three groups: the sick elderly, the medically complicated elderly, and the fit elderly (Table 3.3).

The sick elderly
The sick elderly are those suffering from malignant disease, dementia or other disorders that may be expected to reduce life expectancy or that can be seen to be drastically reducing the patient's quality of life. This category would include patients with severe disabling arthritis, incapacitating emphysema, and any who had failed to recover from a major cerebrovascular event. For these patients, long-term prophylactic therapy given to reduce the risk of a myocardial infarct, sudden death, or a stroke would be inappropriate. Their hypertension should not be treated.

The medically complicated elderly
The medically complicated elderly encompasses a relatively large group of patients with a wide range of medical problems. They suffer from the common disorders of old age, some of which are listed in Table 3.3. Their disability will need to be evaluated and the impact of their disease on their life will need to be assessed. The situation will also be influenced by their personality, their home circumstances, and the support of family and friends. This group of patients will almost certainly be taking drugs for other conditions and the number of

The sick elderly
   Those who also suffer from
   • dementia
   • malignant disease
   • severe chronic disorders

The medically complicated elderly
   Those who also suffer from:
   • chronic bronchitis
   • gout
   • angina
   • heart failure
   • peripheral vascular disease
   • cerebrovascular disease

The fit elderly

Table 3.3
Subgroups of elderly hypertensives.

drugs being taken, the complexity of the regimens, and the importance of compliance and correct dosing will also have a marked impact on the overall assessment. For patients in this group, the potential gain from reducing the risk of vascular complications in the future has to be set against the risk of adding adverse drug reactions to the patient's list of problems and the real possibility that complicating the drug regimen further may lead to failure to take more important medication. Patients taking anticonvulsants, anticoagulants, antiarrhythmic drugs, and hypoglycaemic agents need to take the correct dose of their tablets regularly, and on time.

Having considered all the above, the doctor may well decide that it is not unreasonable for the patient to take a small dose of thiazide diuretic in the real hope that it will reduce the patient's chances of having a stroke, something which could only make a medically complicated patient worse.

The fit elderly

The fit elderly may be a relatively small subgroup of those with hypertension. Nevertheless, there were sufficient for the trial organizers of the SHEP,[3] STOP-hypertension,[4] and MRC Elderly[5] to perform reasonably large-scale studies. Furthermore, the number of relatively well individuals over the age of 75 years is increasing rapidly. For most of these people, the quality of life is good. They hope to stay alive and to remain active. For this group, adequate measures to control blood pressure and reduce the risk of coronary events, sudden death, and particularly stroke are not only reasonable, they may be the most rewarding and cost-effective form of prophylactic medicine available to doctors treating patients in the developed countries of the world today.

Choice of therapy

The drugs available to treat elderly patients with hypertension are the same as those used to treat younger hypertensives. None are absolutely contraindicated, and prescribers will be influenced by their normal prescribing habits and will tend to use drugs with which they are familiar. However, the choice of regimen should be influenced by

- any coexisting disorders (*see* Chapter 13);
- the guidelines below for treating the elderly; and
- the need to avoid the unwanted effects that tend to cause particular problems in the old.

Therapeutic guidelines

When considering the antihypertensive regimen for an elderly hypertensive patient, it would seem prudent to choose one that

- is simple – preferably 1 tablet to be taken once daily;
- is well tolerated – the patient may already have a number of minor medical problems and older people are more prone to suffer from the adverse effects of drugs;
- starts with a low dose – older people do not tolerate rapid changes in blood pressure well and lower doses are almost always better tolerated;
- does not accumulate in the body – renal function deteriorates with advancing age.

Unwanted effects

In addition to these guidelines, the prescriber should take into consideration that the elderly are more prone to suffer from certain medical problems that may be caused by or exacerbated by drug treatment. These include the following conditions.

1. Confusion and impaired higher mental function, which may be provoked by dehydration, electrolyte disturbances, and other metabolic abnormalities.
2. Falls and dizziness, which could be produced by postural hypotension or marked falls in blood pressure.
3. Constipation.
4. Insomnia.
5. Incontinence.

Drugs available

Thiazide diuretics

There is a strong case for considering a low dose of a thiazide diuretic as a first choice for many elderly hypertensive patients. Thiazides have been shown to reduce the incidence of both coronary and cerebrovascular events[3-5] and to be effective in both isolated systolic hypertension[3] and in patients with both systolic and diastolic hypertension.[4,5] Furthermore, the regimen is simple – one tablet to be taken once daily – and the side effects are usually mild and infrequent.[6,7] Occasionally dehydration, electrolyte disturbances, or a deterioration in diabetic control may be encountered, and gout may be precipitated.

Beta-blockers

Beta-blockers tend to have a bad reputation and may be considered unsuitable for use in the elderly. However, atenolol was reasonably well tolerated in two of the major trials,[2,5] and in other investigations, beta-blockers (particularly low doses of beta$_1$-selective agents) have been found to be very acceptable in clinical practice.[6,7,13,14] Their particular advantage is that there is evidence to suggest that they have

the potential to reduce coronary mortality[15,16] and reduce the risk of sudden death[17-19] in patients who have had a myocardial infarction. This is important, as the frequency of coronary events increases with advancing age,[13,20,21] and diuretics have little impact on sudden death.[3,16]

Thus it would be reasonable to argue against non-selective beta-blockers but in favour of once daily beta$_1$-selective regimens. These are effective in reducing blood pressure, and they are the most effective means of reducing the most life-threatening complications of hypertension in the elderly, namely myocardial infarction and sudden death.[3,4,13,22,23] Furthermore, they are well tolerated,[19] and they are unlikely to cause severe falls in blood pressure or any major metabolic disturbances when beta$_1$-selective agents are used.[13,24-26]

Other antihypertensive drugs

Clinical data on the use of the other antihypertensive agents in the elderly are limited.

Calcium antagonists are sometimes put forward as the drug of choice for the management of the elderly hypertensive (Table 3.4). Unfortunately, there are no good clinical data to suggest that these characteristics translate into greater efficacy and tolerability in clinical practice.

Similarly, ACE inhibitors are being used increasingly in the elderly, and experience of their use in patients with heart failure[27,28] and in patients with diabetes mellitus[29,30] is very reassuring. However, it is difficult to produce data from good clinical trials to argue in favour of their use as first-line treatment for elderly hypertensives.

Conclusion

Hypertension in the elderly has ceased to be a disorder best left well alone; it has become a

1. Simple regimen – many calcium antagonists are available as once-daily preparations
2. Tend to correct the underlying problem (i.e. increased peripheral resistance)
3. Suitable for treating patients with
   - chronic obstructive airways disease
   - peripheral vascular disease
   - angina
   - mild heart failure
   - diabetes
   - gout
   - renal impairment
4. Unlikely to cause
   - confusion
   - postural hypotension

Table 3.4
Potential advantages of a calcium antagonist in the management of hypertension in the elderly

therapeutic opportunity in which a relatively well-tried simple remedy may be offered to reduce the risk of a devastating stroke. However, elderly patients require careful assessment to ensure that only those with an otherwise reasonable prognosis are treated and that the drugs chosen do not adversely affect coexisting diseases or interact with other treatments that the patient is already taking. In most instances, a low dose of a thiazide diuretic can be recommended as a cheap, safe and effective treatment.

References

1 Amery A, Birkenhager W, Brixko P et al. Efficacy of antihypertensive drug treatment according to age, sex, blood pressure and previous cardiovascular disease in patient over the age of 60. *Lancet* 1986; ii:589–92.

2 Coope J, Warrender TS. Randomised trial of treatment of hypertension in elderly patients in primary care. *Br Med J* 1986; **293**:1145–51.

3 SHEP Cooperative Research Group. Prevention of stroke by antihypertensive drug treatment in older persons with isolated systolic hypertension. Final results of the Systolic Hypertension in the Elderly Program. *J Am Med Ass* 1991; **265**:3255–64.

4 Dahlof B, Lindholm LH, Hansson L, Schersten B, Ekborm T, Wester PO. Morbidity and mortality in the Swedish Trial in Old Patients with Hypertension (STOP Hypertension). *Lancet* 1991; **338**:1281–5.

5 MRC Working Party. Medical research council trial of treatment of hypertension in older adults: principal results. *Br Med J* 1992; **304**:405–12.

6 Goldstein G, Materson BJ, Cushman WC et al. Treatment of hypertension in the elderly: II. Cognitive and behavioral function. Results of a Department of Veterans Affairs Cooperative Study. *Hypertension* 1990; **15**:361–9.

7 Applegate WB. Hypertension in Elderly Patients. Review. *Ann of Intern Med* 1989; **110**:901–15.

8 Kittler ME. Elderly hypertensives and quality of life: some methodological considerations. *Eur Heart J* 1993; **14**:113–21.

9 Kuramoto K, Matsushita S, Kuwajima I, Murakawi M. Prospective study on the treatment of mild hypertension in the aged. *Jap Heart J* 1981; **22**:75–85.

10 Kaplan NM. Systemic Hypertension in the Elderly Program (SHEP) and Swedish Trial in old Patients with Hypertension (STOP). *Am J Hypertens* 1992; **13**:331–4.

11 Australian National Blood Pressure Management Committee. The Australian therapeutic trial in mild hypertension. *Lancet* 1980; i:1261–7.

12 Hypertension Detection and Follow up Program Cooperative Group. Five year findings of the Hypertension Detection and Follow up Program, II: Mortality by race, sex and age. *JAMA* 1979; **242**:2572–7.

13 Wikstrand J, Westergren G, Berglund G et al. Antihypertensive treatment with metoprolol or hydrochlorothiazide in patients aged 60–75 years. *JAMA* 1986; **255**:1304–10.

14 Jaatela A, Baandrup S, Houtzagers J, Westergren G. The efficacy of low dose metoprolol CR/ZOK in mild hypertension and in elderly patients with mild to moderate hypertension. *J Clin Pharmacol* 1990; **30**:566–71.

15 Green KG. British MRC trial of treatment for mild hypertension – a more favourable interpretation. *Am J Hypertens* 1991; **4**:723–4.

16 Wikstrand J, Kendall MJ. The role of beta blockade in preventing sudden death. *Europ Heart J* 1992; **13** (suppl D):111–20.

17 Norwegian Study Group. Timolol induced reduction in mortality and reinfarction in patients surviving acute myocardial infarction. *N Engl J Med* 1981; **304**:801–7.

18 Beta Blocker Heart Attack Trial Research Group. A randomized trial of propranolol in patients with acute myocardial infarction, 1. Mortality Results. *JAMA* 1982; **247**:1707–13.

19 Olsson G, Wikstrand J, Warnold I et al. Metoprolol induced reduction in post infarction mortality: pooled results from five double blind randomised trials. *Eur Heart J* 1992; **13**:28–32.

20 Kannel WB, Gorton T. Evaluation of cardiovascular risk in the elderly: The Framingham Study. *Bull N Y Acad Med* 1978; **54**:573–91.

21 Byny RL. Hypertension in the Elderly. *Am J Med* 1986; **81**:1055–8.

22 Dollery GT. Does it matter how blood pressure is reduced? *Clin Sci* 1981; **61**:4135–205.

23 Olsson G, Rehnqvist N, Sjogren A et al. Long term treatment with metoprolol after myocardial infarction. Report on three year mortality and morbidity. *J Am Coll Cardiol* 1985; **5**:1428–37.

24 Wilkins MR, Kendall MJ. Beta adrenoceptor blocking drugs and the elderly. *J R Coll Physicians Lond* 1984; **18**:42–5.

25 Neaton JD, Grimm RH, Prineas RS. Treatment of mild hypertension study. Final results. *JAMA* 1993; **270**:713–24.

26 Sawicki P. Guidelines for management of hypertension: Metabolic effects of drug treatment exaggerated. *Br Med J* 1994; **308**:855.

27 The SAVE Investigators. Effect of captopril on mortality and morbidity in patients with left ventricular dysfunction after myocardial infarction. *N Engl J Med* 1992; **327**:669–77.

28 The Acute Infarction Ramipril Efficacy (AIRE) Study Investigators. Effect of ramipril on mortality and morbidity of survivors of acute myocardial infarction with clinical evidence of heart failure. *Lancet* 1993; **342**:821–8.

29 Pollare T, Lithell H, Berne C. A comparison of the effects of hydrochlorthiazide and captopril on glucose and lipid metabolism in patients with hypertension. *N Engl J Med* 1989; **321**:868–73.

30 Bergemann R, Wohler T. Improved glucose regulation and microalbuminuria/proteinuria in diabetic patients treated with ACE inhibitors. A meta analysis of published studies of 1985–1990. *Schweiz Med Wochensch* 1992; **122**:1369–76.

4

Ethnic factors
Norman M Kaplan

Hypertension is more difficult to manage and more dangerous among certain ethnic groups, largely because of their lower socioeconomic status.[1] Most of the information now available about ethnic factors in hypertension comes from studies on African Americans in the USA, and most of this chapter will focus on this group. In addition, recently published data about hypertension in US Mexican Americans will be covered. A few closing comments will be made about hypertension in primitive societies, wherein ethnicity seems to contribute far less than the general lifestyle of the populations.

Prevalence

Hypertension is commoner among African Americans than other ethnic groups. Data from a survey of a large representative sample of the US population performed from 1988 to 1991 demonstrate a higher prevalence of hypertension among elderly African American than among elderly Whites or Mexican Americans (Table 4.1).[2] Previous surveys have shown similarly higher prevalence rates in younger African Americans as well (Figure 4.1).[3]

Although they are generally of as low a socioeconomic status as African Americans, Mexican Americans in San Antonio, Texas, do not have higher incidence rates of hypertension than non-Hispanic whites.[4] However, in a national survey of Mexican American

	Men	Women	Totals
African-American	71.6	71.9	71.8
Whites	54.9	51.2	52.9
Mexican Americans	56.9	53.1	54.9

Table 4.1
Prevalence (percentage) of hypertension in the civilian, non-institutionalized US population, aged 65–74, 1988–1991. (Hypertension is defined as having the average of 3 blood pressure measurements ≥ 140 mmHg (systolic) and/or ≥ 90 mmHg (diastolic) on a single occasion or as taking antihypertensive medication.) (From the Centers for Disease Control and Prevention, National Center for Health Statistics, Hyattsville, Maryland: provided in National High Blood Pressure Education Working Group.[2])

middle-aged men, hypertension was found to be more prevalent among those who were in the middle of the acculturation process than in those who were less or more acculturated.[5] This finding was attributed to higher levels of psychological stress for those who are undergoing acculturation but who have not yet reached the presumed freedom of being fully acculturated.

A long-term prospective study of Japanese men in Japan, Hawaii, and California[6] has

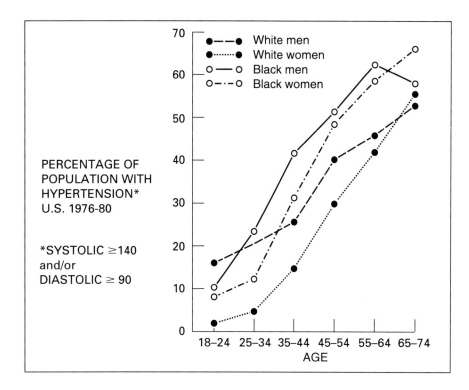

Figure 4.1
The prevalence of hypertension defined as systolic of 140 mmHg and/or diastolic of 90 mmHg or higher, among a representative sample of white and black men and women in the United States measured in the National Health and Nutrition Examination Survey from 1976 to 1980 (from Rowland M and Roberts J).[3]

found that hypertension is about half as common again among those who migrated to mainland USA than among those who remained in Japan or lived in Hawaii. Here again, varying influences of acculturation may be at play.

Complications

Hypertension is not only more common in African Americans, it is also more severe, less well managed and, therefore, more deadly. As best as can be ascertained, African Americans at any given level of blood pressure do not suffer more vascular damage than non-blacks, but rather they display a shift to the right of

the pressure distribution, yielding a higher overall prevalence of hypertension and a higher proportion of severe disease, which is associated with more vascular damage.[7] Moreover, blacks tend to have less of a nocturnal fall in pressure[8] (Fig. 4.2) and this may explain their greater degree of target organ damage.[9]

Much of the excess morbidity and mortality found in African Americans compared to US whites is related to their lower socioeconomic status, but at every level of income, African Americans, at least till age 65, have higher mortality than whites (Fig. 4.3).[10]

Cardiac disease
Although the overall prevalence of coronary heart disease (CHD) is lower among African

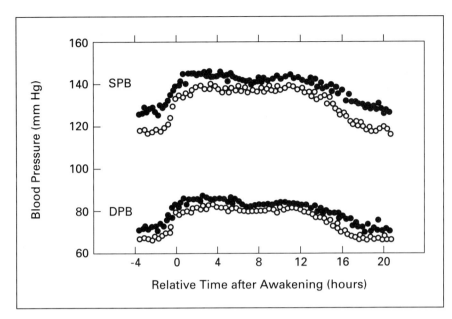

Figure 4.2
Twenty-four-hour profile for systolic (SBP) and diastolic (DBP) blood pressure for 275 black (●) and 246 white (○) individuals not previously treated with antihypertensive drugs. The difference in blood pressure and heart rated is significant (p < 0.001). Time 0 corresponds to the awakening time of each individual, as determined by diary (from Gretler DD et al).[8]

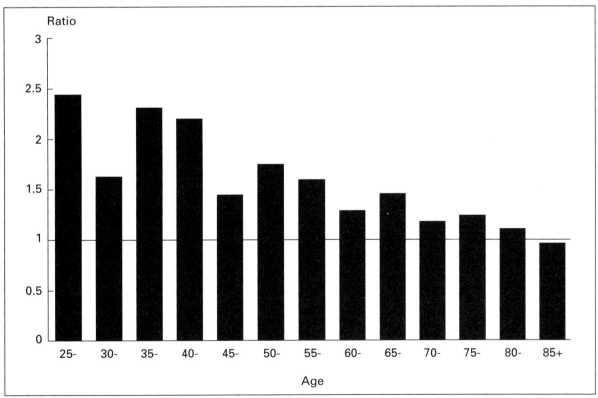

Figure 4.3
Income-adjusted ratio of black:white death rates from all causes (from Sorlie P et al).[10]

	Whites (N=380)	Blacks (N=47)
Diastolic blood pressure (mmHg)	98	104
Left ventricular mass (g/m²)	105	119
Prevalence of LVH (%)	19	41
Prevalence of concentric remodeling (%)	12	21

Table 4.2
Left ventricular mass and geometry by echocardiography. (Adapted from Koren et al.)[12]

Americans than US whites, mortality rates from CHD are similar. This probably reflects more severe disease and less adequate health care among African Americans.[11] In particular, African Americans have a lower incidence of myocardial infarction than US whites but have higher myocardial infarction fatality rates and a 2- to 3-fold greater risk of sudden cardiac death.[12]

These higher rates of mortality may reflect the fact that for the same degree of hypertension, blacks have a greater degree of left ventricular hypertrophy (LVH) than whites. Koren et al[12] found twice the prevalence of LVH and concentric remodeling among blacks with uncomplicated hypertension who were seen at the New York Hospital Hypertension Center than among whites with slightly lower average blood pressure (Table 4.2).

Cerebrovascular disease

Blacks have more strokes and die more frequently from them than non-blacks. Age-specific stroke mortality among African Americans were 3- to 4-fold higher than for non-blacks in all age groups under 65 years old.[14]

Renal disease

Although it is only the 3rd commonest serious consequence of hypertension, progressive renal damage that eventuates in end-stage renal disease (ESRD) is even more disproportionately represented among black hypertensives than coronary or cerebrovascular diseases. When various known precursors are taken into account (including age, prevalence of hypertension, severity of hypertension, diabetes, and level of education), blacks still have a 4.5 times greater risk for ESRD than non-blacks.[15] This, too, may reflect their lesser fall in blood pressure during sleep.[9] Moreover, even when they are treated as effectively as non-blacks, renal function in black hypertensives may continue to deteriorate, whereas it remains stable or improves in non-blacks.[16]

Mechanisms of hypertension in blacks

In order to manage more effectively the more dangerous hypertension seen among blacks, help may be obtained from an understanding of possible mechanisms involved in their higher prevalence and severity of hypertension. As in non-blacks, multiple factors are likely to be involved (Table 4.3).[17]

Genetics

Members of a single ethnic group would be expected to have more genes in common than

Genotype
- Candidate genes unique to blacks

Intermediate phenotype
- Enhanced sodium sensitivity
- Altered cation transport
- Suppressed renin–angiotensin–aldosterone
- Lower kallikrein–kinin, prostaglandin
- Increased adrenergic reactivity
- Hyper-responsiveness to growth factors

Phenotype
- Greater left ventricular hypertrophy
- Increased peripheral vascular resistance
- More advanced nephrosclerosis
- Less nocturnal fall in pressure

Table 4.3
Pathogenesis of hypertension in blacks. (Adapted from Falkner B.)[17]

people of different origins. Data support genetic associations of hypertension among blacks, but these genetic associations do not appear to differ quantitatively from those reported in non-blacks. This may reflect the genetic admixture that has occurred within black populations.

Sodium sensitivity

A higher degree of responsiveness of the blood pressure to both abrupt and chronic manipulations of sodium intake has been noted in normotensive and hypertensive blacks compared to non-blacks.[19] In those who had a pressor response to a sodium load, the renal excretion of the sodium was delayed and correlated with lower plasma renin levels.

Sodium transport

Abnormalities in sodium transport across vascular smooth muscle cells may be involved in the pathogenesis of most hypertension. Black normotensives and hypertensives have been found to have multiple differences from non-blacks in various cell transport measures.[20] These differences may be either secondary to volume expansion arising from a defect in renal excretory capacity, or they may be primary cellular defects which induce peripheral vascular constriction.

Stress

A large literature attests to an association between the stresses of low socioeconomic status and hypertension. As applied to African Americans, the association is likely to explain a considerable portion of their increased prevalence of hypertension but not all of it.[21] Even with equal levels of education, blacks have a higher prevalence of hypertension than whites.[22] A good example of the likely interaction between low socioeconomic status and a genetic trait is the finding that raised blood pressure levels were significantly associated with darker skin color in those blacks in the lower levels of socioeconomic status but not in those of higher status.[23]

Increased vascular responsiveness

Blacks have been shown, in various ways, to have a greater degree of vascular responsiveness to pressor stimuli. Examples include higher blood pressures in black children in third grade at school than in their non-black classmates during a stress video game,[24] and increased blood pressure response to various active coping tests in blacks with borderline hypertension.[25]

Diet

Particularly among older black women, the higher prevalence of hypertension is closely correlated with obesity.[26] Although they have greater sensitivity to sodium, blacks do not appear to ingest more sodium than do non-blacks, but their intake of both potassium and calcium is lower.[1]

Insulin resistance

Insulin resistance may be of considerable importance in the overall pathophysiology of hypertension. Few data are available concerning its relation to hypertension in blacks. Falkner et al[27] found increased resistance to exogenous insulin in hypertensive blacks similar to that as observed in hypertensive non-blacks. The hyperinsulinemia that results from insulin resistance was closely correlated with their blood pressure sensitivity to sodium.

Responsiveness to growth factors

Dustan[28] has hypothesized an increased responsiveness to vascular growth factors comparable to that noted in fibroblasts that form keloids. This could help to explain the increased prevalence of severe hypertension in blacks. She relates such hypertrophy to the finding of a different histological pattern – myointimal hyperplasia – in renal tissue from blacks with severe hypertension compared to the typical fibrinoid necrosis seen in non-blacks.[29]

Mechanisms in other ethnic groups

Other ethnic groups in the USA probably share both genetic and environmental exposures in a manner similar to African Americans. However, much less is known about their special characteristics, so that only a few generalizations will be provided rather than an attempt to examine other ethnic groups in detail.

Primitive versus acculturated

Groups of any race living a rural, more primitive life-style tend to ingest less sodium, remain less obese, and have less hypertension than other groups. When they migrate into urban areas and adapt more modern life-styles, they ingest more sodium, gain weight, and develop more hypertension.[30] Dramatic changes in the prevalence of hypertension and the nature of cardiovascular complications have been seen when formerly isolated ethnic groups adapt modern life-styles. An example is the rise in blood pressure among Asians who migrate into the USA.[31]

Of more serious consequence is the lack of even rudimentary health care in impoverished countries. As an example, 317 hypertensives were seen over a 2 year period in a hospital in Burkina Faso, a country in sub-Saharan Africa[32]. Of these, 43% had a diastolic blood pressure above 130 mmHg and 38% renal insufficiency. One-fifth of the patients died during their hospital stay. This situation is similar to that seen before the advent of effective antihypertensive therapies in more wealthy countries. The difficulty is obvious: without therapy, hypertension can progress and cause major morbidity and mortality.

Persistence of ethnic differences

Although environmental changes often alter blood pressure and other cardiovascular risks, some ethnic groups preserve characteristics that presumably reflect stronger genetic influences. For example, Amerindian descendants, such as Mexican Americans in San Antonio, have a lower prevalence of hypertension despite their high prevalence of obesity and diabetes with insulin resistance.[33] Thus, ethnic origins may work in both ways, to increase the propensity toward hypertension or to protect against the threat.

Increased sodium sensitivity
Lower intake of potassium
Lower intake of calcium
Greater prevalence of obesity
Greater prevalence of alcohol abuse
Greater prevalence of smoking

Table 4.4
Reasons for the need for life-style modifications in black hypertensives

Treatment

Modifications in life-style may be even more effective in lowering blood pressure among ethnic groups – in particular blacks – who carry more of the genetic and environmental burdens that lead to their higher prevalence of hypertension than it is among whites (Table 4.4). Although there is no evidence that the changes in life-style needed to correct these burdens are any more effective in black hypertensives, they should nevertheless be vigorously encouraged. In particular, reduction in

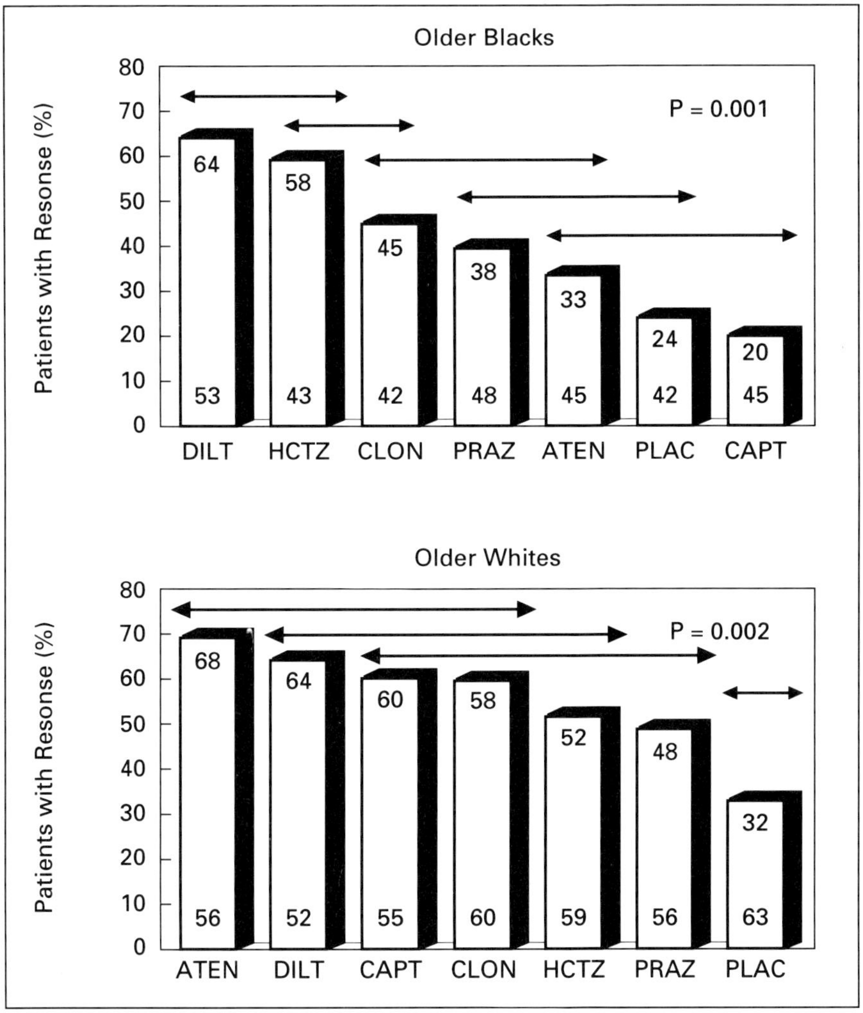

Figure 4.4.
The percentage of responders among older black and white patients in the VA Cooperative Study to placebo or one of six antihypertensive agents. Dilt – diltiazem; HCT – hydrochlorothiazide; Clon – clonidine; Praz – prazosin; Aten – atenolol; Plac – placebo; Capt – captopril. (From Materson et al.)[37]

body weight for the large percentage of black hypertensive women who are obese and moderate restriction of sodium for all blacks should be pursued.

When given equal access to the same treatment, blacks respond in a similar manner and may experience an even lower incidence of cardiovascular disease than whites.[34] However, the higher prevalence of poverty and obesity among African American hypertensives impede the control of their hypertension.[35] Similar cultural and socioeconomic barriers may explain the lower level of control of hypertension found among Mexican Americans in San Antonio.[36]

Antihypertensive drugs

The response to various antihypertensive drugs may differ between blacks and other ethnic groups.[37] In general, blacks have less response to beta-blockers and angiotensin converting enzyme (ACE) inhibitors, perhaps because they tend to have lower renin levels. On the other hand, they respond as well as whites to diuretics, calcium channel blockers, and alpha$_1$-receptor blockers (Fig. 4.4).[38]

In this Veterans Administration cooperative study, 1292 hypertensive men with a diastolic blood pressure of 95 to 109 mmHg on placebo, 48% black, were randomly assigned to one of 6 drugs or a placebo. The drug doses were titrated to a goal of a diastolic blood pressure less than 90 mmHg and therapy was continued for at least one year. The responses to the representative drugs of each of the 6 major classes were influenced both by the age and

race of the patients. In particular, both younger (average age 50) and older (average age 66) blacks responded best to the calcium entry blocker, diltiazem, and least well to the ACE inhibitor, captopril. The older blacks responded better to the diuretic and less well to the beta-blocker than did the younger blacks.

Despite their somewhat lesser response to beta-blockers and ACE inhibitors, these agents should be given to those hypertensive blacks who have specific indications for them, e.g. a beta-blocker should be used after an acute myocardial infarction, and an ACE inhibitor should be used in the presence of diabetic nephropathy. Moreover, the antihypertensive efficacy of these agents can be enhanced by the addition of a small dose of diuretic. This may be either because the diuretic activates the renin–angiotensin system so that the renin-suppressing drugs are more effective, or because the diuretic corrects the relatively greater volume expansion that characterizes the black hypertensive.

Therapy may need to be more vigorous in blacks to slow the progress of renal damage which is so much more prevalent in them than in non-blacks even with similar degrees of hypertension[39]. A goal of less than 130/85 may be appropriate since even when their pressures were reduced to below 95 mmHg in the MRFIT trial, renal function tended to continue to decline in the blacks[40].

It is obvious that the ethnic factors described in this chapter will engender more of the accelerated and unresponsive types of hypertension described in subsequent chapters.

References

1 Kaplan NM. Primary hypertension: natural history, special populations, and evaluation. In: Kaplan NM, ed. *Clinical Hypertension* 6th edn. Baltimore: Williams and Wilkins, 1994:109–143.

2 National High Blood Pressure Education Program Working Group. National High Blood Pressure Education Program Working Group report on hypertension in the elderly. *Hypertension* 1994; 23:275–85.

3 Rowland M, Roberts J. Blood pressure levels and hypertension in persons aged 6–74 years. United States, 1976–80. *NCHS Advance Data, No. 84, Vital and Health Statistics of the National Center for Health Statistics.* Washington DC: US Department of Health and Human Services, 8 October 1982.

4 Haffner SM, Mitchell BD, Valdez RA, Hazuda HP, Morales PA, Stern MP. Eight-year incidence of hypertension in Mexican Americans and non-Hispanic whites. The San Antonio Heart Study. *Am J Hypertens* 1992; 5:147–53.

5 Markides KS, Lee DJ, Ray LA. Acculturation and hypertension in Mexican Americans. *Ethnicity Dis* 1993; 3:70–4.

6 Yano K, Reed DM, Kagan A. Coronary heart disease, hypertension and stroke among Japanese–American men in Hawaii: The Honolulu Heart Program. *Hawaii Med J* 1985; 44:297–312.

7 Cooper RS, Liao Y. Is hypertension among blacks more severe or simply more common [Abstract]. *Circulation* 1992; 85:12.

8 Gretler DD, Fumo MT, Nelson KS, Murphy MB. Ethnic differences in circadian hemodynamic profile. *Am J Hypertens* 1994; 7:7–14.

9 Harshfield GA, Pulliam DA, Alpert BS. Ambulatory blood pressure and renal function in healthy children and adolescents. *Am J Hypertens* 1994; 7:282–5.

10 Sorlie P, Rogot E, Anderson R, Johnson NJ, Backlund E. Black–white mortality differences by family income. *Lancet* 1992; 340:346–50.

11 Keil JE, Sutherland SE, Knapp RG, Lackland DT, Gazes PC, Tyroler HA. Mortality rates and risk factors for coronary disease in black as compared with white men and women. *N Engl J Med* 1993; 329:73–8.

12 Koren MJ, Mensah GA, Blake J, Laragh JH, Devereux RB. Comparison of left ventricular mass and geometry in black and white patients with essential hypertension. *Am J Hypertens* 1993; 6:815–23.

13 Mayet J, Shahi M, Thom S, Poulter N, Sever PS, Foale RA. Why do black hypertensives fare worse [Abstract]? *Circulation* 1993; 2:1–511.

14 Caplan LR. Strokes in African-Americans. *Circulation* 1993; 83:1469–71.

15 Whittle JC, Whelton PK, Seidler AJ, Klag MJ. Does racial variation in risk factors explain black–white differences in the incidence of hypertensive end-stage renal disease? *Arch Intern Med* 1991; 151:1359–64.

16 Walker WG, Neaton JD, Cutler JA, Neuwirth R, Cohen JD. Renal function change in hypertensive members of the Multiple Risk Factor Intervention Trial. *JAMA* 1992; 268:3085–91.

17 Falkner B. Differences in blacks and whites with essential hypertension: biochemistry and endocrine. State of the art lecture. *Hypertension* 1990; 15:681–6.

18 Savage DD, Watkins LO, Grim CE, Kumanyika SK. Hypertension in black populations. In: Laragh JH, Brenner BM, eds. *Hypertension: Pathophysiology, Diagnosis, and Management.* New York: Raven Press, 1990; 1837–52.

19 Luft FC, Miller JZ, Grim CE et al. Salt sensitivity and resistance of blood pressure. *Hypertension* 1991; 17(Suppl I):I-102–I-108.

20 Kimura M, Cho JH, Lasker N, Aviv A. Differences in platelet calcium regulation between African Americans and Caucasians: implications for the predisposition of African Americans to essential hypertension. *J Hypertension* 1994; 12:199–207.

21 Fray JCS. Hypertension in blacks: physiological, psychosocial, theoretical, and therapeutic challenges. In: Fray JCS, Douglas JG, eds. *Pathophysiology of Hypertension in Blacks*. New York: Oxford University Press, 1993:3–22.

22 Tyroler HA. Socioeconomic status, age, and sex in the prevalence and prognosis of hypertension in blacks and whites. In: Laragh JH, Brenner BM, eds. *Hypertension: Pathophysiology, Diagnosis, and Management*. New York: Raven Press, 1990:159–74.

23 Klag MJ, Whelton PK, Coresh J, Grim CE, Kuller LH. The association of skin color with blood pressure in US blacks in low socioeconomic status. *JAMA* 1991; **265**:599–602.

24 Murphy JK, Alpert BS, Walker SS. Consistency of ethnic differences in children's pressor reactivity 1987 to 1992. *Hypertension* 1994; **23**(Suppl I):I-152–I-155.

25 Light KC, Obrist PA, Sherwood A, James SA, Strogatz DS. Effects of race and marginally elevated blood pressure on responses to stress. *Hypertension* 1987; **10**:555–63.

26 Anderson NB, Myers HF, Pickering T, Jackson JS. Hypertension in blacks: psychosocial and biological perspectives. J *Hypertension* 1989; **7**:161–72.

27 Falkner B, Hulman S, Kushner H. Hyperinsulinemia and blood pressure sensitivity to sodium in young blacks. *J Am Soc Nephrol* 1992; **3**:940–6.

28 Dustan HP. Growth factors and racial differences in severity of hypertension and renal diseases. *Lancet* 1992; **339**:1339–40.

29 Muirhead EE, Pitcock JA. Histopathology of severe renal vascular damage in blacks. *Clin Cardiol* 1989; **12**(Suppl IV):IV-58–IV-65.

30 Poulter NR, Khaw KT, Hopwood BEC et al. The Kenyan Luo migration study: observations on the initiation of a rise in blood pressure. *Br Med J* 1990; **300**:967–72.

31 Munger RG, Gomez-Marin O, Prineas RJ, Sinaiko AR. Elevated blood pressure among Southeast Asian refugee children in Minnesota. *Am J Epidemiol* 1991; **133**:1257–65.

32 Laville M, Lengani A, Sermé D, Fauvel J-P, Ouandaogo BJ, Zech P. Epidemiological profile of hypertensive disease and renal risk factors in Black Africa. *J Hypertension* 1994; **12** (839–43).

33 Ferrannini E, Haffner SM, Stern MP et al. High blood pressure and insulin resistance: influence of ethnic background. *Eur J Clin Invest* 1991; **21**:280–7.

34 Ooi WL, Budner NS, Cohen H, Madhavan S, Alderman MH. Impact of race on treatment response and cardiovascular disease among hypertensives. *Hypertension* 1989; **14**:227–34.

35 Shea S, Misra D, Ehrlich MH, Field L, Francis CK. Predisposing factors for severe, uncontrolled hypertension in an inner-city minority population. *N Engl J Med* 1992; **327**:776–81.

36 Haffner SM, Morales PA, Hazuda HP, Stern MP. Level of control of hypertension in Mexican Americans and non-Hispanic whites. *Hypertension* 1993; **21**:83–8.

37 Wright JT Jr, Douglas JG. Drug therapy in black hypertensives. In: Fray JCS, Douglas JG, eds. *Pathophysiology of Hypertension in Blacks*. New York: Oxford University Press, 1993:271–91.

38 Materson BJ, Reda DJ, Cushman WC et al. Single-drug therapy for hypertension in men. A comparison of six antihypertensive agents with placebo. *N Engl J Med* 1993; **328**:914–21.

39 Tracy RE, Guzman MA, Oalmann MC, Newman WP III, Strong JP. Nephrosclerosis in three cohorts of black and white men born 1925 to 1944, 1934 to 1953, and 1943 to 1962. *Am J Hypertens* 1993; **6**:185–92.

40 Walker WG, Neaton JD, Cutler JA, Neuwirth R, Cohen JD. Renal function change in hypertensive members of the Multiple Risk Factor Intervention Trial. *JAMA* 1992; **268**:3085–91.

SECTION II

THE TYPE

5

Secondary hypertension

Neil JL Gittoes and Michael C Sheppard

Secondary hypertension is defined as high blood pressure resulting from identifiable, and thus potentially treatable causes. In the general population the overall prevalence is 0.1–0.2%, and in hypertensive patients this rises to not greater than 5%.[1] The causes of secondary hypertension along with their respective frequencies are shown in Table 5.1.

Patients with secondary hypertension tend to be younger and may have specific symptoms suggesting the cause. Once the possibility of secondary hypertension is considered, the patient should be investigated appropriately, although the yield of true positive results tends to be low. Nevertheless, those few patients diagnosed as having secondary hypertension can often be offered a potential cure before end organ damage occurs.

The various pathologies responsible for secondary hypertension interfere with the normal homoeostatic mechanisms of blood pressure control. In this way they provide useful insights into potential aetiological factors for the generation and perpetuation of essential hypertension.

Endocrine causes of hypertension

Phaeochromocytoma

Of all the causes of secondary hypertension, the pathophysiology of phaeochromocytoma is the best understood, its diagnosis potentially the easiest and its treatment the most sure. The pathology in this condition is related to episodic secretions of large quantities of catecholamines which, through stimulation of alpha- and/or beta-adrenergic receptors, are temporally related to characteristic symptoms and signs. The relationship between paroxysmal hypertension and the finding of adrenal tumours at post-mortem was first noted in 1922.[2] Within years of the discovery of phaeochromocytoma, the first successful

Causes of hypertension	Frequency (%)	
Primary hypertension		95.3
Secondary hypertension		4.7
Renoparenchymal	2.4	
Renovascular	1.0	
Coarctation	0.1	
Endocrine	0.4	
Drugs	0.8	

Table 5.1
Frequency of hypertension in the general population. Adapted from Danielson and Dammstrom.[1]

reports of their removal were announced.[3,4] Histologically these tumours were found to have a distinctive brownish colour when stained with chromium salts.[5]

Phaeochromocytomas are the cause of hypertension in 0.1–0.2% of all newly diagnosed hypertensive patients, although the condition accounts for a larger proportion of hypertensive crises and malignant hypertension. The overall incidence in the general population is between 1 in 4000 and 1 in 5000.[6]

The tumours are derived from primitive neuroectodermal cells (sympathogonia) which have the capacity to synthesize and secrete catecholamines. These cells are known as APUD (amine precursor uptake and decarboxylation) cells and are found in the adrenal medulla, along the sympathetic chain and in the organs of Zuckerkandl (a collection of para-aortic, paraganglionic cells around the inferior mesenteric artery). Tumours arising outside the adrenal medulla are sometimes referred to as paraganglionomas.[7] The prevalence of the anatomical locations of phaeochromocytomas is shown in Table 5.2.

Multiple tumours tend to be associated with the multiple endocrine neoplasia (MEN) syndrome type II, Sipple's syndrome.[8] Between 5 and 15% of phaeochromocytomas are malignant. Malignancy can only be determined on the basis of distant metastases, as even benign tumours show local invasion.[9] Malignant phaeochromocytomas do, however, tend to be slow growing and can be associated with long survival.[10]

Phaeochromocytomas usually secrete some adrenaline along with noradrenaline. Catecholamines are produced from tyrosine and this pathway can be interrupted by pharmacological means (Fig. 5.1). If the tumour is of extra-adrenal origin, adrenaline is only rarely secreted.[12] Small tumours tend to secrete more catecholamines than larger ones since the latter have greater storage capacity and can metabolize the catecholamines to inactive forms.

Location of tumour	Frequency (%)
Intra-abdominal	97–99
Single adrenal tumour	50–70
Single extra-adrenal tumour	10–20
Multiple tumours (multiple endocrine neoplasia)	15–40
Bilateral tumours	5–25
Multiple extra-adrenal tumours	5–15
Extra-abdominal	1–3
Intrathoracic (posterior mediastinum)	2
Neck	< 1

Table 5.2
Frequency of anatomical location of phaeochromocytomas.

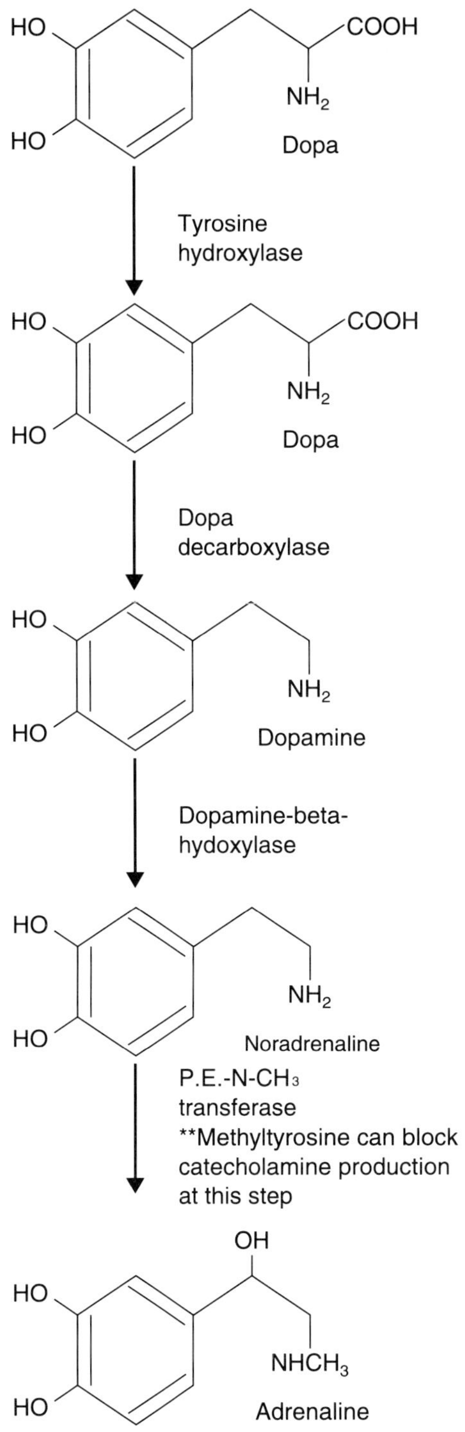

Figure 5.1
The biosynthesis of catecholamines

Clinical presentation

The specific catecholamine secretory products of phaeochromocytomas determine the clinical presentation. If mainly adrenaline is secreted then hypertension tends to be predominantly systolic,[13] owing to increased cardiac output associated with tachycardia, sweating, flushing and tremor. There may even be instances of hypotension due to the disproportionate activity of adrenaline on beta$_2$ receptors,[14] causing peripheral vasodilatation and hence hypotension. Noradrenaline, however, has a similar action at alpha$_1$, alpha$_2$ and beta$_1$ receptor sites, with an overall effect of raising systolic and diastolic blood pressure[15] with little effect on heart rate. Renal beta-receptors are also stimulated by high concentrations of circulating catecholamines, which causes release of renin from the juxtaglomerular cells of the kidney and a further increase in arterial pressure by activating the circulating renin–angiotensin system.

Most patients presenting with phaeochromocytoma tend to be over 40 years of age (excluding familial cases) and there are a number of important differential diagnoses to consider (Table 5.3). Occasionally symptoms may be provoked by an exogenous source, e.g. exercise, bending, defaecation, micturition, anaesthaesia, or abdominal palpation. In such cases, these specific symptoms may suggest both the diagnosis and localization of the tumour, e.g. palpitations and headaches on micturition with a bladder phaeochromocytoma.[16]

Clinical features of phaeochromocytoma

Headache	Palpitations	Anxiety	Sweating
Tremor	Weight loss	Nausea	Abdominal or chest pain
Vomiting	Constipation	Polyuria/polydipsia	Heat intolerance
Hypotension	Cold extremities	Raynaud's phenomenon	Hypertension
Pallor	Tachycardia	Bradycardia	Arrhythmias
Glycosuria	Fever		

Conditions simulating above clinical features

Anxiety	Hypoglycaemia	Diabetes	Migraine
Thyrotoxicosis	Endocarditis	Menopause	Eclampsia
Carcinoid	Porphyria		

Important associations

Neurofibromatosis	Multiple endocrine neoplasia	Cardiomyopathy

Table 5.3
List of symptoms and signs of phaeochromocytoma with important differential diagnoses shown. Rare associations with phaeochromocytoma are also shown.

Diagnosis

There should be a low threshold for further investigations in patients who have hypertension, or more specifically fluctuating hypertension, with a compatible history. Sensitive and specific biochemical measures of plasma and urine catecholamines and their principal metabolites are available, and these indicate the presence of a phaeochromocytoma. Once the diagnosis has been established, the location of the tumour should be sought using appropriate imaging techniques.

Biochemical assessment

Three 24-hour urine collections for catecholamine metabolites (metanephrines) are still widely used as an initial assessment. Most (60–75%) patients with phaeochromocytoma excrete large quantities of catecholamine metabolites, making this test a very useful primary screening investigation.

The measurement of noradrenaline and adrenaline in urine and plasma has recently become widely available and offers a sensitive and specific test for diagnosing those 20–30% of patients who excrete smaller concentrations of catecholamine metabolites.[17] Despite the availability of these assays, there is a minority of patients who have normal or non-diagnostic levels of adrenaline and noradrenaline.

Although plasma renin levels are elevated in phaeochromocytoma, through stimulation of renal renin, the levels are so variable that they are of no use diagnostically.[18]

In addition to catecholamine and metanephrine secretion, phaeochromocytomas may also produce a variety of other compounds:

- peptides
  enkephalins
  neuropeptide Y
  atrial natriuretic peptide

- proteins
    chromogranin A
    dopamine beta-hydroxylase

Chromogranin A,[19] neuropeptide Y,[20,21] and atrial natriuretic peptide[22] can be detected in plasma. Some patients with malignant phaeochromocytomas have very high plasma levels of neuropeptide Y,[20] with paradoxically less mRNA for this peptide than benign tumours.[23] This observation may in the future help distinguish between benign and malignant phaeochromocytomas, a task that is at present histologically very difficult.

Imaging
Most phaeochromocytomas are intra-abdominal, and of these 80–90% are intra-adrenal. Tumours measuring more than 4 cm in diameter can be seen by routine imaging with computerized tomography or ultrasonography, however, these modalities are not tissue specific. Magnetic resonance imaging using T2-weighted spin imaging, on the other hand, has become especially useful in specifically enhancing tumour tissue.[24,25]

The property of chromaffin cells to concentrate [meta-^{125}I]iodobenzylguanidine (MIBG) is utilized in the MIBG scan.[26] This is particularly useful for detecting small, extra-abdominal tumours and also in post-operative surveillance for detecting recurrent tumours, as the local anatomy may be distorted after surgery.

Transoesophageal echocardiography may be used to image the very rare entity of intracardiac or pericardial phaeochromocytoma.[27]

Treatment of Phaeochromocytomas
Pharmacological treatment of phaeochromocytomas is always necessary before considering definitive surgical treatment (Table 5.4).

When it is possible that a patient has a phaeochromocytoma, beta-blocking drugs should

Alpha-receptor antagonists
    phenoxybenzamine, phentolamine
Beta-receptor antagonists
    metoprolol, atenolol
Combined alpha- and beta-receptor antagonists
    labetalol
Tyrosine hydroxylase inhibitor
    methyltyrosine

Table 5.4
Drugs used in the management of adrenomedullary hypertension.

not be given alone. In this case beta-blockade without alpha-blockade may result in worsening of hypertension, owing to a relative increase in alpha-stimulation, which can cause intense vasoconstriction and severe hypertension. Initially, therefore, alpha-blocking drugs or combined alpha- and beta-blocking drugs should be used. Alpha-receptor blockers reduce arterial pressure by relieving the vasoconstrictor effects of catecholamines. Conventionally, phenoxybenzamine is started at a dose of 10 mg and increased by 10 mg daily to a dose of around 1–2 mg/kg per day in 2 divided doses. Phentolamine can be administered intravenously to control blood pressure rapidly. Alternatively, labetalol at an initial dose of 100 mg twice daily increasing to a maximum of 2.4 g/day in 3–4 divided doses may be prescribed. This drug will block both alpha- and beta-receptors, and can be administered intravenously or orally.

Beta-receptor blockers may be useful in controlling the symptoms attributable to tachycardia. Should hypertension remain a problem despite alpha- and beta-blockade, the problem may be related to a stimulated renin–angiotensin system. In these cases, an ACE inhibitor may prove effective.

Surgery is often curative,[28] but it should only be contemplated once adequate alpha- and, if necessary, beta-blockade is complete. Intraoperative and perioperative management of blood pressure is often difficult. Recurrence occurs in 10–15% of cases and, although it may be benign, malignant transformation should always be considered. Clinical, biochemical, and radiographic evidence of recurrence may take years to become evident.

When a tumour is inoperable and blocking drugs are inadequate to relieve symptoms, methyltyrosine, a tyrosine hydroxylase inhibitor, may be used effectively to inhibit the synthesis of catecholamines (see Fig. 5.1).

Recent chemotherapeutic combinations have been shown to be effective in reducing tumour bulk in malignant phaechromocytoma and this produces a concurrent decrease in the production of catecholamines and their metabolites.[29] MIBG in large doses has also been successfully used experimentally – it acts as a carrier that selectively delivers therapeutic doses of radioactivity to malignant phaeochromocytomas.[30,31]

Conn's syndrome

True Conn's syndrome is primary hyperaldosteronism caused by an adrenocortical adenoma. It is an uncommon cause of secondary hypertension. Aldosterone is normally secreted from the zona glomerulosa and acts at the distal nephrons to promote sodium reabsorption in exchange for potassium and hydrogen ions. As the result of this action, when aldosterone is being produced in excess the characteristic biochemical picture of hypokalaemic alkalosis develops. Physiologically aldosterone is under the control of the renin–angiotensin system (Fig. 5.2), although in Conn's syndrome the secretion

of aldosterone is autonomous. Primary hyperaldosteronism may occasionally be due to the presence of an adrenal or ovarian carcinoma.[32]

The adrenal adenomas responsible for Conn's syndrome are usually small (< 2 cm) and they protrude from the gland. On sectioning, the tumour has a characteristic golden yellow colour.

Clinical presentation

Hypertension secondary to Conn's syndrome usually presents with the manifestations of hypokalaemia, i.e. weakness, polyuria, nocturia, polydipsia, paraesthesiae, tetany, and paralysis. The age at presentation is 30–50 years; females are affected more often than males. Hypertension tends to be mild although occasionally the presenting problem is malignant hypertension.[33] The mechanism of hypertension is related to sodium retention, plasma expansion, and hence increased cardiac output (see Fig. 5.2).

The biochemical features of Conn's syndrome are:

High aldosterone	Hypokalaemia
Low renin	Metabolic alkalosis (high HCO_3, high pH)
Low angiotensin II	Hypernatraemia

Aldosterone levels normally rise when a person adopts an erect posture, through activation of the renin–angiotensin system. With autonomous secretion of aldosterone (Conn's syndrome), the level stays constant or even falls. This fact is of importance diagnostically.

In one third of patients who have biochemical Conn's syndrome (hypertension, excess aldosterone and low plasma renin), there is bilateral adrenal hyperplasia but no adrenal tumour apparent on imaging. This quite distinct clinical entity is termed idiopathic hyperaldosteronism.

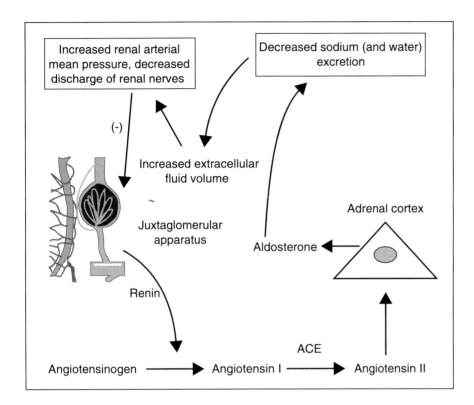

Figure 5.2
Flow diagram of renin–angiotensin system activation.

The aldosterone level in this situation remains under control of the renin–angiotensin system (i.e. it is not autonomous).

On closer examination of the adrenal glands of patients with idiopathic hyperaldosteronism, there is diffuse or occasionally focal hyperplasia and occasional nodule formation. The nodules tend to be multiple and bilateral, with arteriopathic changes in the capsular vessels. This condition occurs in older patients and was originally thought to be the result of vascular disease associated with essential hypertension.[34] However, it is now accepted that idiopathic hyperaldosteronism represents a truly distinct pathology, probably caused by the action of an aldosterone stimulating factor released from the anterior pituitary. Hypersecretion of this stimulating factor is proposed to cause hyperplasia of the zona glomerulosa and increased sensitivity of aldosterone to angiotensin II. The treatment of idiopathic hyperaldosteronism differs from that of true Conn's syndrome.

Investigations
The possibility of Conn's syndrome is usually suggested as the result of finding hypokalaemia in a hypertensive patient. A useful screening test is to perform supine and erect renin and aldosterone levels. Plasma aldosterone is measured at 08:00 h after an overnight period of bed rest followed by a repeat sample at 12:00 h after 4 hours of being ambulant. In the case of idiopathic aldosteronism, the response to posture is the same as that encountered physiologically (i.e. raised aldosterone on standing). As mentioned above, with autonomous secretion the level of aldosterone stays constant or even falls.

More recently, erect and supine aldosterone estimations have been superseded by the calculation of the ratio of random plasma aldosterone (measured in pmol/l) to plasma renin activity (measured in ng/ml/hr). The rationale of this test relies on the fact that the ratio of normal plasma aldosterone to plasma renin activity will be abnormal at all times and under all situations in patients with primary hyperaldosteronism. A ratio of greater than 290 is diagnostic of primary hyperaldosteronism.[35]

Once the diagnosis has been made, the tumour must be localized. High resolution CT or MRI offer a simple and non-invasive technique for detecting tumours, even when they are small.

Adrenal vein sampling and venography can also be useful in localizing tumours, although technically this investigation is very difficult to perform. The adrenal veins are cannulated and aldosterone levels are measured from both sides. Once the pathological side has been identified, then retrograde flush of contrast can be injected which may outline an adenoma if it is more than 1 cm in diameter. Complications of this procedure are thrombus formation within the adrenal vein, and extravasation, which may cause adrenal insufficiency.

Adrenal scintillation scanning uses radiolabelled (^{131}I) 19-iodocholesterol uptake into the adrenal glands. Scanning is carried out sequentially over 2 weeks and the presence of a 'hot spot' indicates the presence of an adrenal tumour.[36] This technique is rarely used in clinical practice.

Treatment

Pharmacological treatment is suggested, at least at first, for all types of hyperaldosteronism.[37] The aldosterone antagonist, spironolactone, is often helpful in controlling hypertension and symptoms due to hypokalaemia. An initial dose of 100 mg daily should be commenced but can be increased to 400 mg/day if necessary for control of blood pressure. Hypokalaemia tends to be corrected before the hypertension, which may take as long as 4–8 weeks to correct. The dose of spironolactone can often be reduced after several months of therapy to as little as 50 mg/day.

One of the side effects of spironolactone is gynaecomastia; hence the drug of choice for men is a potassium-sparing diuretic, such as amiloride at an initial dose of 5 mg twice daily increasing if necessary to a maximum daily divided dose of 30 mg. Potassium supplementation should not be given during treatment with spironolactone or amiloride, owing to the risk of hyperkalaemia.

In the presence of idiopathic hyperaldosteronism, spironolactone alone or amiloride alone is often not sufficient to control blood pressure adequately. In such instances, second line adjunctive treatment with calcium channel blockers, ACE inhibitors or thiazides have all proved effective.[38,39]

Patients with the rare entity of primary aldosteronism due to adrenal carcinoma should be treated with surgery. Unilateral adrenalectomy for true Conn's syndrome caused by a unilateral adrenal adenoma is associated with a good cure rate (68–83%).[40] There have recently been reports of successful laparoscopic adrenalectomies for primary aldosteronism.[41] In the presence of bilateral adrenal hyperplasia (idiopathic hyperaldosteronism), results from surgery are disappointing (18–35% cured).[40] This discrepancy presumably reflects the different aetiologies of these conditions.

Cushing's syndrome

The description of the classical symptoms and signs of hypercortisolism was first published in 1912 by Harvey Cushing.[42] Among the well-recognized array of profound metabolic consequences of steroid excess, 9 of the 12 patients

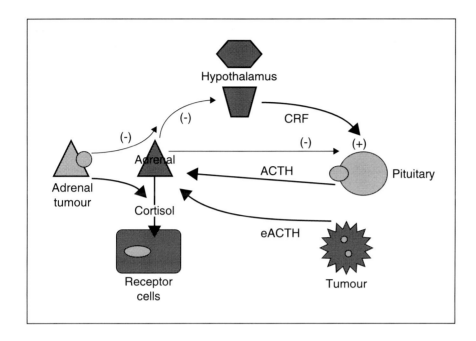

Figure 5.3
Hypothalamic–pituitary–adrenal axis showing causes of Cushing's syndrome. (ACTH – Adrenocorticotrophic hormone, eACTH – ectopic ACTH, CRF – corticotrophin releasing factor.)

in the original series were found to have hypertension. In the hypertensive population, Cushing's syndrome represents around 0.1% of all cases. Hypercortisolism may be due to excess production of either adrenocorticotrophic hormone (ACTH) or of cortisol itself (Fig. 5.3).

Type of hypercortisolism	Hypertension (%)
Pituitary dependent	88
Adrenal tumour	85
eACTH	55
Iatrogenic (steroids)	17

Table 5.5
Frequency of hypertension seen in various causes of Cushing's syndrome.

Elevated blood pressure is seen in patients with all forms of Cushing's syndrome, including Cushing's disease (pituitary-dependent Cushing's), although the frequency of hypertension varies for each subgroup (Table 5.5). Whatever the underlying cause of the hypercortisolism, the hypertension seen in Cushing's syndrome is very resistant to conventional antihypertensive treatment.

Non-pituitary-dependent Cushing's syndrome
Non-pituitary-dependent Cushing's syndrome encompasses primary adrenal tumours, ectopic ACTH production and exogenous administration of glucocorticoids (see Fig. 5.3). Autonomous secretion of endogenous steroids arises from solitary adrenocortical tumours that may be benign or malignant. Ectopic ACTH (eACTH) may be secreted from any malignant tumour, although the commonest source is small cell (oat cell) carcinoma of the bronchus. With approximately 5 million

patients in the United States taking oral steroids at any one time, the quantitative importance of iatrogenic Cushing's syndrome is clear.

Pituitary Cushing's

Pituitary-dependent Cushing's (Cushing's disease) arises from excess secretion of ACTH from pituitary microadenomas. This in turn causes bilateral adrenal hyperplasia and excess cortisol secretion.

Clinical presentation

The usual presentation of Cushing's syndrome is with a history of change in appearance; however, complications of hypertension may be present at the time of diagnosis or may even be the sole presenting feature (e.g. cardiac failure, cerebrovascular event). Cushing's syndrome secondary to eACTH secretion is classically associated with a hypokalaemic alkalosis that is usually absent in other forms of the condition. Patients with this condition also tend to be pigmented. Adrenal carcinoma is likely to be the aetiology of Cushing's syndrome when virilization or hirsutism are prominent features.

Mechanisms of hypertension

The pathogenesis of hypertension in Cushing's is poorly understood. Originally the explanation was thought to be related to sodium retention secondary to the action of mineralocorticoid excess. However, Ritchie et al[43] have shown that there is no rise in exchangeable sodium; that sodium depletion does not help the hypertension, and that there is no correlation between exchangeable sodium and blood pressure.

This study also revealed normal catecholamine levels; normal renin–angiotensin system activity, and normal sympathetic receptor density, but demonstrated increased cardiac sensitivity to catecholamines.[43] Others have shown that steroids increase the density of beta-receptors on granulocytes[44] and lymphocytes,[45] although not on myocardial cells. Increased cardiac sensitivity to both the positive chronotropic and inotropic effects of catecholamines results in increased cardiac output, which may be partly responsible for the hypertension seen in Cushing's.

Investigations

The classical dexamethasone suppression tests are still widely used in the diagnosis of Cushing's; they also help to distinguish the origin of the hypercortisolism. For screening purposes, a single midnight dose of 1 mg of dexamethasone will detect 98% of Cushing's patients, with 5% false positives.[46] Normally the plasma cortisol level at 09:00 h is suppressed to less than 180 nmol/l. This test can be done on an out-patient basis.

If the cortisol level does not suppress after an overnight dexamethasone suppression test, the patient should be admitted for low- and high-dose dexamethasone suppression. The rationale of these investigations is based on the observation that cortisol secretion is not suppressed by dexamethasone in patients with adrenal tumours or eACTH even when high doses (2 mg 4 times a day for 2 days) are given, whereas such doses do inhibit ACTH-driven secretion in patients with Cushing's disease. Low-dose dexamethasone (0.5 mg) suppresses in neither instance. A false-positive low-dose dexamethasone suppression test may occur in patients who are obese or depressed.

ACTH levels can be assayed and tend to be suppressed to undetectable levels (less than 10 ng/l) in non-ACTH dependent Cushing's. The levels in pituitary-dependent and eACTH-related Cushing's tend to be high (> 200 ng/l).

A chest x-ray is mandatory in order to search for an occult malignancy underlying the cause of eACTH. CT or MRI scanning of the adrenal glands may show discrete adenomas or carcinomas. Similar imaging of the pituitary fossa may show signs of a pituitary tumour. Very occasionally, selective venous catheterization of the inferior petrosal sinuses is required to determine a pituitary origin of Cushing's.[47]

A powerful and relatively new diagnostic tool used in the determination of the cause of hypercortisolism is the CRF stimulation test. Administration of bovine CRF stimulates elevation of ACTH and cortisol levels in patients with pituitary dependent Cushing's disease. There is no effect on these levels in patients with eACTH syndrome.[48] The differential diagnostic accuracy of the test in this context is 85%. Patients with Cushing's syndrome of adrenal aetiology have low or undetectable levels of ACTH, and these levels do not rise after exogenous administration of CRF.

Treatment
Left untreated, Cushing's has a poor prognosis with death occurring from hypertension, ischaemic heart disease, infection, and heart failure. All treatment modalities are directed at the underlying aetiology. Prior to definitive treatment, cortisol hypersecretion may need to be suppressed using metyrapone (0.25–6.0 g per day depending on cortisol secretion), an enzyme blocking agent that prevents synthesis of endogenous steroids. An alternative to metyrapone is aminoglutethamide. Adrenal adenomas should be excised surgically after preparation with this drug. Owing to suppression of the unaffected gland by the tumour in the contralateral adrenal, postoperatively it is necessary to provide supplementation with hydrocortisone (20 mg morning, 10 mg evening) and fludrocortisone 0.1 mg per day until the secretory role of the normal gland returns, as indicated by a successful short synacthen test (cortisol > 550 nmol at 30 minutes).

Adrenal carcinomas and eACTH-related Cushing's can be associated with very high levels of cortisol secretion. As an interim measure before surgery, drugs should be used to reduce the secretion of adrenal hormones. Mitotane ($o,p'DDD$) is an adrenolytic agent that reduces the bulk and activity of the adrenal glands. After preoperative preparation with mitotane, adrenal carcinomas should ultimately be surgically removed. With troublesome Cushing's due to eACTH, bilateral adrenalectomy may be required if the source of the ectopic secretion cannot be found.

Pituitary-dependent Cushing's should be treated by trans-sphenoidal adenomectomy. Using the combination of the CRF test and bilateral simultaneous inferior petrosal sinus sampling to lateralize the disorder, the surgical cure rate of Cushing's disease can be around 95%.[49] Yttrium radioactive needles have been implanted successfully but this is rarely carried out today. External beam radiotherapy as a primary form of treatment is slow and is effective in only 20–50% of cases.

The rare problem of Nelson's syndrome may arise when a patient has had bilateral adrenalectomy and subsequently develops a pituitary tumour secondary to unsuppressed ACTH secretion. The treatment for this condition is hypophysectomy and external beam radiotherapy.

Hypertension in patients with all forms of Cushing's tends to be refractory to conventional antihypertensive medications. In a recent study, only 4 of 28 patients achieved normalization of blood pressure on diuretics, calcium antagonists, and ACE inhibitors, whether administered as single agents or in combination.[50] Subsequently, ketoconazole, an inhibitor of steroidogenesis, was added to the treatment regime and all but 1 of the patients achieved good blood pressure control. A separate group of 12 patients was given ketoconazole alone, and again very successful blood pressure control was achieved in all but 1 instance. It therefore appears that hypertensive patients with Cushing's syndrome only achieve good blood pressure control after reduction or normalization of the hypercortisolism. Specific antihypertensive agents may not be required if this goal can be achieved.

Acromegaly

The basic pathology in this condition is sustained excess growth hormone secretion from the anterior pituitary. Cardiovascular abnormalities are well described, and 20–40% of patients have hypertension,[51,52] the severity of the elevated blood pressure being directly related to the activity of the acromegaly. Patients have double the mortality rate of normal individuals and the vast majority of this discrepancy is related to cardiovascular pathology.

Clinical features

In adults, excess growth hormone causes typical bony and soft tissue abnormalities (Table 5.6). The dominant clinical findings at presentation are large hands and feet and coarsening of facial features with frontal bossing and prognathism. Classically, patients complain of rings getting too small, shoes not fitting, sweating, headaches; joint pains, or symptoms relating to the pituitary tumour itself (i.e. visual field defects).

Mechanisms of hypertension

The pathophysiology of hypertension in acromegaly is related to sodium retention, and hence fluid retention and a concomitant rise in extracellular fluid volume and plasma volume.[43] There appears to be a direct effect of growth hormone on the kidney and this promotes sodium and water retention.[53] There is also some evidence that the usual rise in plasma atrial natriuretic factor levels in response to acute intravenous saline loading is blunted in acromegaly.[54] This effect tends to perpetuate an elevated extracellular fluid volume and hypertension.

Investigations

Patients with features suggestive of acromegaly should have a standard 75 g oral glucose tolerance test with half-hourly measurements of glucose and growth hormone. Physiologically, growth hormone levels are suppressed by glucose loading. In the presence of acromegaly, however, this response is lost and quite often there is a paradoxical rise in growth hormone

Visual field defect	Macroglossia	Goitre	Galactorrhoea
Hirsutism	Carpal tunnel syndrome	Large hands and feet	Proximal myopathy
Arthropathy	Oedema	Frontal bossing	Prognathism
Interdental spacing	Heart failure	Hypertension	Thick greasy skin
Glycosuria	'Hypopituitarism'		

Table 5.6
Classical signs of acromegaly.

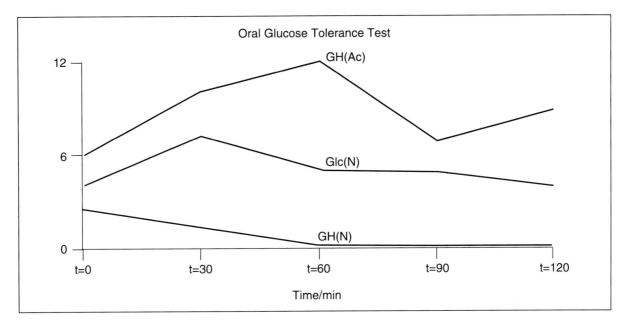

Figure 5.4
Schematic representation of growth hormone response to oral glucose load in a normal subject (suppression) and a patient with acromegaly (no suppression or paradoxical rise). GH(Ac)–Growth hormone levels in acromegalic, Glc(N)–normal glucose profile, GH(N)–normal growth hormone response.

(Fig. 5.4). Measurement of a single 'insulin-like growth factor 1' (IGF1) level is useful, as this tends to be elevated in individuals with acromegaly.[55]

Imaging of the pituitary fossa with CT or MRI may show evidence of a pituitary tumour.

Treatment

The underlying pituitary pathology can be treated by trans-sphenoidal surgery,[56] radiotherapy,[57] dopamine agonist drugs (bromocriptine),[58] or somatostatin analogues such as octreotide.[59] There have been reports of hypertension resolving with successful treatment of the underlying acromegaly, although in practice it may be difficult to attain a 'biochemical cure'.[60] If hypertension remains despite specific treatment of the

acromegaly, there are theoretical reasons for using diuretics as a first line treatment because of the sodium and extracellular fluid volume overload seen in this condition.

Primary hyperparathyroidism

Primary hyperparathyroidism may be due to parathyroid adenomas, hyperplasia, or rarely carcinoma. Parathyroid hormone is secreted from C cells within the parathyroid glands situated in the substance of the thyroid gland. The cardinal feature of this condition is hypercalcaemia. The original work on hyperparathyroidism showed 70% of patients to be hypertensive,[61] although others have found the value closer to 30%.[62] Elevated blood pressure tends to be mild, although hypertension and its sequelae account for approximately 50% of the mortality rate in primary hyperparathyroidism.[61]

Clinical features

The symptoms are those seen in hypercalcaemia. Patients may complain of general malaise and depression, bone pain, and abdominal pain, sometimes related to peptic ulceration. Renal calculi may form and cause typical renal colic and haematuria.

Mechanisms of hypertension

Elevated levels of calcium are associated with hypertension, and conversely reducing the level of hypercalcaemia may cause a concomitant reduction in blood pressure. The final pathway in this mechanism is unknown, although many pressor agents and effectors (e.g. angiotensin, ACTH, and smooth muscle contractility) have calcium as their 'second messenger', which may in part help explain the observed relationship between hypercalcaemia and hypertension.

Investigations

The diagnosis can be made on the basis of hypercalcaemia and hypophosphataemia in association with a non-suppressed or elevated parathyroid hormone (PTH) level. Localization of the tumour should be sought using ultrasound, high resolution CT scanning, subtraction thallium–technetium scanning and if necessary parathyroid vein sampling for PTH.

Treatment

Treatment is surgical if calcium levels remain above 3 mmol/l and are associated with symptoms. Hypercalcaemia can be controlled with the use of bisphosphonates, and blood pressure may be reduced using this class of drug alone.

If surgery is necessary, the parathyroid glands may be difficult to localize anatomically and can prove demanding to excise while preserving normal functioning glands.

Theoretical benefits from using calcium antagonists in this condition have been proposed but in practice this is unproven.

Dysthyroidism

Both hyperthyroidism and hypothyroidism are associated with elevated blood pressure. In thyrotoxicosis, the hypertension tends to be predominantly systolic. The mechanism of hypertension in the presence of thyroid dysfunction is thought to be mediated through a modulatory role of thyroid hormones on the effects of catecholamines.[63] In treating this type of hypertension, a beta-blocker is useful in the thyrotoxic patient as symptomatic relief may also be obtained. Reversal of hypertension in thyrotoxicosis is seen when the underlying hyperthyroidism is treated.[64]

Coarctation of the aorta

This defect represents 5–10% of congenital cardiovascular anomalies. It was first described by Menke in 1750,[65] although it was not for another 2 centuries that the first successful surgical correction was reported.[66] Without treatment, significant coarctation can result in early death (mean age 35 years[67]), which is usually secondary to cardiac failure, cerebral haemorrhage, aortic dissection, or subacute bacterial endocarditis.

Pathology

The basic pathology in this condition is a localized deformity of the aortic wall giving a classical external hour glass appearance. The defect can occur anywhere along the length of the thoracoabdominal aorta, although it most commonly affects the area just distal to the origin of the left subclavian artery (Fig. 5.5). There is an association with bicuspid aortic valves and patent ductus arteriosus. The aetiology is not fully understood though the defect is likely to occur *in utero*. Rarely, coarctation can be caused by arteritis or neurofibromatosis.[68]

The haemodynamic consequences of coarctation are dependent on the site of the coarctation and the degree of narrowing. If the stenosis is only mild then collateral vessels tend to dilate slowly and thus allow re-establishment of adequate blood supply to the lower limbs. Often, however, aortic obstruction progresses rapidly in the perinatal period, which results in cardiac decompensation and failure. With the onset of cardiac failure, the initial upper body elevated blood pressure often drops to normal levels.

There have been various proposed mechanisms for the hypertension seen in this condition. The mechanical theory maintains that coarctation of the aorta, by definition, offers increased resistance to the left ventricle. To overcome this obstructive lesion the prestenotic blood pressure must rise so as to improve flow to the lower limbs at the expense of causing upper body hypertension. This hypothesis seems plausible but there are no clinical data to support it.

The renal theory is based on the results of animal experiments and proposes that coarctation reduces renal perfusion thereby rendering the kidneys relatively ischaemic. This process would then result in activation of the renin–angiotensin system, and thus elevation of the systemic blood pressure would occur in an attempt to improve renal perfusion. This hypothesis is supported by the fact that infrarenal coarctation does not result in hypertension.[69] Also, in animal models, transplantation of a kidney from a site below a coarctation to above the constriction results in normalization of elevated blood pressure.[70]

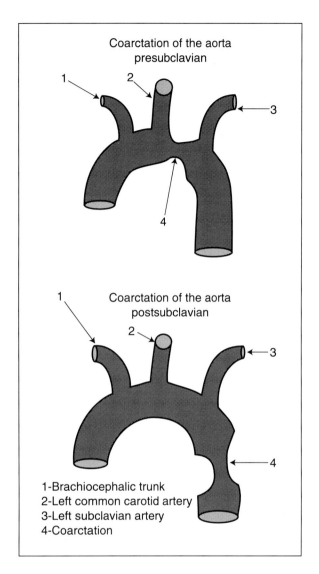

Figure 5.5
Common sites for coarctation of the aorta.

There is some evidence that the true origin of the hypertension is a combination of the 2 proposed mechanisms. In clinical practice, resection of a coarctation results in an immediate drop in blood pressure, which may be due to the mechanical factors. With time, however, there is a further drop in blood pressure, which may be related to the reversal of the renal component of hypertension.

Presentation

Most patients with coarctation present in the first year of life. Blood pressure is lower in the legs than the arms and the femoral pulses may be weak or impalpable. Radiofemoral delay may be evident on palpation, as may clinical features of congestive cardiac failure. Murmurs may not be apparent if the stenosis is significant, owing to poor flow.

In patients presenting at an older age, the degree of narrowing is less and clinical progression is slower. Patients are usually asymptomatic and hypertension is often a coincidental finding. Unlike in young children, these patients invariably have a systolic murmur, which is loudest at the left sternal edge and frequently radiates through to the back. Bruits may be heard over the collateral vessels in the chest, and the radiographic evidence of this is rib notching.

Investigations

Electrocardiography in children shows a pattern of right ventricular hypertrophy; in adults, it shows left ventricular hypertrophy. Digital subtraction angiography is the investigation of choice and will give useful information regarding the extent of the narrowing and the precise anatomical location.

Treatment

Treatment is surgical. Blood pressure should be controlled preoperatively with conventional antihypertensive medications. Infants with congestive cardiac failure secondary to coarctation should be dealt with urgently. Once the diagnosis has been made, referral should be immediate so that end-organ damage is minimized. Sometimes, hypertension may persist postoperatively and indeed coarctation may even recur.

Renal causes of hypertension
Renal parenchymatous disease

Primary renal parenchymatous disease of any aetiology can cause hypertension. Conversely, long-standing moderate to severe essential hypertension may also cause impaired renal function and nephrosclerosis. Glomerulonephritis is quantitatively the most important aetiological factor in the generation of secondary hypertension. Even mild glomerular disease can cause raised blood pressure, which resolves following successful treatment of the glomerulopathy. Patients presenting with glomerulonephritis often have haematuria, proteinuria or microscopic proteinuria, oedema, and hypertension. The diagnosis is reliably established with carefully performed phase-contrast microscopy of urine to detect red cells of bizarre morphology, red cell casts, and oval fat bodies. Microscopic haematuria and proteinuria are not caused by hypertension except in the malignant phase, when they reflect acute vascular and glomerular lesions. In this case, the glomerular changes and the urine abnormalities both disappear within 2 weeks of effective control of blood pressure. Renal abnormalities persisting beyond this time indicate underlying primary renal disease and renal biopsy must be performed.

Pyelonephritis

There is no associated elevation in blood pressure with acute pyelonephritis. With persistent or recurrent urinary tract infections, as in the presence of vesicoureteric obstruction, parenchymal scars occur, and these have been implicated aetiologically with hypertension. Vesicoureteric reflux is common in children and is found to be the underlying cause of hypertension in 64% of children with elevated blood pressure.[71] Removal of the affected kidney often results in normalisation of blood pressure.

Analgesic nephropathy

The pathogenesis of the hypertension seen in this condition is related to necrosis of the interstitial cells within the renal medulla, which, through the production of prostaglandins, have an antihypertensive function. Destruction of this important region is thus associated with a rise in blood pressure.

Diabetic nephropathy

Hypertension is present in 60–78% of patients with diabetes. The renal pathology is glomerulosclerosis and the degree of involvement is proportional to the degree of blood pressure elevation.

Polycystic kidney disease

Hypertension is universal in adult polycystic kidney disease (an autosomal dominant condition). Half of the patients develop cardiovascular pathology (myocardial infarction, cerebrovascular accidents, and cardiac failure) which is secondary to the hypertension. As more renal parenchyma is destroyed owing to increasing cyst formation, the hypertension worsens.

Renin secreting tumours

These are very rare tumours of the juxtaglomerular apparatus. They cause severe hypertension despite their small size. Hypertension resolves after complete excision.[72]

Hypertension with other renal tumours

Wilms' tumour causes hypertension, probably because of excess renin secretion. Hypernephroma also causes hypertension, owing to cortical ischaemia. The treatment for both conditions is excision.

Hydronephrosis

It is unusual to develop hypertension with hydronephrosis. The mechanism is thought to be related to stretching of the interlobular arteries as they pass around the distended calyces, causing relative segmental renal ischaemia. There have been reported cases of hypertension being cured on nephrectomy of the involved kidney.

Scleroderma

The renal lesions in scleroderma are very similar to those seen in malignant hypertension. Patients are often normotensive, only to present with an acute fulminant episode of malignant hypertension (often precipitated by pregnancy) which is refractory to treatment. This results in incipient renal failure. The aetiopathogenesis is related to rapid narrowing of interlobular arteries causing microinfarctions.

Polyarteritis nodosa

Most patients with polyarteritis nodosa who have renal involvement are hypertensive. As with scleroderma, the mechanism of hypertension is thought to be related to areas of ischaemic necrosis in the renal cortex due to arteritis.

Renovascular hypertension

This form of hypertension is defined as hypertension secondary to an obstruction of one or both renal arteries or one of its branches or to a cortical infarct caused by embolus or trauma.

Pathology

Renal artery obstruction or stenosis leading to hypertension may be caused by atherosclerotic plaques or fibromuscular dysplasia. The former is the commonest, affects older individuals and occurs in the proximal third of the renal artery. It is more often seen on the left than the right, though it is bilateral in 30% of cases. Fibromuscular dysplasia can be inherited as an autosomal dominant condition and is found in younger people. It affects females 5 times as often as males and it is often bilateral. It tends to affect the middle third of the renal artery.

The hypertension caused by these problems is induced by activation of the renin–angiotensin system. Renal perfusion is reduced, and this causes renin release from the juxtaglomerular apparatus, conversion of angiotensin I to angiotensin II (the most potent pressor agent known), and increased levels of aldosterone. The combined effect is therefore to increase total peripheral resistance and hence blood pressure. However, the presence of renal artery stenosis does not automatically render an individual hypertensive. Holley et al[73] have performed post-mortem examinations on normotensive subjects and hypertensive patients with a mean age of 58 years and found that 49% had severe renal artery obstruction or stenosis. These findings have been verified by others.[74] Why there should be a discrepancy between the incidence of renal artery stenosis and the finding of hypertension is not clear, although there does appear to be a critical degree of stenosis that is required before provoking renin hypersecretion and hypertension.

Clinical features
Patients tend to be asymptomatic, although they may describe nocturia in association with the hypokalaemia that is sometimes seen secondary to aldosterone excess. Other findings are bruits in the paraumbilical regions and persistent bacteriuria.

Investigations
Plain abdominal x-rays may show calcification in atherosclerotic plaques of renal artery lesions. Rapid sequential intravenous pyelography offers a useful screening test. With renal artery stenosis, the typical radiographic findings are delayed appearance of contrast in the kidneys; increased density of contrast with delayed excretion, and reduced renal size.

The ability of the kidneys to selectively concentrate and slowly excrete 99mTc-labelled DTPA (technetium chelate) is used in the DTPA scan. The renal scintigrams produced provide information on renal size and the presence of tumours, cysts, or infarcts of the renal parenchyma.

Renal arteriography is the investigation of choice for diagnosing renal artery stenosis. It is the only test available that accurately assesses the degree of stenosis and localizes the lesion. The variables that can be measured are:

- gradient of pressure across the stricture, if stenosis is > 60%;
- degree of poststenotic dilatation;
- thickness of the renal cortex (in both kidneys) – normal is 6 mm, but if < 5.5 mm, this is an indication of severe disease;
- renal size;
- presence of collaterals (in severe stenosis).

Arteriosclerotic obstructive lesions occur in the proximal renal artery and tend to be hourglass shaped. Stenoses due to dysplasia occur in the middle third of the renal artery, may be multiple, and may appear as strings of beads or represent localized areas of narrowing. Dysplastic strictures can occur in other large vessels such as the coeliac, mesenteric, carotid, axillary, and iliac arteries.

Management
Once the presence of renal artery stenosis has been established, any causal relationship to hypertension should be sought: renal artery stenosis is often a coincidental finding in

patients with essential hypertension. Patients with true renovascular hypertension have exaggerated plasma renin activity in response to upright posture, sodium depletion, administration of thiazides, hydralazine, nitroprusside, or diazoxide. Plasma renin activity is increased on the side of the stenosis, and this can be demonstrated using selective renal vein sampling. The above facts can be utilized in the differential renal function tests for plasma renin activity, and diagnostic accuracy can be further increased by administering a single dose of captopril. This test is dealt with in detail elsewhere.[75]

Surgery is the treatment of choice. The prognosis is best in young people with dysplastic strictures of the renal artery. The risks of surgery in the elderly may be great, considering the possibility of diffuse atheromatous disease of the coronary and carotid or cerebral vessels.

If there is a distal renal artery obstruction or stenosis of one of the branches of the renal artery, surgery may be impracticable. In this instance, if the hypertension is severe, nephrectomy should be considered.

Surgery offers a potential cure. Hunt[76] has shown that, up to 10 years after follow-up, 84% of patients treated with surgery survive, compared with 60% of those treated by medical intervention alone. Postoperatively, renal artery stenosis may recur in those patients with atherosclerotic lesions.

The medical management of the hypertension associated with renal artery stenosis is related to overactivity of the renin–angiotensin system. ACE inhibitors fulfil their theoretical use in such situations and prove very effective in clinical practice. It is important, however, to be aware that ACE inhibition in the presence of bilateral renal artery stenosis can prove dangerous. In such circumstances, renal perfusion pressures can be reduced to levels that are inadequate for effective glomerular filtration and hence risk renal failure. This risk does apply in the presence of unilateral renal artery stenosis but is far less significant a problem.

There has been some success using angioplasty techniques in dilating stenosis in the renal arteries.[77]

References

1 Danielson M, Dammstrom B. The prevalence of secondary hypertension. *Acta Med Scand* 1981; **209**:451–5.

2 L'Abbe M, Tinel J, Doumer E. Crises solaires et hypertension paroxystique en rapport avec une tumeur surrenale. *Bull Soc Med Hop* 1922; **46**:982.

3 Mayo C. Paroxysmal hypertension with tumour of retroperitoneal nerve. Report of a case. *J Am Med Assoc* 1927; **89**:1047.

4 Shipley A. Paroxysmal hypertension associated with tumour of suprarenal. *Ann Surg* 1929; **90**:742.

5 Manasse P. Histologie und Histogenese der primaren Nierengeschwulste. *Virchows Arch Pathol Anat* 1896; **145**:113.

6 Manger W, Gifford R. *Phaeochromocytoma.* New York: Springer Verlag, 1977.

7 Glenner G, Grimley P. Tumours of the extra adrenal paraganglion system (including chemoreceptors). In: *Atlas of Tumour Pathology* 2nd Series, Fasc 9. Washington DC: Armed Forces Institute of Pathology, 1974:90.

8 Sipple J. The association of phaeochromocytoma with carcinoma of the thyroid gland. *Am J Med* 1961; **31**:163–6.

9 Neville A. The adrenal medulla. In: Symington T, ed. *Functional Pathology of the Human Adrenal Gland.* Edinburgh: Livingstone, 1969:219.

10 Scharf Y, Mahir A, Better O et al. Prolonged survival in malignant phaeochromocytoma of the organ of Zuckerkandl with pharmacological treatment. *Cancer* 1973; **31**:746.

11 Watson R, Stallard T, Flinn R. Factors determining direct arterial pressure and its variability in hypertensive man. *Hypertension* 1980; **56**:303–9.

12 Fries J, Chamberlin J. Extra-adrenal phaeochromocytoma: literature review and report of a cervical phaeochromocytoma. *Lancet* 1968; **1**:609.

13 Clutter W, Bier D, Shah S et al. Epinephrine plasma metabolic clearance rates and physiologic thresholds for metabolic and hemodynamic actions in man. *J Clin Invest* 1980; **66**:94.

14 Lees G. A hitch-hikers guide to the galaxy of adrenoreceptors. *Br Med J* 1981; **283**:173.

15 Allwood M, Cobbold A, Ginsburg J. Peripheral vascular effects of noradrenaline, isopropylnoradrenaline and dopamine. *Br Med Bull* 1963; **19**:132.

16 Higgins P, Tressider G. Phaeochromocytoma of the urinary bladder. *Br Med J* 1966; **2**:274.

17 Duncan M, Compton P, Lazarus L et al. Measurement of norepinephrine and 3,4-dihydroxyphenylglycol in urine and plasma for the diagnosis of phaeochromocytoma. *N Engl J Med* 1988; **319**:136–42.

18 Krakoff L, Garbowit D, Adreno-medullary hypertension: a review of syndromes, pathophysiology, diagnosis, and treatment. *Clin Chem* 1991; **37**:1849–53.

19 O'Conner D, Bernstein K. Radioimmunoassay of chromogranin A in plasma as a measure of exocytic sympathoadrenal activity in normal subjects and patients with phaeochromocytoma. *N Engl J Med* 1984; **311**:764–70.

20 Grouzman E, Comoy E, Bohoun C. Plasma neuropeptide Y concentrations in patients with neuroendocrine tumours. *J Clin Endocrinol Metab* 1989; **68**:808–13.

21 Takahashi K, Mouri T, Itoi K et al, Increased plasma immunoreactive neuropeptide Y concentrations in phaeochromocytoma and chronic renal failure. *J Hypertens* 1987; **5**:749–53.

22 Vesely D, Arnold W, Winters C et al. Increased circulating concentration of the N-terminus of the atrial natriuretic factor prohormone in persons with phaeochromocytomas. *J Clin Endocrinol Metab* 1990; **71**:1138–46.

23 Helman L, Cohen P, Averbush S et al. Neuropeptide Y expression distinguishes malignant from benign phaeochromocytoma. *J Clin Endocrinol Metab* 1989; **7**:1720–5.

24 Quint L, Glazer G, Francis I et al. Phaeochromocytoma and paragangioma:

comparison of MR imaging with CT and I-131 MIBG scintigraphy. *Radiology* 1987; **165**:89–93.

25 Schmedtje J Jr, Sax S, Pool J et al. Localization of ectopic phaeochromocytomas by magnetic resonance imaging. *Am J Med* 1987; **116**:1785–9.

26 Shapiro B. Imaging of catecholamine-secreting tumours: uses of MIBG in diagnosis and treatment. *Clin Endocrinol Metab* 1993; **7**:491–507.

27 Jebara V, Uva M, Farge A et al. Cardiac pheochromocytomas. *Ann Thorac Surg* 1992; **53**(2):356–61.

28 Orchard T, Grant C, Van-Heerden J et al. Pheochromocytoma – continuing evolution of surgical therapy. *Surgery* 1993; **114**:1153–8.

29 Averbuch S, Steakley C, Young R et al. Malignant phaeochromocytoma: effective treatment with a combination of cyclophosphamide, vincristine, and dacarbazine. *Ann Intern Med* 1988; **109**:267–73.

30 Shapiro B, Sisson J, Wieland D et al. Radiopharmaceutical therapy of malignant phaeochromocytoma with ^{131}I-metaiodobenzylguanidine: results from ten years of experience. *J Nucl Biol Med* 1991; **35**(4):269–76.

31 Sisson J, Shapiro B, Bierwaltes W et al. Radiopharmaceutical treatment of malignant phaeochromocytoma. *J Nucl Biol Med* 1984; **25**:197–206.

32 Todesco S, Terribile V, Borsatti A et al. Primary aldosteronism due to a malignant ovarian tumour. *J Clin Endocrinol Metab* 1975; **41**:809.

33 Sunman W, Rothwell M, Sever P. Conn's syndrome can cause malignant hypertension. *J Hum Hypertens* 1992; **6**(1):75–6.

34 Dobbie J. Adrenocortical nodular hyperplasia: the ageing adrenal. *J Pathol* 1969; **99**:1.

35 McKenna T, Sequeira S, Hefferman A et al. Diagnosis under random conditions of all disorders of the renin–angiotensin–aldosterone axis, including primary hyperaldosteronism. *J Clin Endocrinol Metab* 1991; **73**:952–7.

36 Beierwaltes W, Lieberman L, Ansari A et al. Visualization of human adrenal glands in vivo by scintillation scanning. *JAMA* 1971; **216**:275.

37 Young W, Hogan M, Klee G et al. Primary aldosteronism: Diagnosis and treatment. *Mayo Clinic Proc* 1990; **65**:96–110.

38 Bravo E, Fouad F, Tarazi R, Calcium channel blockade with nifedipine in primary hyperaldosteronism. *Hypertension* 1986; **8**(suppl I):I191–I194.

39 Griffing G, Sindler B, Aurecchia S et al. The therapeutic effect of a new angiotensin converting enzyme inhibitor, enalapril maleate, in idiopathic hyperaldosteronism. *Clin Res* 1983; **31**:271A [abstract].

40 Weinberger M, Grim C, Hollifield J et al. Primary aldosteronism: Diagnosis, localisation and treatment. *Ann Intern Med* 1979; **90**:386–95.

41 Go H, Takeda M, Takahashi H et al. Laparoscopic adrenalectomy for primary aldosteronism: a new operative method. *J Laparoendosc Surg* 1993; **3**(5):455–9.

42 Cushing H. The basophil adenomas of the pituitary body and their clinical manifestations (pituitary basophilism). *Bull Johns Hopkins Hosp* 1932; **50**:137–95.

43 Ritchie C, Sheridan B, Fraser R et al. Studies on the pathogenesis of hypertension in Cushing's disease and acromegaly. *Q J Med* 1990; **280**:855–67.

44 Davies A, Lefkowitz R. In vitro desensitisation of beta adrenergic receptors in human neutrophils: attenuation by corticosteroids. *J Clin Invest* 1980; **71**:565–71.

45 Sano V, Ford L, Begley M et al. Effect of in vitro anti-asthma drugs on human leukocyte beta adrenergic receptors. *Clin Res* 1980; **28**:431A.

46 Crapo L. Cushing's syndrome: a review of diagnostic tests. *Metabolism* 1979; **28**:955.

47 Oldfield E, Doppman J, Nieman L et al. Petrosal sinus sampling with and without corticotropin releasing hormone for the differential diagnosis of Cushing's syndrome. *N Engl J Med* 1991; **325**:897.

48 Chrousos G, Schulte H, Oldfield E et al. The corticotropin releasing factor stimulation test: An aid in the differential diagnosis of Cushing's syndrome. *N Engl J Med* 1984; **310**:622.

49 Oldfiel D, Chrousos G Jr, Schulte H et al. Preoperative lateralisation of ACTH secreting

pituitary microadenomas by bilateral and simultaneous inferior petrosal sinus sampling. *N Engl J Med* 1985; **312**:100.

50 Fallo F, Paoletta A, Tona F et al. Response of hypertension to conventional antihypertensive treatment and/or steroidogensis inhibitors in Cushing's syndrome. *J Intern Med* 1993; **234**(6):595–8.

51 McGuffin W, Sherman B, Roth J et al. Acromegaly and cardiovascular disorders. A prospective study. *Ann Intern Med* 1974; **81**:11–18.

52 Popovici D, Buteiskis A, Handoca A et al. Cardiovascular pathology in acromegaly and some effects of the 90 yttrium implant in the hypophysis. *Endocrinologie* 1978; **16**:223–8.

53 Biglieri E, Watlington C, Forsham P. Sodium retention with human growth hormone and its subtractions. *J Clin Endocrinol Metab* 1961; **21**:361–70.

54 McKnight J, McCance D, Hadden D et al. Basal and saline-stimulated levels of plasma atrial natriuretic factor in acromegaly. *Clin Endocrinol* 1989; **31**:431–8.

55 Dohan O, Goth M, Szabolcs I et al. The place of insulin like growth factor I in the diagnosis of acromegaly. *Orv Hetil* 1993; **134**(42):2301–3.

56 Fahlbusch R, Honegger J, Buchfelder M. Surgical management of acromegaly. *Endocrinol Metab Clin North Am* 1992; **21**:669–92.

57 Eastman R, Gorden P, Glatstein P et al. Radiation therapy of acromegaly. *Endocrinol Metab Clin North Am* 1992; **21**:693–712.

58 Wass J, thorner M, Morris D et al. Long term treatment of acromegaly with bromocriptine. *Br Med J* 1977; **1**:875–8.

59 Barkan A, Kelch R, Hopwood N et al. Treatment of acromegaly with the long acting somatostatin analogue SMS 201-995. *J Endocrinol Metab* 1988; **66**:16–23.

60 Wass J. Acromegaly: treatment after 100 years. *Br Med J* 1993; **307**:1505–6.

61 Hellstrom J, Birke J, Edvall C. Hypertension in hyperparathyroidism. *Br J Urol* 1958; **30**:13–24.

62 Scholtz D. Hypertension in hyperparathyroidism. *Arch Intern Med* 1977; **137**:1123–5.

63 Bilezikian J, Loeb J, Gammon D. The influence of hyperthyroidism and hypothyroidism on the beta-adrenergic responsiveness of the turkey erythrocyte. *J Clin Invest* 1979; **63**:184–92.

64 Gasiorowski W, Plazinska M. Arterial hypertension associated with hyper and hypothyroidism. *Pol Tyg Lek* 1992; **47**(44–45):1009–10.

65 Jarcho S, Coarctation of the aorta (Meckel 1750, Paris 1791). *Am J Cardiol* 1961; **7**:844.

66 Crafoord C, Nylin G. Congenital coarctation of the aorta and its surgical treatment. *J Thorac Cardiovasc Surg* 1945; **14**:347.

67 Campbell J. Natural history of coarctation of the aorta. *Br Heart J* 1970; **32**:633.

68 Schuerg W, Messerli F, Genest J et al. Arterial hypertension and neurofibromatosis: renal artery stenosis and coarctation of abdominal aorta. *Can Med Assoc J* 1975; **113**:879.

69 Groenewald J, Van Zijl J. Acute renal and systemic effects after experimental coarctation of the aorta in the baboon. *Invest Urol* 1970; **7**:299.

70 Harrison R, Alton J. The renal factor in the hypertension of experimental coarctation of the aorta. *Surg Forum* 1955; **30**:206.

71 Still J, Cottom D. Severe hypertension in childhood. *Arch Dis Child* 1967; **42**:34–9.

72 Robertson P, Klidjian A, Harding L et al. Hypertension due to renin-secreting renal tumour. *Am J Med* 1967; **43**:963–76.

73 Holley K, Hunt J, Brown A. Renal Artery Stenosis. A clinical-pathologic study in normotensive and hypertensive patients. *Am J Med* 1964; **37**:14–22.

74 Dustan H, Humphries A, de Wolfe V et al. Normal arterial pressure in patients with renal artery stenosis. *JAMA* 1964; **187**:1028–9.

75 Re R, Novelline R, Escourrou M et al. Inhibition of angiotensin-converting enzyme for diagnosis of renal artery stenosis. *N Engl J Med* 1978; **298**:582–6.

76 Hunt J, Sheps S, Harrison E. Renal and renovascular hypertension. A reasoned approach to diagnosis and management. *Arch Intern Med* 1974; **133**:988–99.

77 Schwartes D. In: Narins R, ed. *Controversies in Nephrology and Hypertension*. New York: Churchill Livingstone, 1984:161.

6

The J-curve phenomenon: inverse relation between achieved diastolic blood pressure and risk of acute myocardial infarction

Ulf Lindblad, Lennart Råstam and Lars Rydén

High blood pressure is the most important risk factor for stroke,[1–5] and it is also a major risk factor for acute myocardial infarction.[4–8] Clinical trials demonstrate that pharmacological treatment of hypertension can prevent stroke[9] with an achieved risk reduction in correspondence with that expected from observational studies.[10,11]

Based upon observational evidence, treatment of hypertension would have a similar impact on the risk of acute myocardial infarction.[5,10] In this respect, however, clinical trials have generally failed to provide the expected results.[9–12] While the reason for this discrepancy is unresolved, several possible explanations have been suggested:

Confounding
According to this hypothesis, hypertension is not in itself causally related to risk, but is merely a marker for one or more other risk factors. For example, there may be a correlation between blood pressure and certain blood lipids[13,14] or between blood pressure and insulin resistance as in the metabolic syndrome.[15,16]

Negative effects of medication
This hypothesis suggests that treatment of hypertension *per se* decreases risk, but this is counteracted by side effects from the medication, such as disturbances in the electrolyte balance, in glucose metabolism, or in lipid metabolism.[9,17–20]

Concomitant risk
This hypothesis suggests that a possible benefit from treatment is counteracted by other risk factors, such as smoking, hypercholesterolemia, or impaired glucose tolerance, which are over-represented among hypertensives.[17,21,22]

Treatment is started too late
According to this theory, many patients have their antihypertensive medication started after several years of undetected hypertension, which has already initiated organ damage.[23,24]

Insufficient blood pressure reduction
In clinical trials of the treatment of hypertension, the achieved difference in blood pressure between cases and controls is often smaller than what is expected from estimations of statistical power when the trial is designed.[25,26]

The J-curve phenomenon
According to this theory, there is a hazard with too great a blood pressure reduction: when diastolic blood pressure is lowered beyond a critical level, the risk for myocardial infarction no longer decreases but increases.[27]

The aim of this chapter is to review the scientific foundation for the theory behind the

J-curve phenomenon. Supporting and contradicting epidemiological, clinical-trial-based and physiological foundations will be explored. A practical solution to the inherent therapeutic dilemma is also suggested.

Achieved blood pressure and risk of acute myocardial infarction

The relation between the blood pressure level that is achieved when a patient is treated for hypertension and the risk of acute myocardial infarction has been under scrutiny for some years. It is important to remember that, even bearing in mind some of the hypotheses listed above, there is little doubt that lowering severe hypertension is beneficial. The problem is not whether to treat these patients or not. The intriguing question is what happens when patients approach the low end of the distribution curve, i.e. when a high pressure is pharmacologically reduced to a low or very low level. Three main hypotheses may be put forward, each supported by some empirical evidence that will be reviewed in this chapter (Fig. 6.1).

Alternative A in Fig. 6.1 is a J-shaped risk function. Its clinical implication is that if the diastolic blood pressure is lowered too much, the treatment by itself will counteract its main aim to reduce risk. According to this hypothesis, the increased risk at a low level of blood pressure is linked to the blood pressure *per se*. Side effects of the treatment also need to be borne in mind.

Alternative B in Fig. 6.1 suggests that there is little point in lowering blood pressure beyond a certain level as no further risk reduction is

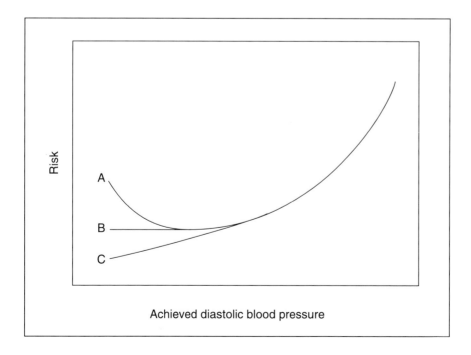

Figure 6.1
Outline of the J-curve relation between achieved diastolic blood pressure and the risk of acute myocardial infarction (A), and two alternative relations (B and C).

achieved. In contrast to alternative A, however, there is no increased harm, apart from the fact that side effects and cost of medication may increase with more extensive medication.

Alternative C in Fig. 6.1 is in accord with the classical clinical thinking 'the lower the better'. If this is true, all lowering of blood pressure within the 'normal' range should potentially benefit the patient. From this perspective, the clinician's effort should always be to lower a patient's blood pressure as much as possible, with due regard to pharmacological side effects.

As explained below, there is strong physiologic evidence that the diastolic blood pressure should be the focus of interest. Unless otherwise indicated, diastolic phase 5 is referred to.

Observational studies

Studies in support of alternative A

The goal 'the lower the better' for the treatment of hypertension was first questioned by Anderson in 1978.[28] Framingham data had provided evidence for a linear relationship between achieved blood pressure in treated patients and the incidence of cardiovascular events.[29] Anderson, however, observed that the original data were statistically smoothed, and he suspected that a non-linear relationship could have been overlooked. He re-analysed the data and was able to demonstrate that, below 90 mmHg, the occurrence of cardiovascular events did not continue to decline – rather it tended to increase with decreasing diastolic blood pressure.

Further early support for a non-linear relation was added by Stewart in 1979 with data from 120 men and 49 women treated for uncomplicated severe hypertension over 6 years.[30] Mean pretreatment diastolic blood

pressure was 124 mmHg. In patients who had their diastolic blood pressure decreased beyond 90 mmHg, the relative risk of myocardial infarction was more than five times that of patients with reduction into the range of 105–109 mmHg.

Surprisingly little attention was paid to these results, and it was not until Cruickshank published his data in 1987 that any real interest in a possible J-curve phenomenon emerged. He presented a follow-up of 902 men and women who attended a hospital clinic for treatment of hypertension.[31] They had moderate to severe hypertension which was treated with the beta-blocker atenolol, either alone or in combination. Pretreatment blood pressure was not related to mortality, but there was a non-linear relation between achieved diastolic blood pressure and death from myocardial infarction, independent of age. Mortality was lowest in patients with diastolic blood pressure lowered to 85–90 mmHg, with higher mortality rates both above and below (Fig. 6.2).

The higher mortality in the lowest range (< 85 mmHg) was confined to 342 subjects with evidence of ischaemic heart disease or other atherosclerotic manifestations (previous myocardial infarction, angina pectoris, intermittent claudication, or electrocardiographic evidence of myocardial ischaemia; see Fig. 6.2). There was, by contrast, a strong positive linear relation between achieved systolic blood pressure and mortality from acute myocardial infarction; i.e. there was no evidence of a non-linear component.

Similar results were reported from the Swedish Gothenburg Primary Prevention Trial.[32] The screening program identified 686 hypertensive men (aged 47–54 years) without a history of myocardial infarction. They were treated and followed for 12 years at the hospital hypertension clinic.[33] When incidence rates of coronary heart disease were related to

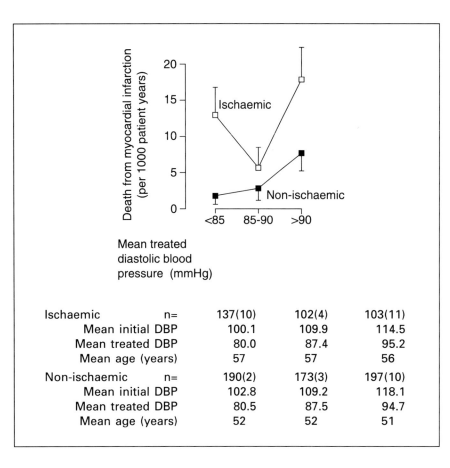

Ischaemic

Non-ischaemic

Death from myocardial infarction (per 1000 patient years)

<85   85-90   >90

Mean treated diastolic blood pressure (mmHg)

Ischaemic n=	137(10)	102(4)	103(11)
Mean initial DBP	100.1	109.9	114.5
Mean treated DBP	80.0	87.4	95.2
Mean age (years)	57	57	56
Non-ischaemic n=	190(2)	173(3)	197(10)
Mean initial DBP	102.8	109.2	118.1
Mean treated DBP	80.5	87.5	94.7
Mean age (years)	52	52	51

Figure 6.2
Main results from Cruickshank's first paper on the J-curve phenomenon. (The number of deaths are given in parentheses.) (From Cruickshank et al.[31])

achieved blood pressure following adjustment for differences in coronary heart disease risk at entry, a non-linear relationship was confirmed, as a quadratic term added to the Cox regression was statistically significant, with the nadir at 81 mmHg.[34] Among subjects in the lower quintiles of achieved diastolic blood pressure who developed coronary heart disease, a majority had clinical signs of cardiac ischaemia at the annual check-up that preceded the development of the coronary heart disease.

Cruickshank's results and those of the Gothenburg group rapidly received support by two British studies. In one, a multicentre study including 1075 men and 1070 women, the influence of the mean diastolic blood pressure achieved during a 3–12 month period was used to predict survival during a mean follow-up period of 4 years.[35] The lowest fifth (< 86 mmHg) had an ischaemic heart disease mortality that equalled that of the highest fifth (> 103 mmHg). The lowest event rate was observed in the range of 86–91 mmHg. The findings were, however, not statistically significant.

In the other British study, conducted at the Glasgow Blood Pressure Clinic, 3350 male and female hypertensives were followed for a mean 6.5 years.[36] Coronary heart disease mortality in the highest fifth of achieved diastolic blood pressure was twice that of the lowest fifth. The lowest rate occurred in the middle quintile, which comprised patients in the range of 91–98 mmHg. The shape of the curve was similar in men and women, and in patients with and without pre-existing coronary heart disease. After adjustment for age, gender, initial diastolic blood pressure, smoking, prevalent coronary heart disease, and signs of left ventricular hypertrophy plus strain in the baseline ECG, a non-linear component of the relation was statistically significant.

An early trial of 884 elderly patients (60–79 years) gave similar findings.[37–39] There were J-shaped relations between mean achieved diastolic blood pressure and myocardial infarction in both the treatment group and the control group. The lowest rates occurred at 80–89 mmHg in the former and at 90–99 mmHg in the latter group.

In the EWPHE trial, 840 patients aged 60 years and above with sitting blood pressure 160–239/90–119 mmHg were randomized to receive placebo or active treatment.[40] A follow-up visit at 9 months was completed by 339 subjects on placebo and 352 on active drug. Mortality related to tertiles both of treated systolic and diastolic blood pressure was lower in those on active treatment than in those on placebo. In the placebo group, there was a U-shaped relationship between mortality and diastolic blood pressure, whereas in those on active drug, there was a linear inverse association. In both groups, however, there were similar trends for cardiovascular and non-cardiovascular mortality. Differences in outcome could not be explained by differences in the morbidity pattern at entry or by a greater fall in diastolic blood pressure from the start. However, body weight and haemoglobin

concentration decreased significantly among patients in the lower tertiles in both groups compared to the two upper tertiles. Thus, some deterioration of general health was suggested as a contributing cause of the increased mortality associated with low blood pressure.

Recently, a population-based case-control study reported similar findings among 912 subjects aged 30–79 years with no signs of previous coronary heart disease. They received standard clinical treatment for hypertension within a US health maintenance organization. The relationship between the achieved diastolic blood pressure and the risk of a first myocardial infarction was J-shaped.[41]

Studies in support of alternative B

Three trials suggest a non-linear relationship, but no directly negative impact of lowering the blood pressure too far.

The Australian therapeutic trial in mild hypertension involved 3427 men and women.[42] No firmly J-shaped relation between achieved diastolic blood pressure and the incidence of trial end-points (ischaemic heart disease and cerebrovascular accidents combined) was demonstrated.[43] Rather, the observed curve flattened at approximately 90 mmHg and below in the actively treated group and below 95 mmHg in the placebo-treated group. Data on myocardial infarction only was not presented.

In the IPPPSH study[44] 6,357 men and women with uncomplicated essential hypertension were randomized to treatment with a beta-blocker or placebo alone or, if necessary, in combination with other drugs, and subsequently followed for 3–5 years. Morbidity rates in the 2 groups showed the same pattern: lower blood pressure during treatment was associated with lower rates of cardiac events (myocardial infarction and sudden death), but with a levelling off below 90–95 mmHg. There was, however, no level at which a lower treated diastolic blood pressure was associated with higher incidence rate.

The MRC trial in mild hypertension enrolled 17 354 previously untreated men and women aged 35–64 years with diastolic blood pressures of 90–109 mmHg and systolic blood pressure below 200 mmHg.[45] Patients were randomly allocated to treatment with either a diuretic, a beta-blocker or placebo. In both sexes there was a statistically significant non-linear (quadratic) relation between treated diastolic blood pressure and morbidity from myocardial infarction.[46] In men there was no upturn in coronary heart disease with low treated diastolic blood pressure, whereas there was a borderline significant J-shaped quadratic effect in women (p=0.05).[46] However, the upward slope in women was small as was the event rate, which mainly was confined to the placebo group.[46]

Studies in support of alternative C

One study supports alternative C. This is the SHEP trial, which randomized patients aged 60 and older with isolated systolic hypertension (systolic blood pressure above 160 mmHg and diastolic blood pressure less than 90 mmHg) to active treatment (n=2365) or matching placebo (n=2371).[47] Initial mean blood pressure was 170/77 mmHg in both groups and after five years it was 155/72 mmHg in the placebo group and 143/68 mmHg in the actively treated group. No J-shaped or U-shaped relation between diastolic blood pressure and coronary risk was reported despite the low initial and treated diastolic blood pressure. This trial has been held as evidence against the existence of a threshold.[48] However, these subjects had no diastolic hypertension from the start, which is an otherwise common feature

for those studies in which a J-curve has been demonstrated.

Meta-analyses

One meta-analysis, published in 1991, provides support for alternative A.[27] The analysis was done after an extensive literature search through 1989. Thirteen studies that met specific selection criteria (stratified cardiovascular outcomes by at least 3 achieved blood pressure levels) were identified.[30,31,33,35–37,40,43,44,46,49–51] A more or less consistently J-shaped relation between diastolic blood pressure after treatment and cardiac events was found. The meta-analysis excluded studies that reported cardiac events by change in blood pressure,[49,50] and studies in which the levels of stratification of achieved diastolic blood pressure was unclear from the publication or in which cardiac events were not related to treated diastolic blood pressure.[40,43,46] One very small study dealt exclusively with patients treated for severe hypertension and was also not included.[51] With the results of the 7 remaining studies,[30,31,33,35–37,44] a summary curve for the relation between achieved diastolic blood pressure and risk of coronary heart disease was produced. It was a J-shaped expression with the nadir of the curve at 84 mmHg (Fig. 6.3).[27] The curvature of the relation was statistically significant.

In contrast, a recently published meta-analysis of 9 observational studies that included a large number of subjects denied the existence of a curvilinear relation between diastolic blood pressure and coronary heart disease.[5] However, the methods and results of this meta-analysis have been criticized, mainly because high-risk subjects were omitted.[52–55] In the same concept, a meta-analysis of 14 randomized clinical trials including 36 908 hypertensive subjects were presented.[11] With a calculated mean difference of 5–6 mmHg in

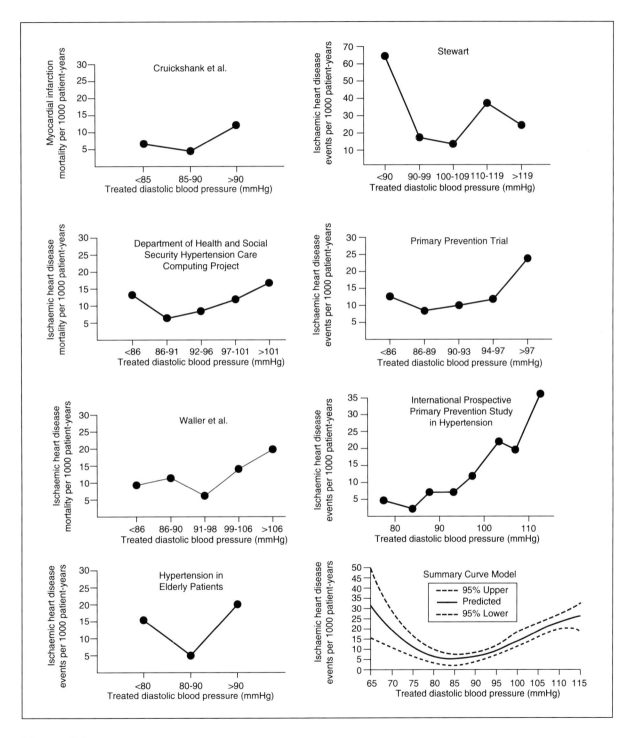

Figure 6.3
Summary of studies involved in the meta-analysis (From Farnett L et al.[27])

diastolic blood pressure between intervention and control groups in these trials, it was estimated that almost all stroke and about half of the CHD events expected from observational studies[5] were rapidly (in about five years) and statistically significantly reduced. However, analyses were based on comparisons of observed and expected event rates in the intervention groups and hence achieved diastolic blood pressure was not accounted for. Previous meta-analyses that have addressed the issue of prevention of cardiovascular complications by treatment in mild to moderate hypertension have not demonstrated any significant effect on morbidity from coronary heart disease.[9,10,12] The significant findings in the present meta-analysis could be explained by the inclusion of trials enrolling subjects with more severe hypertension.[55] This meta-analysis have also been criticized by other authors.[52–54]

Clinical trials

To our knowledge, only two studies have been initiated to test the hypothesis of increasing risk with extensive lowering of blood pressure. The Swedish BBB study (Behandla Blodtryck Bättre – Treat Hypertension Better) was launched in 1987.[56] It is now terminated but its results have been published only as an abstract.[57]

The objectives of the study were 'to evaluate the feasibility and the possible reduction in hypertension-associated morbidity and mortality by more intensive lowering of the diastolic blood pressure by treatment'. Patients with treated hypertension and diastolic blood pressure in the range of 90–100 mmHg were randomized to receive either unaltered antihypertensive treatment or more intense treatment with the goal of reaching a blood pressure of ≤ 80 mmHg. It was estimated that 3 years of

follow-up of approximately 2000 patients would provide the necessary statistical power.

The trial finally included 2213 patients with no history of ischaemic heart disease and with a normal electrocardiogram. They were followed for 44 months. Table 6.1 summarizes the findings, taken from the abstract.[57] No statistically significant results were obtained. One reason for that may be that the resulting difference in diastolic blood pressure was lower than expected. Based upon the available results, it may be concluded that the results of the BBB study does not contradict the J-curve hypothesis.

The Hypertension Optimal Treatment (HOT) study is an on-going multinational trial, also co-ordinated from Sweden.[26] Patients are randomized to three groups with different therapeutic goals for diastolic blood pressure: ≤ 90 mmHg, ≤ 85 mmHg, and ≤ 80 mmHg. Unfortunately, the protocol may be less well suited to test the current hypothesis. All patients are started on 5 mg felodipine daily. Further treatment (if necessary) includes the addition of an ACE-inhibitor and/or a beta-blocker and/or a diuretic. Thus, those randomized to achieve the lower therapeutic goals will be treated to a greater extent with medications that possess documented cardioprotective effect.[58–62] Consequently, a harmful effect from extensive lowering of the diastolic blood pressure could be compensated by the different treatment.

The problems with designing a trial to test the J-curve hypothesis are evident from this. As discussed below, the pathophysiology of the coronary circulation and factors associated with the autoregulation and coronary flow reserve appear crucial for the risk of coronary heart disease in hypertensive subjects. Thus, these characteristics should be considered in clinical trials, e.g. by stratifying the patients by the most important factors. The interaction

	Intensified treatment	Unchanged treatment
Number of subjects (Total 2213)	n/a	n/a
Goal diastolic blood pressure (mmHg)	≤ 80	90–100
Achieved diastolic blood pressure (mmHg)*	83	90
Achieved systolic blood pressure (mmHg)*	142	152
Myocardial infarction (number)	20	18
Clinical myocardial infarction (number)	18	13
Silent myocardial infarction (number)	2	5
Stroke (number)	8	11
*(mean; SD not given)		

Table 6.1
Characteristics and results from the BBB study. (Adapted from Hansson et al.[57])

between such patient characteristics and treatment regimen have to be given special concern.

Is change in blood pressure with treatment important?

The bulk of studies on the J-curve phenomenon have dealt with the absolute level of achieved blood pressure. Two studies did, however, primarily address the alternative hypothesis of a prognostic impact of the change in diastolic blood pressure that was induced by treatment.[49,50]

In the Hypertension Detection and Follow-up Program, the relation between diastolic blood pressure reduction and mortality was analysed using subjects from both stepped care and referred care.[49] The change in blood pressure from the baseline examination to the first annual follow-up in 10 053 participants was used to predict 568 deaths that occurred over 4 years. The findings support a curvelinear relation with an evident J-shape. The

authors do, however, suggest caution in the interpretation, owing to large standard errors.

The impact of treatment-induced blood pressure reduction on the risk of myocardial infarction was investigated in a US study of 1765 previously untreated hypertensives with blood pressure ≥ 160 and/or 95 mmHg.[50] During 4 years follow-up, morbidity was related to a small (≤ 6 mmHg), moderate (7–17 mmHg) or large (≥ 18 mmHg) fall in diastolic blood pressure. The risk was lowest with a moderate fall and significantly higher in the other two.

Other studies have failed to demonstrate such a relationship[33,36] and, therefore, there is so far only weak evidence that the absolute fall in blood pressure should be considered in the treatment of mild and moderate hypertension.

The impact of cardiac status

At least two of the studies reviewed above suggest that deprived cardiac status among the patients increases the likelihood that a J-shaped relation is found.[31,34] Recently, we published data from a Swedish cohort that was able to investigate this hypothesis in some detail.[63] The study supports an interaction between coronary flow reserve and blood-pressure-related risk of acute myocardial infarction in treated hypertensives.

The cohort was established in Skaraborg county, Sweden, in 1977, when a program for the detection and management of hypertensives was implemented in primary care.[64] By 1981, 1121 men and 1453 women aged 40–69 years had completed their first annual check-up without any evidence of a previous myocardial infarction.[63]

The achieved blood pressure at this first annual check-up was used to predict a first myocardial infarction, with adjustment for differences in age, sex, body mass index, serum cholesterol, smoking, diabetes mellitus, and left ventricular hypertrophy.[63] Smoking, left ventricular hypertrophy (both sexes) and serum cholesterol (men only) were significantly related to risk. In men, but not in women, there was a negative linear relation between achieved diastolic blood pressure and risk of a first acute myocardial infarction.

This striking finding was further explored in two subgroups of men according to the characteristics of their baseline electrocardiograms. In

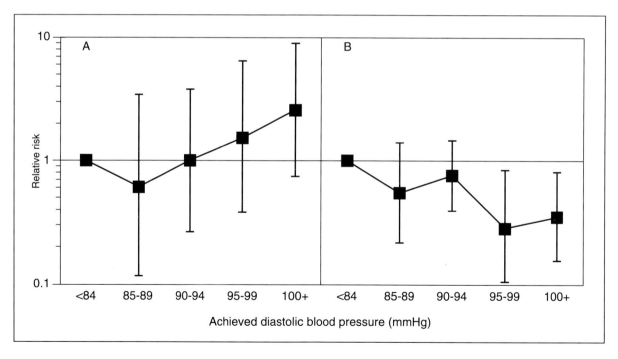

Figure 6.4
Relative risks (95% confidence intervals) for a first acute myocardial infarction among men with (A) normal electrocardiogram and (B) men with ischaemic/hypertrophic electrocardiogram. (The Skaraborg Hypertension Project. Adapted from Lindblad U et al.[63])

those 345 men who had an entirely normal electrocardiogram, the risk decreased significantly and linearly with decreasing diastolic blood pressure (Fig. 6.4).

The opposite was found in the subset of 499 men who had ST-depression and/or negative T-waves and/or high voltage (ECG signs that coincide with myocardial hypertrophy and/or ischaemia).[65] In these patients, the risk increased significantly with decreasing diastolic blood pressure. The relative risk in such men with a diastolic blood pressure of 95–99 mmHg and those with a diastolic pressure above 100 mmHg was about one third of that in men with the lowest blood pressure (< 85 mmHg) (see Fig. 6.4). Interestingly, all other characteristics of the groups were similar, and therefore the explanation of the findings seems to rest in the achieved diastolic blood pressure level. No similar relationship was found for women or for systolic blood pressure.

The results of this study suggest that men with normal electrocardiograms would benefit from treatment-induced lowering of the diastolic blood pressure, at least down to 85 mmHg. In men with abnormal (ischaemic or hypertrophic) electrocardiograms the results are consistent with the hypothesis that reduction of the diastolic blood pressure below a critical level is harmful in subjects who probably have impaired coronary flow.[66]

The pathophysiology of coronary complications

An important question that arises at this point is whether there is any pathophysiological relevance in a J-shaped relationship between achieved diastolic blood pressure and the risk of myocardial infarction.

The risk of severe cardiac complications such as myocardial infarction, sudden death, and arrhythmias increases when myocardial circulation is impaired. The availability of oxygen in the myocardium depends on the myocardial demand on the one hand, and the supply on the other, the latter in part determined by coronary flow.[66–70] Due to autoregulatory mechanisms, coronary flow at rest can be increased as much as fivefold by relaxation of the coronary artery bed when needed, i.e. there is a flow reserve of 5.[70] Coronary perfusion occurs in diastole. As oxygen extraction is nearly maximal at rest,[67] increased oxygen demand must be compensated by increased coronary flow. When perfusion pressure changes within the autoregulatory range, coronary flow thus adapts to maintain the circulation in the myocardium.[66–70]

In hypertensive patients, coronary flow reserve can be impaired by different causes. First, coronary flow at rest, as well as the ability to dilate the coronary artery bed on demand, is decreased when the coronary artery lumen is narrowed by an arteriosclerotic stenosis and/or when the coronary vessels are narrowed by hypertrophy of the vascular wall.[31,68,71–75] Both these conditions are common sequelae to diastolic hypertension.

Secondly, in hypertensive patients, the lower end of the autoregulatory curve is shifted to the right,[71–76] even before any signs of left ventricular hypertrophy are seen.[71–75] In the additional presence of left ventricular hypertrophy, oxygen demand will increase[66–70,77] and coronary flow reserve is further depressed.[78] These upward shifts of the autoregulatory curve will decrease the coronary flow reserve synergistically, placing the lower end where the perfusion pressure maintains coronary flow at a higher level.[66–70] The negative impact of the low coronary perfusion pressure will thus be more evident in the case of combined coronary artery disease and left ventricular hypertrophy.[75,79] From a clinical standpoint electrocardiographic signs of ischaemia reflects increased susceptibility to a decrease in coronary perfusion pressure.[75] A low coronary flow may increase blood viscosity and platelet adhesiveness and, as a consequence, the risk of thrombus formation.[66] Between ischaemic and well perfused areas of the myocardium, metabolic gradients may develop, thereby increasing the risk of arrhythmias.[66]

The relation between these different factors and the chain of events leading to a CHD event are summarized by Berglund (Fig. 6.5).[66] This model also explains why the occurrence of a J-shaped relation between treated diastolic blood pressure and risk of CHD is confined to hypertensive subjects with coronary heart disease and/or left ventricular hypertrophy.

As a further support for the hazards of decreasing the diastolic blood pressure in hypertensive subjects, there is a circadian variation with increased risk of subendocardial myocardial infarction during the night when diastolic blood pressure is lowest.[80] In treated hypertensives, blood pressure decreases more during the night than in untreated subjects. Thus, the coronary pressure could fall below the level where autoregulation maintains the coronary flow, especially in subjects with coronary stenosis or left ventricular hypertrophy, and the risk

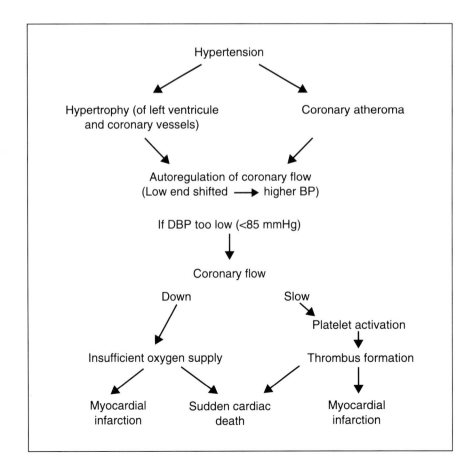

Figure 6.5
Outline of the pathophysiologic events leading to acute myocardial infarction in hypertensive patients. (From Berglund G.[66])

of myocardial infarction increases.[80] It has also been proposed that low diastolic blood pressure during the night may cause ischaemia through an imbalance between left ventricular work load and coronary perfusion pressure.[81]

Is there a J-curve phenomenon?

The hypertensive populations in the studies reviewed are not homogeneous. A denominator in most studies that provide support for a J-curve phenomenon (type A) is that they recruited hypertensives both with and without impaired cardiac function. The cohorts that demonstrated a relationship of type B or C were all derived in clinical trials that more or less completely excluded subjects with any signs of impaired coronary flow reserve. The Skaraborg findings, in which a negative relation between achieved diastolic blood pressure and the risk of myocardial infarction was confined to patients with impaired coronary flow reserve, provides a valid explanation for this discrepancy. The J-curve may simply be a combination of a negative linear regression in these patients and a positive linear regression among those with an unaffected myocardium.

It is, however, important to keep in mind that the lower range of the achieved diastolic blood pressure includes outliers in different respects, including respects other than blood pressure reaction (e.g. disease prevalence). Although the J-shaped curve is a consistent finding in trials with a potential to identify such an effect, the cause of the J-shaped curve may vary with the characteristics of the population under study. Thus, a J-shaped curve has also been identified in untreated controls,[38-40,43,46] and in populations other than hypertensives.[82,83] The cause probably differs between different populations under study. In other words, the causes of the J-curve phenomenon are complex and it may well be that in each population of hypertensives it is caused by a combination of factors with different weight. Another contributing explanation of the J-curve phenomenon might be that in some patients, a large blood pressure reduction induced by treatment could be due to poor neuroendocrine mechanisms counteracting the fall in blood pressure. The lack of this defence mechanism could reflect impaired health and other factors that may also be associated with increased risk of coronary heart disease.[66,84,85]

A trial designed to explore the causality of the potential harm by lowering the blood pressure is obviously needed, but the design problems are evident. Patients who are randomized to achieve different treatment goals are expected to have similar baseline characteristics. Any patient randomized to achieve a lower pressure will therefore necessarily have to use a more efficient medication than the subject randomized to a higher level. Therefore, in a trial, there is no simple way of separating effects of differing medication from that of the difference in blood pressure.

Clinical implications

While waiting for the perfect trial, one has to rely on observational evidence. The best support for the theory of a J-curve phenomenon is the consistency of the findings with what is expected from the pathophysiological properties of the myocardium. With this background, in combination with the strong negative impact suggested in the Skaraborg Project, it is now justified to suggest some change in the general recommendations for treatment of patients with hypertension and impaired coronary flow reserve.[75]

Current guidelines recommend that blood pressure lowering treatment is chosen and ordered individually after considering each patient's blood pressure, other risk factors, and intercurrent diseases.[86] However, following the awareness of a J-shaped curve and the potential harm of lowering the coronary perfusion pressure in some hypertensives, it is advocated that treatment goals should also be formed individually.

So far no study has demonstrated any benefits of lowering the diastolic blood pressure below 85 mmHg in subjects with diastolic hypertension. In general, and certainly in patients with no established ischaemic heart disease or left ventricular hypertrophy, this goal seems justified, not the least because of the lowered risk of stroke, cardiac failure, and renal failure. The aims may be set at lower levels for this category, in case it can be achieved without violation of the other threats to impact of treatment (e.g. side effects of treatment affecting glucose metabolism, lipid metabolism, and electrolyte balance) suggested in the introduction to this chapter.

For hypertensive patients with symptomatic ischaemic heart disease or electrocardiographic findings consistent with left ventricular hypertrophy or myocardial ischaemia, it now seems realistic to use a different strategy. A realistic goal in these patients may be to aim at 95 mmHg, where the risk of acute myocardial infarction is lowest. With respect to the risk of stroke, this may imply some sacrifice, though this treatment goal is still justified, as the incidence of cerebral events in the population is less than that of myocardial infarction.

So far, only diuretics and beta-blockers have demonstrated a positive impact of blood pressure lowering, and consequently they should be regarded first choice medication in most cases. However, as ACE-inhibitors have a capability of restoring left ventricular function,[59–62] they should be used as first choice in the patients with impaired coronary flow reserve. This is recommended with the reservation that we have nothing but indirect proof that treatment with these agents will reduce stroke incidence to an extent that is comparable with that of the older drugs.

It is evident that clinical trials are warranted to test the feasibility and impact of these guidelines. In such trials it will be important to include patients with impaired myocardial function, and also to stratify based upon such traits.

References

1 Kannel WB, Wolf PA, Verter J et al. Epidemiologic assessment of the role of blood pressure in stroke, The Framingham study. *JAMA* 1970; **214**:301–10.

2 Dyken ML, Wolf PA, Barnett HJM et al. A statement for physicians by the sub-committee on risk factors and stroke of the stroke council. *Stroke* 1984; **15**:1105–11.

3 Bonita R. Epidemiology of stroke. *Lancet* 1992; **339**:342–4.

4 Dawber TR. *The Framingham Study: The Epidemiology of Atherosclerotic Disease.* Cambridge: Harvard University Press, 1980.

5 MacMahon S, Peto R, Cutler J et al. Blood pressure, stroke, and coronary heart disease. Part 1: prolonged differences in blood pressure: prospective observational studies corrected for the regression dilution bias. *Lancet* 1990; **335**:765–74.

6 Inter-Society Commission for Heart Disease Resources, Atherosclerosis Study Group, Epidemiology Study Group. Primary prevention of the atherosclerotic diseases. *Circulation* 1970; **42**:A55–A94.

7 Reid DD, Hamilton PJS, McCartney P et al. Smoking and other risk factors for coronary heart disease in British civil servants. *Lancet* 1976; **ii**:979–84.

8 The Pooling Project Research Group. Relationship of blood pressure, serum cholesterol, smoking habit, relative weight and ECG abnormalities to incidence of major coronary events: Final report of the Pooling Project. *J Chron Dis* 1978; **31**:201–306.

9 MacMahon SW, Cutler JA, Furberg CD et al. The effects of drug treatment for hypertension on morbidity and mortality from cardiovascular disease: A review of randomized controlled trials. *Prog Cardiovasc Dis* 1986; **29**(suppl 1):99–118.

10 MacMahon SW, Cutler JA, Neaton JD et al. Relationship of blood pressure to coronary and stroke morbidity and mortality in clinical trials and epidemiological studies. *J Hypertens* 1986; **4**(suppl 6):S14–S17.

11 Collins R, Peto R, MacMahon S et al. Blood pressure, stroke, and coronary heart disease. Part 2: short-term reductions in blood pressure: overview of randomised drug trials in their epidemiological context. *Lancet* 1990; **335**:827–35.

12 Holme I. Drug treatment of mild hypertension to reduce the risk of CHD: is it worthwhile? *Stat Med* 1988; **7**:1109–20.

13 Criqui MH, Barrett-Connor E, Holdbrook MJ et al. Clustering of cardiovascular disease risk factors. *Prev Med* 1980; **9**:525–33.

14 Bønaa K, Thelle D. Association between blood pressure and serum lipids in a population: The Tromsø Study. *Circulation* 1991; **83**:1305–14.

15 Reaven GM, Hoffman BB. Hypertension as a disease of carbohydrate and lipoprotein metabolism. *Am J Med* 1989; **87**(suppl 6A):2S–6S.

16 Ferranini E, Buzzigoli G, Bonnadonna R et al. Insulin resistance in essential hypertension. *N Engl J Med* 1987; **317**:350–7.

17 Multiple Risk Factor Intervention Trial Research Group. Multiple risk factor intervention trial: Risk factor changes and mortality results. *JAMA* 1982; **248**:1465–77.

18 Pollare T, Lithell H, Berne C. A comparison of the effect of hydro-chlorothiazide and captopril on glucose and lipid metabolism in patients with hypertension. *N Engl J Med* 1989; **321**:868–73.

19 Multiple Risk Factor Intervention Trial Research Group. Mortality after 10½ years for hypertensive participants in the multiple risk factor intervention trial. *Circulation* 1990; **82**:1616–28.

20 Black HR. The coronary artery disease paradox: The role of hyperinsulinemia and insulin resistance and implications for therapy. *J Cardiovasc Pharmacol* 1990; **15**(suppl 5):S26–S38.

21 Kannel WB. Status of risk factors and their consideration in antihypertensive therapy. *Am J Cardiol* 1987; **59**:80A–90A.

22 Samuelsson O, Wilhelmsen L, Andersson OK et al. Cardio-vascular morbidity in relation to change in blood pressure and serum cholesterol levels in treated hypertension. Results from the primary prevention trial in Göteborg, Sweden. *JAMA* 1987; **258**:1768–76.

23 Samuelsson O. Hypertension in middle-aged men: Management, morbidity and prognostic factors during long-term hypertensive care. *Acta Med Scand Suppl* 1985; **702**:1–79.

24 Dunn FG, McLenachan J, Isles CG et al. Left ventricular hypertrophy and mortality in hypertension: an analysis of data from the Glasgow Blood Pressure Clinic. *J Hypertens* 1991; **8**:775–82.

25 Hansson L, Dahlöf B. What are we really achieving with long-term antihypertensive drug therapy? In: Laragh LH, Brenner BM, eds. *Hypertension: Pathophysiology, diagnosis and management.* New York: Raven, 1990:2131–41.

26 The HOT Study Group. The Hypertension Optimal Treatment Study (The HOT Study). *Blood Pressure* 1993; **2**:62–8.

27 Farnett L, Mulrow CD, Linn WD et al. The J-Curve phenomenon and the treatment of hypertension. Is there a point beyond which pressure reduction is dangerous? *JAMA* 1991; **265**:489–95.

28 Anderson TW. Re-examination of some of the Framingham blood pressure data. *Lancet* 1978; **11**:1139–41.

29 Kannel WB, Gordon T, Schwartz MJ. Systolic vs diastolic blood pressure and risk of coronary heart disease. *Am J Cardiol* 1971; **27**:335–46.

30 Stewart IMcDG. Relation of reduction in pressure to first myocardial infarction in patients receiving treatment for severe hypertension. *Lancet* 1979; **1**:861–5.

31 Cruickshank JM, Thorpe JM, Zacharias FJ. Benefits and potential harm of lowering high blood pressure. *Lancet* 1987; **1**:581–4.

32 Berglund G, Samuelsson O. Lowered blood pressure and the J-shaped curve. *Lancet* 1987; **i**:1154–5 [letter].

33 Samuelsson O, Wilhelmsen L, Anderson OK et al. Cardiovascular morbidity in relation to change in blood pressure and serum cholesterol levels in treated hypertension: results from the Primary Prevention Trial in Göteborg, Sweden. *JAMA* 1987; **258**:1768–76.

34 Samuelsson OG, Wilhelmsen LW, Pennert KM et al. The J-shaped relationship between coronary heart disease and achieved blood pressure level in treated hypertension: further analyses of 12 years of follow-up of treated hypertensives in the Primary Prevention Trial in Gothenburg, Sweden. *J Hypertens* 1990; **8**:547–55.

35 Fletcher AE, Beevers DG, Bulpitt CJ et al. The relationship between a low treated blood pressure and IHD mortality: a report from the DHSS Hypertension Care Computing Project. *J Hum Hypertens* 1988; **2**:11–15.

36 Waller PC, Isles CG, Lever AF et al. Does therapeutic reduction of diastolic blood pressure cause death from coronary heart disease? *J Hum Hypertens* 1988; **2**:7–10.

37 Coope J, Warrender TS. Randomized trial of treatment of hypertension in elderly patients in primary care. *Br Med J* 1986; **293**:1145–8.

38 Cooper J, Warrender TS. Lowering blood pressure. *Lancet* 1987; **i**:1380 [letter].

39 Coope J, Warrender TS. Lowering blood pressure. *Lancet* 1987; **ii**:518 [letter].

40 Staessen J, Bulpitt C, Clement D et al. Relation between mortality and treated blood pressure in elderly patients with hypertension: report of the European Working Party on High Blood Pressure in the Elderly. *Br Med J* 1989; **298**:1552–6.

41 McCloskey LW, Psaty BM, Koepsell TD et al. Level of blood pressure and risk of myocardial infarction among treated hypertensive patients. *Arch Int Med* 1992; **152**:513–20.

42 Report by the Management Committee, The Australian Therapeutic Trial in Mild Hypertension. *Lancet* 1980; **1**:1261–7.

43 The Management Committee of the Australian Therapeutic Trial in Mild Hypertension. Untreated mild hypertension. *Lancet* 1982; **1**:185–91.

44 The IPPPSH Collaborative Group. Cardiovascular risk and risk factors in a randomized trial of treatment based on the beta-blocker oxprenolol: the International Prospective Primary Prevention Study in Hypertension (IPPPSH). *J Hypertens* 1985; **3**:379–92.

45 Medical Research Council Working Party. MRC trial of mild hypertension: principal results. *Br Med J* 1985; **291**:97–104.

46 Medical Research Council Working Party. Stroke and coronary heart disease in mild hypertension: risk factors and the value of treatment. *Br Med J* 1988; **296**:1565–70.

47 SHEP Cooperative Research Group. Prevention of stroke by antihypertensive drug treatment in older persons with isolated systolic hypertension. Final results of the systolic hypertension in the elderly program (SHEP). *JAMA* 1991; **265**:3255–64.

48 Fletcher AE, Bulpitt CJ. How far should blood pressure be lowered? *N Engl J Med* 1992; **326**:251–4.

49 Cooper SP, Hardy RJ, Labarthe DR et al. The relation between degree of blood pressure reduction and mortality among hypertensives in the Hypertension Detection and Follow-up Program. *Am J Epidemiol* 1988; **127**:387–402.

50 Alderman MH, Ooi WL, Madharan S, Cohen H. Treatment induced blood pressure reduction and the risk of myocardial infarction. *JAMA* 1989; **262**:920–4.

51 Pererra GA. Antihypertensive drug vs symptomatic treatment in primary hypertension: effect on survival. *JAMA* 1960; **173**:11–13.

52 Jenkinson ML. *Lancet* 1990; **335**:1093 [letter].

53 Cruickshank JM, Fox K, Collins P. *Lancet* 1990; **335**:1092 [letter].

54 Alderman MH. *Lancet* 1990; **335**:1092 [letter].

55 Kaplan NM. *Lancet* 1990; **335**:1093 [letter].

56 The BBB Study Group. The BBB study: a prospective randomized study of intensified antihypertensive treatment. *J Hypertens* 1988; **6**:693–7.

57 Hansson L, Dahlöf B, Abelin J. Cardiovascular morbidity and mortality in the BBB study, *6th European Meeting on Hypertension, Milan* 1993; S435(abstr 87).

58 Kendall MJ, Wikstrand J. Hypertension and coronary artery disease: impact of beta blockers. *Cardiovascular Risk Factors* 1991; **1**:527–35.

59 The SOLVD Investigators. Effect of enalapril on survival in patients with reduced left ventricular ejection fractions and congestive heart failure. *N Engl J Med* 1991; **325**:293–302.

60 Pfeffer MA, Braunwald E, Moyé LA et al. Effect of captopril on mortality and morbidity in patients with left ventricular dysfunction after myocardial infarction. Results of the survival and ventricular enlargement trial. *N Engl J Med* 1992; **327**:669–77.

61 The SOLVD Investigators. Effect of enalapril on the mortality and the development of heart failure in asymptomatic patients with reduced left ventricular ejection fractions. *N Engl J Med* 1992; **327**:685–91.

62 Yusuf S, Pepine CJ, Garces C et al. Effect of enalapril on myocardial infarction and unstable angina in patients with low ejection fractions. *Lancet* 1992; **340**:1173–8.

63 Lindblad U, Råstam L, Rydén L et al. Control of blood pressure and risk of first myocardial infarction: Skaraborg hypertension project. *Br Med J* 1994; **308**:681–6.

64 Berglund G, Isacsson SO, Rydén L. The Skaraborg Project: a controlled trial regarding the effect of structured hypertension care. *Acta Med Scand* 1979; **205**(suppl 626):64–8.

65 Sokolow M, Lyon TP. The ventricular complex in left ventricular hypertrophy as obtained by unipolar precordial and limb leads. *Am Heart J* 1949; **37**:161–86.

66 Berglund G. Goals of antihypertensive therapy. Is there a point beyond which pressure reduction is dangerous? *Am J Hypertens* 1989; **2**:586–93.

67 Strandgaard S, Haunsø S. Why does antihypertensive treatment prevent stroke but not myocardial infarction? *Lancet* 1987; **1**:658–61.

68 Cruickshank JM. Coronary flow reserve and the J curve relation between diastolic blood pressure and myocardial infarction. *Br Med J* 1988; **297**:1227–30.

69 Frohlich ED, Apstein C, Chobanian A et al. The heart in hypertension. *N Engl J Med* 1992; **327**:998–1008.

70 Klocke FJ. Measurements of coronary flow reserve: defining pathophysiology versus making decisions about patient care. *Circulation* 1987; **76**:1183–9.

71 Vogt M, Motz W, Strauer BE. Coronary haemodynamics in hypertensive heart disease. *Eur Heart J* 1992; **13**(suppl D):44–9.

72 Lucarini AR, Picano E, Salvetti A. Coronary microvascular disease in hypertensives. *Clin Exp Hypertens* 1992; **A14**(1,2):55–66.

73 Brush JE Jr, Cannon RO, Schenke WB et al. Angina due to coronary microvascular disease in hypertensive patients without left ventricular hypertrophy. *N Engl Med J* 1988; **319**:1302–7.

74 Lucarini AR, Eugenio P, Lattanzi F et al. Dipyramidole echocardiography stress testing in hypertensive patients. Targets and tools. *Circulation* 1991; **83**:III68–III72.

75 Cruickshank JM. Blood pressure and myocardial infarction. Low blood pressure can be hazardous. *Br Med J* 1994; **308**:1301–2 [letter].

76 Leschke M, Schoebel FC, Vogt M et al. Reduced peripheral and coronary vasomotion in systemic hypertension. *Eur Heart J* 1993; **13**(suppl D):96–9.

77 Polese A, De Cesare N, Montorsi P et al. Upward shift of the lower range of coronary flow autoregulation in hypertensive patients with hypertrophy of the left ventricle. *Circulation* 1991; **83**:845–53.

78 Houghton JL, Frank MJ, Carr AA, von Dohlen TW, Prisant LM. Relations among impaired coronary flow reserve, left ventricular hypertrophy and thallium perfusion defects in hypertensive patients without obstructive coronary artery disease. *J Am Coll Cardiol* 1990; **15**:43–51.

79 Cruickshank JM. Clinical importance of coronary perfusion pressure in the hypertensive patient with left ventricular hypertrophy. *Cardiology* 1992; **81**:283–90.

80 Floras JS. Antihypertensive treatment, myocardial infarction, and nocturnal myocardial ischemia. *Lancet* 1988; **ii**:994–6.

81 Mansour P, Boström PÅ, Mattiasson I, Lilja B, Berglund G. Low blood pressure levels and signs of myocardial ischemia: importance of left ventricular hypertrophy. *J Hum Hypertens* 1993; **7**:13–18.

82 Dágostino RB, Belanger AJ, Kannel WB et al. Relation of low diastolic blood pressure to coronary heart disease death in presence of myocardial infarction: the Framingham study. *Br Med J* 1991; **303**:385–9.

83 Coope J, Warrender TS, McPherson K. The prognostic significance of blood pressure in the elderly. *J Hum Hypertens* 1988; **2**:79–88.

84 Coope J. Hypertension: the cause of the J-curve. *J Hum Hypertens* 1990; **4**:1–4.

85 Coope J, Warrander TS. Caution in left ventricular hypertrophy. *Br Med J* 1994; **308**:1302 [letter].

86 Subcommittee of WHO/ISH Mild Hypertension Liaison Committee. Summary of 1993 World Health Organisation–International Society of Hypertension guidelines for the management of mild hypertension. *Br Med J* 1993; **307**:1541–6.

7

Resistant Hypertension

Iftikhar U Haq, Ian G Chadwick, Wilfred W Yeo, Peter R Jackson and Laurence E Ramsay

Resistant hypertension is here used to mean hypertension that fails to be reduced to target blood pressure on an adequate regimen of 3 antihypertensive drugs. However, as Frohlich has pointed out,[1] failure to control blood pressure is sometimes due to deficiencies in management on the part of doctors, or to the reluctance of patients to follow the advice proffered. These aspects of difficult hypertension will be discussed briefly at the end of the chapter.

Definition

Hypertension has generally been defined as resistant when it remains uncontrolled despite a 'good' regimen of 3 anti-hypertensive drugs at full dosage.[1-8] Definitions have differed in detail because various target blood pressures have been used, but control would now be considered inadequate if the systolic pressure exceeded 160 mmHg or the diastolic 90 mmHg.[9] A 'good' regimen would generally include a thiazide diuretic, a beta-blocker, and an ACE inhibitor or a calcium antagonist. Recently, Setaro and Black[10] have suggested that hypertension should be considered resistant when it remains uncontrolled by a regimen of only 2 drugs, on the grounds that newer antihypertensive drugs are more effective and better tolerated than the older drugs. We do not believe that this is justified. The newer drugs are neither more effective in lowering

blood pressure nor better tolerated than those such as thiazides and beta-blockers, that have long been available.[11,12] The plan of investigation and management laid out below has evolved from observations and studies in patients who were not adequately controlled by 3 drugs, and there is little doubt that specialist referral and detailed investigation of such patients is soundly based. Redefining resistant hypertension as '2-drug failure' will lead to referral and investigation of a much larger proportion of hypertensive patients, and there is no evidence that this is either necessary or beneficial. It is a retrograde step towards a policy of investigating in detail all hypertensive patients – a policy that was correctly abandoned because the yield of abnormalities and the benefit to patients were negligible.

Prevalence

Resistant hypertension is relatively common in hypertension clinics because of selection by referral, and it is seen in 13–20% of such patients.[6,13,14] It has been considered uncommon in the general population of hypertensive patients,[15,16] but this may be incorrect. For example, in the Australian Therapeutic Trial, 19% of patients with mild hypertension needed treatment with three drugs,[17] and despite this 4% of all patients had diastolic pressures averaging 100 mmHg or higher, and no less than 25% averaged 90 mmHg or higher.[18]

The same trial also illustrated the importance of resistant hypertension by showing that it confers a bad prognosis.[19] Patients with diastolic pressures averaging 100 mmHg or higher despite treatment had vascular complications at a rate of 8.5% per year, and those averaging 90–99 mmHg had a rate of 5.0% per year, compared to a rate of only 1.3% per year in those who attained the target (<90 mmHg).[18] Treatment-resistant patients are also much more likely to have evidence of end-organ damage such as left ventricular hypertrophy, cardiomegaly, renal impairment and proteinuria.[2,4]

Treatment resistance damages patients' peace of mind as well as their cardiovascular system – it cannot be fun to have your blood pressure measured every month only to be told that 'it is not good enough'. It also causes doctors considerable discomfort because many are uncertain how to deal with the problem. As discussed later, resistant hypertension is best approached with an explicit differential diagnosis that leads naturally to a logical plan of management.

Clinical features

Many factors have been proposed as contributing to treatment resistance, but much that has been written is a mixture of clinical impression, uncontrolled observations, and extrapolation from hypertensive subjects without treatment resistance. Weight is given in the account below to the relatively few studies of resistant hypertension that have included an appropriate control group.[2,4,20,21]

Patients with resistant hypertension clearly differ from other hypertensive subjects in three important ways:

- they have more severe hypertension to start with;
- they have more end-organ damage;
- and they are more likely to have an identifiable underlying cause for hypertension.

As regards the severity of hypertension, Isaksson et al[4] reported blood pressures at referral of 188/111 mmHg in those who became resistant to treatment compared to 165/102 mmHg in control patients. Toner et al[2] reported a mean arterial pressure averaging 153 mmHg at entry to a hypertension clinic in patients who became resistant, compared to 135 mmHg in control hypertensive subjects, and this was despite use of more antihypertensive drugs by those who proved resistant. Patients with resistant hypertension more often had left ventricular hypertrophy, renal impairment, and proteinuria,[2] and they were much more likely to have had accelerated (malignant phase) hypertension in the past (17% in resistant cases, 2% in controls).[2] It is not clear whether the higher prevalence of renal impairment in treatment resistance is a consequence of previous accelerated phase hypertension or whether it signals primary renal disease that was not formally diagnosed because renal biopsy is not commonly performed in such patients.[2]

Patients with treatment resistance are more likely to have an underlying cause for hypertension, with estimates of the frequency varying from 10–36%.[2,4,10,13,22,23] Of these causes the commonest is renovascular disease, with an incidence as high as 15–25%.[2,4,23] It is also the most important cause, because it is now potentially correctable by transluminal angioplasty, and the hypertension is therefore potentially curable. Renoparenchymal disease and obstructive uropathy were each found in 5% of patients with resistant hypertension,[23] but it is unclear from controlled studies whether the prevalence of these abnormalities is higher than that observed in all hypertensive subjects.[2,4]

Causes of hypertension other than renal disorders are less common. In various series,[2,4,10,13,22] there are reports of primary hyperaldosteronism (0–4%), Cushing's disease (0–2%) and aortic coarctation (0–1%) associated with treatment resistance. Phaeochromocytoma is an occasional cause of treatment resistance, but it seldom features in reported series presumably because the tumour is removed immediately upon diagnosis.

Apart from these features, patients with resistant hypertension have few distinctive clinical characteristics. Isaksson et al[4] reported that diabetes was common in resistant hypertension, with a prevalence 12% higher than that in control patients, possibly because of diabetic nephropathy. A curious observation in the same study[4] was a large excess of chronic musculoskeletal pain in treatment-resistant patients which was not caused by non-steroidal anti-inflammatory drugs. The authors speculated that chronic pain might itself cause poor blood pressure control. The patients with resistant hypertension in this study were much more likely than controls to be manual workers and to have psychological morbidity, and these confounding factors could have been responsible for the apparent association between chronic pain and treatment resistance.

Personal and dietary factors

Some factors have been linked with resistant hypertension, for example older age[24] and regular alcohol use,[25,26] when in fact there is little supporting evidence. Two controlled studies[2,4] showed no relation of treatment resistance to age, sex, or heavy alcohol use. One of these studies[2] showed no relation of obesity to treatment resistance, but in the other,[4] resistant patients weighed significantly more than controls. This association was confined to those resistant patients who did not have renovascular disease,[4] raising the possibility that there may be 2 populations of patients with resistant hypertension – those with idiopathic hypertension who are overweight, and those with an underlying cause for their hypertension who are not overweight.

The relationship of smoking to resistant hypertension is unclear. In 1 study, resistant hypertension was related significantly to cigarette smoking,[2] and it was proposed that cigarette smoking might predispose to treatment resistance through its recognized relations to accelerated phase hypertension[27–29] and renovascular disease.[30,31] However, Isaksson et al showed no relation of treatment resistance to smoking.[4]

Heavy salt intake raises blood pressure in patients with so-called salt-sensitive hypertension, particularly in black and elderly subjects and in those with renal insufficiency, and has been cited as a cause of treatment resistance.[10,15] However we are unaware of any evidence supporting this. One controlled study did not support a role for dietary salt,[2] but sodium intake was not measured directly.

Caffeine ingestion has a pressor effect, but there is no relation of caffeine use alone to treatment resistance.[2] The combination of cigarette smoking and caffeine ingestion causes a substantial and prolonged pressor effect,[32] and this may possibly contribute to treatment resistance.[2]

Isaksson et al[4,21] found that patients with resistant hypertension were significantly more likely to have low occupation status than control hypertensive subjects, with 76% of their treatment-resistant hypertensive patients having manual or unskilled non-manual employment compared to 42% in the reference group. The explanation for this observation, which requires confirmation, is unclear.

Psychological factors

It is not clear whether psychological factors play a role in resistant hypertension. Isaksson et al studied the psychological and social characteristics of hypertensives resistant to treatment[4] and found a higher prevalence of nervous complaints and mental distress.[21] They had an impaired ability to channel emotions, especially anger, and they experienced less joy. Treatment-resistant patients reported fewer important life events, and significantly fewer positive life events over the previous 10-year period. As noted above, the findings of this study were confounded by a large difference in socioeconomic status between resistant patients and controls.

In contrast to these findings, Toner et al found no excess of affective disorder in those with resistant hypertension when compared to controls, as measured by the Crown-Crisp experiential index questionnaire.[2] Scores for anxiety and depression were slightly but not significantly higher in resistant patients. Those with resistant hypertension also did not differ from control patients as regards anxiety when attending the clinic; their attitudes to the clinic, doctor or treatment; perception of the need for and value of treatment; or general well-being.[2]

Causes of resistant hypertension

The causes of resistant hypertension are listed in Table 7.1.

Drug interactions

Dramatic drug interactions, for example those between tricyclic antidepressants and adrenergic blockers such as guanethidine, are now largely of historic interest. However many

Drug interactions
Non-compliance
Measurement artefact
Secondary hypertension
False tolerance

Table 7.1
Causes of resistant hypertension.

drugs now in common use have more subtle effects on blood pressure control, largely through drug–disease interactions – meaning that they elevate blood pressure even in the absence of antihypertensive drugs. Drugs likely to elevate blood pressure are shown in Table 7.2.

It is therefore important to take a detailed drug history from patients with resistant hypertension, with particular attention to over-the-counter preparations such as nasal decongestants or cold cures containing sympathomimetic drugs, which are readily overlooked. Also easy to overlook are drugs used illicitly such as anabolic steroids or cocaine, which elevated blood pressure. Oestrogens in combined oral contraceptive preparations are associated with hypertension, but those used for hormone replacement therapy appear to have no detrimental effect on blood pressure[33] and are not contraindicated. They may in fact reduce overall cardiovascular risk.

Of the drugs listed in Table 7.2 the non-steroidal anti-inflammatory drugs are the most important in terms of frequency of prescribing and their effect on blood pressure.[34,35] They inhibit the action of intrarenal vasodilating prostaglandins and, through this mechanism, they impair natriuresis and cause volume

Non-specific interactions
  non-steroidal anti-inflammatory drugs
    (e.g. indomethacin, ibuprofen)
  sympathomimetic drugs in cold cures
    (e.g. phenylpropanolamine, pseudoephedrine)
  synthetic oestrogens (in oral contraceptive preparations)
  corticosteroids
  carbenoxolone sodium
  sodium-containing preparations (e.g. sodium bicarbonate)
  cyclosporin
  erythropoeitin
  anabolic steroids
  cocaine
 	
Specific interactions
  amitriptyline and adrenergic blockers (e.g. guanethidine)
  amitriptyline and centrally acting drugs (e.g. methyldopa,
    clonidine)

Table 7.2
Drugs that may reduce the effect of antihypertensive treatment.

expansion, and thus elevate blood pressure. Their pressor effect appears to be independent of the class of antihypertensive drug taken and indeed independent of drug therapy. We always consider stopping non-steroidal anti-inflammatory drugs in patients with resistant hypertension, but have had limited success because the patients usually seem to need them.[35]

Non-compliance

Failure to follow the prescribed drug regimen is an important cause of apparent treatment resistance, with estimates of the incidence of non-compliance ranging from 10–50% of cases.[1,3,4,7,10,22,36] In 1 study, which used low-dose phenobarbitone as a marker, non-compliance appeared to explain or to contribute to treatment resistance in 25% of patients.[36] Treatment-resistant patients do not seem more likely to forget to take their tablets.[2] Compliance should always be assessed formally in patients with refractory hypertension.

Measurement artefact

In some patients with apparent resistant hypertension, the persistent elevation of blood pressure is a consequence of measurement artefact. At the simplest level this may be due to the use of an inappropriately small cuff on an arm of large diameter. Every surgery, outpatient clinic, and hospital ward should have sphygmomanometer cuffs appropriate for large arms – but in ordinary practice large cuffs are remarkably difficult to find. More complex forms of measurement artefact are a white-coat element to treatment resistance, pseudohypertension, and cuff-inflation hypertension. Before discussing these, note again that patients with hypertension resistant to treatment when measured by conventional methods have a very high rate of vascular complications.[18] This does not rest easily with the notion that measurement artefact is a very common cause of apparent treatment resistance. There is some danger that treatment resistance may be attributed too readily to measurement artefact, and patients may thus be left inadequately treated and at high risk of cardiovascular disease.

White-coat phenomenon

White-coat hypertension is a term used to describe persistently elevated clinic or surgery measurements when blood pressure is clearly normal when measured by ambulatory recording. Although usually considered in the context of mild untreated hypertension there is evidence for a white-coat element in some patients with treatment-resistant hypertension. These patients are not actually normotensive, but their blood pressure control is more satisfactory than it appears. A group of patients with blood pressures that remained persistently elevated despite aggressive antihypertensive treatment, but who did not show the expected degree of target organ damage, had ambulatory blood pressures much lower than their clinic pressures.[37] Patients with clinic pressures as high as 180/120 mmHg had ambulatory and home pressures that were unequivocally normal.[37] Mejia et al[5] studied 15 patients with refractory hypertension. Eight had elevated blood pressure by direct intra-arterial measurement, and had true treatment resistance, whereas 7 had normal resting mean intra-arterial blood pressure. These patients had minimal or no target organ involvement. Six of these patients had a white-coat element to their treatment resistance, defined as clinic systolic blood pressures at least 20 mmHg higher than home systolic pressures. These small studies in selected patients leave no doubt that there is a white-coat element in some patients, but give no indication of its prevalence in all patients with resistant hypertension.

Although ambulatory blood pressure recording is said to have no role in the routine management of hypertension,[9] it is evident that it is now widely used to evaluate resistant hypertension.[7,38–42] In our own experience, some patients with resistant hypertension do have an important white-coat element (Fig. 7.1). However, we have some unease about the use of ambulatory blood pressure recording in resistant cases. It is possible, for example, that patients may restrict their activities greatly during monitoring and by doing so return a misleadingly low pressure record. Ambulatory recording should be performed during a day of normal activity. Even then the results have to be interpreted carefully. Inclusion of night-time measurements, which are characteristically low, when calculating the 24-hour blood pressure may lead to an overoptimistic assessment of blood pressure control. Even if daytime measurements alone are used, as we believe they should be, the 'target' blood pressure should be a daytime average below 145/80 mmHg and not below the 160/90 mmHg level that is appropriate for clinic measurements. Finally, it is far from clear how patients deemed to have a white-coat element to their resistant hypertension should be monitored during follow-up. Should surgery and clinic measurements be abandoned entirely? Should ambulatory recording be repeated at 3-month intervals, 1-year intervals, or what?

Pseudohypertension

In pseudohypertension, blood pressure measured indirectly by cuff methods overestimates the true intra-arterial pressure.[5,43–48] Precise definitions have been proposed by Zweifler and Shahab.[45] In most cases the measurement discrepancy is thought to be due to rigid sclerotic vessels that cannot be compressed by the sphygmomanometer cuff.

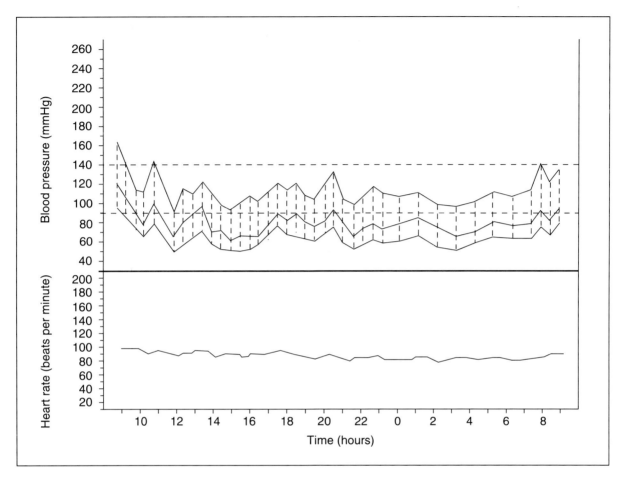

Figure 7.1

Mr BH, a 55-year-old man, was referred to the hypertension clinic after his blood pressure was found to be 240/120 mmHg, measured when he was admitted to hospital for an elective hip replacement. He was seen frequently over a period of a few months as control was proving to be very difficult. Investigations revealed no evidence of target organ damage, nor was a secondary cause found. There was no evidence of non-compliance assessed by tablet count. When on 3 antihypertensive agents, he began to develop symptoms suggestive of hypotension. However, his blood pressure in the clinic remained persistently elevated, and 24-hour ambulatory blood pressure monitoring was performed. The initial reading of 166/102 mmHg was taken in the clinic on his antihypertensive treatment. The blood pressure gradually falls to normal levels with a mean daytime level of 120/68 mmHg. Repeat 24-hour monitoring produced a similar result indicating an element of white-coat hypertension.

Cuff inflation hypertension is a less common variant of pseudohypertension in which intra-arterial blood pressure rises substantially during cuff inflation.[5,45] Mejia et al[5] reported this in 2 of 15 patients with resistant hypertension, with 1 patient showing a rise in intra-arterial blood pressure of 40/36 mmHg during cuff inflation.

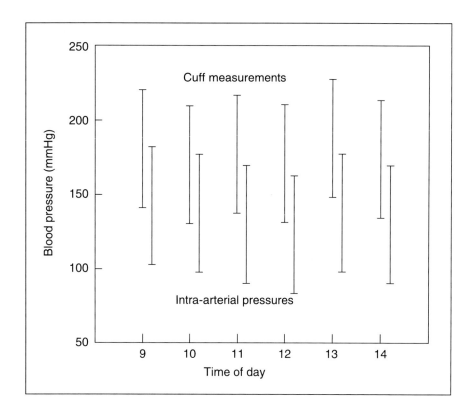

Figure 7.2
These readings were obtained from a 53-year-old lady with pseudohypertension. The graph shows readings measured by a sphygmomanometer cuff of appropriate dimensions using a dynamap semiautomated recorder and readings measured intra-arterially. The sphygomanometer cuff readings are consistently higher than the intra-arterial readings by a factor of about 40/40 mmHg.

There is no doubt from small studies that pseudohypertension does occur in patients with resistant hypertension,[5,44] and a striking example from our own clinic is illustrated in Fig. 7.2. However the prevalence in unselected patients with resistant hypertension has not been determined.

Pseudohypertension is extremely difficult to diagnose. A non-invasive method, the Osler manoeuvre,[45] involves assessment of the state of the radial artery distal to the point of occlusion by a sphygmomanometer cuff. A palpable ('Osler-positive') artery was thought to indicate a stiff sclerotic vessel. Unfortunately, the method has low predictive value and is poorly reproducible.[46-48] The diagnosis of pseudohypertension requires direct measurement of intra-arterial pressure, which is invasive and not widely available. It should be considered when hypertension is severe and resistant, when attempts to increase therapy cause symptoms suggesting hypotension, and when there is a marked discrepancy between blood pressure measurements and evidence of end-organ damage in the absence of a white-coat element.

Diagnosing pseudohypertension is only the beginning of the problem – how should the blood pressure be monitored and how should treatment be adjusted after it is diagnosed? It is obviously not practicable to repeat intra-arterial measurements at frequent intervals. In the patient illustrated in Fig. 7.2, we have continued to measure clinic pressure in the normal way and subtracted the mean difference between cuff and direct measurements (40/40 mmHg) from the readings – but we do not feel entirely comfortable with this procedure!

Secondary hypertension

As discussed earlier, an underlying cause for treatment-resistant hypertension can be identified in 10–36% of patients.[2,4] Of these underlying causes, renovascular disease is the most important numerically[2,4] and also in terms of possible correction, leading to cure or improvement of the hypertension.[49] Other causes of hypertension to be considered in resistant patients are shown in Table 7.3, and a scheme of investigation is given later.

Renal
    renal artery stenosis
    renal parenchymal disease – unilateral
                                          – bilateral
    renal obstruction

Endocrine
    phaeochromocytoma
    primary hyperaldosteronism (Conn's
        syndrome)
    Cushing's syndrome

Other
    coarctation of the aorta
    heavy ingestion of liquorice

Table 7.3
Underlying causes of hypertension.

False tolerance

The phenomenon termed false tolerance has long been recognized as a common cause of resistant hypertension in compliant patients,[50,51] but has received little attention. Many antihypertensive drugs such as vasodilators, alpha-blockers, adrenergic neurone blockers, and centrally acting agents tend to expand the plasma and extracellular fluid volume, and this volume expansion attenuates the antihypertensive effect.[50,51] It is not known whether newer drugs such as ACE inhibitors and calcium antagonists can cause the same phenomenon. Important points about false tolerance are that it may occur despite full dosage of a thiazide diuretic, there may be no evidence of overt fluid retention such as ankle oedema, and it may occur in patients with normal renal function.[20,50–52] An increase in body weight may be the only clue to false tolerance.

False tolerance can be overcome by adding frusemide[20,50,52] or spironolactone[20,52,53] to the regimen, and this causes a decrease in blood pressure that is often dramatic.[20] In contrast, increasing the dosage of a thiazide has no important effect on blood pressure.[20] In a controlled study, most patients with carefully documented resistant hypertension became strictly normotensive (lying mean arterial pressure < 110 mmHg) after the addition of frusemide or spironolactone, and this response persisted for at least 3 months.[20] Others[22] have found the addition of diuretic therapy amongst the most successful interventions in resistant hypertension, and have commented that doctors and patients have become unnecessarily wary of using these drugs because of unwarranted concerns about their supposed adverse effects. Because false tolerance has no characteristic physical signs and because no simple diagnostic test is available, its presence should be assumed in any compliant patient whose blood pressure remains uncontrolled on full triple therapy.

Management

Resistant hypertension is often managed by haphazard changes in treatment and by relatively inexperienced doctors with little or no continuity of follow-up. It is best approached with a systematic management plan based on the explicit differential diagnosis reviewed above. The steps in management are summarized in Table 7.4. This plan should be implemented by a single experienced physician who ensures that there is continuity of follow-up.

Exclude drug interactions

All drugs taken by the patient should be reviewed, with emphasis on over-the-counter treatments, and potentially interacting drugs (see Table 7.2) should be discontinued whenever possible. When it is necessary to continue an interacting drug, as is often the case with non-steroidal anti-inflammatory drugs, it should preferably be prescribed at a constant dosage.

Simplify treatment and assess compliance

A full triple therapy regimen should now need at most 6 tablets per day in two doses (morning and evening) if the drugs and tablet strength are chosen carefully. Patients who appear resistant to a more complex regimen should have their treatment simplified to meet these criteria. Non-compliance is a contributory factor in about a quarter of patients with apparent resistance to treatment.[36] It may be suspected if a patient does not show the expected evidence of drug ingestion, such as a slow heart rate with beta-blockers. However, it should be excluded formally in all patients with resistant hypertension, irrespective of their education or social background, and regardless

1. Review all treatment including self-medication: remove interacting drugs whenever possible.
2. Simplify treatment and assess compliance.
3. Exclude white-coat element to treatment resistance by 24 hour ambulatory BP monitoring.
4. Review history, examination and initial investigations for clues to an underlying cause.
5. Exclude renal abnormality (by rapid sequence intravenous urogram) and phaeochromocytoma.
6. Add frusemide 40 mg to regimen for false tolerance, titrate as required, with strict biochemical monitoring.
7. Use drugs of high potency.
8. Exclude pseudohypertension, and perform renal arteriography simultaneously even if earlier investigations normal.
9. Reset blood pressure target.

Table 7.4
Plan for managing resistant hypertension.

of whether or not the doctor suspects non-compliance. It has been shown repeatedly that the ability of doctors to predict compliance in individual patients is no better than tossing a coin.[54]

Formal assessment of compliance should begin with skilful non-judgmental questioning ('have you managed to take all of the tablets?'). The next step is to prescribe a known excess of tablets and count the number of tablets returned at the following visit. Provided the patient has only one source of tablets the return of too many tablets proves non-compliance. If the tablets are in the bottle they are not in the patient, i.e. this simple method has a specificity of 100%. However, it has a low sensitivity (perhaps 50%) because return of the correct number of tablets does not prove compliance. A determined patient can easily fiddle the tablet count. If compliance is still in question, it can be assessed further by measurement of a drug, metabolite, or marker in blood or urine.

When incomplete compliance is diagnosed the reasons should be explored sympathetically with the patient. Further information on the importance of treating hypertension, the reasons for treatment, and the possible consequences of inadequate blood pressure control should be provided. However, any discussion of risk should be honest and realistic and not couched in exaggerated or threatening terms designed to 'force' treatment on the patient. It should therefore be tailored to the situation of the individual patient. Someone with malignant hypertension who declines treatment has good reason to be frightened, whereas a patient with uncomplicated mild hypertension who declines treatment is choosing to forgo a very small benefit. A few patients at high risk appear to understand fully the risks and benefits involved, yet still choose not to take all their medication. They can often be persuaded to follow a simple regimen comprising 1 or 2 drugs taken once daily. It is important to bear in mind that partial control of blood pressure is better than no treatment at all, because it prevents a large majority of cardiovascular complications in patients with severe hypertension.[55]

Formal assessment of compliance seems to be performed rarely in ordinary practice, perhaps because it is considered time consuming. It is not as time consuming as the alternative, which is to prescribe 1 antihypertensive drug after another while the patient may be taking little or none of the medication prescribed. It should also be recognized that non-compliant patients get locked in to an impossible situation. A patient who is supposed to be taking full dosage of (say) 4 drugs, but who is in fact taking no treatment at all, will inevitably develop severe problems if he suddenly decides to take all the treatment.

Exclude white-coat element

Twenty-four-hour ambulatory blood pressure monitoring should be considered, after compliance has been established, to exclude a white-coat element in the treatment resistance. It is particularly appropriate when there is no evidence of end-organ damage despite apparently severe hypertension. Some disadvantages have been discussed earlier, particularly the lack of established algorithms for diagnostic and therapeutic decision making. In addition, the equipment is expensive and the procedure is considered uncomfortable by some patients. It is important that the equipment employed should meet the standards set by the British Hypertension Society protocol.[56] The results of ambulatory monitoring should be assessed critically and with reference to the normal values for the method and not for clinic measurements. They should not be used as an excuse for inaction when the blood pressure control is in fact inadequate.

Exclude underlying cause

As discussed earlier, the probability of identifying a correctable cause of hypertension is higher in treatment-resistant patients, and the benefits from cure of the hypertension are also larger. The next step in management is therefore to review the history, examination, and initial investigations for a clue to an underlying cause for hypertension, with particular attention to the points in Table 7.5. The emphasis should be upon those causes that are correctable, particularly renovascular disease. Less common correctable causes include unilateral renoparenchymal disease, obstructive uropathy, adrenal causes (Cushing's, Conn's, and phaeochromocytoma) and liquorice ingestion. Appropriate investigations should be pursued as outlined in Table 7.6. Phaeochromocytoma should be excluded by a screening test for urinary catecholamines even in the absence of suggestive clinical features, unless another cause for treatment resistance is evident.

Exclusion of renovascular disease is of particular importance because of the success of transluminal angioplasty, but there has been considerable debate about the investigation of choice.[23] Many who have written on the subject have missed a crucial point – the investigation of resistant hypertension does not require a test that is specific only for renovascular disease. What is required is a general

---

History
  • Paroxysmal features (phaeochromocytoma)
  • Renal disease – current symptoms
                    – past history
                    – family history (polycystic kidneys)
  • Liquorice use
Examination
  • General appearance (Cushing's)
  • Kidneys palpable (polycystic, hydronephrosis, neoplasm)
  • Abdominal or loin bruit (renal artery stenosis)
  • Radiofemoral delay (coarctation of the aorta)
Investigation
  Review
    • Serum creatinine (renal disease)
    • Urine protein, blood (renal disease)
    • Serum potassium (Conn's syndrome, liquorice use)
  Arrange
    • Screen for phaeochromocytoma (e.g. urine vanillylmandelic acid)
    • Rapid sequence intravenous urogram (referral to a physician with a special interest in hypertension is recommended at this stage)

Table 7.5
Points to review in patients with resistant hypertension.

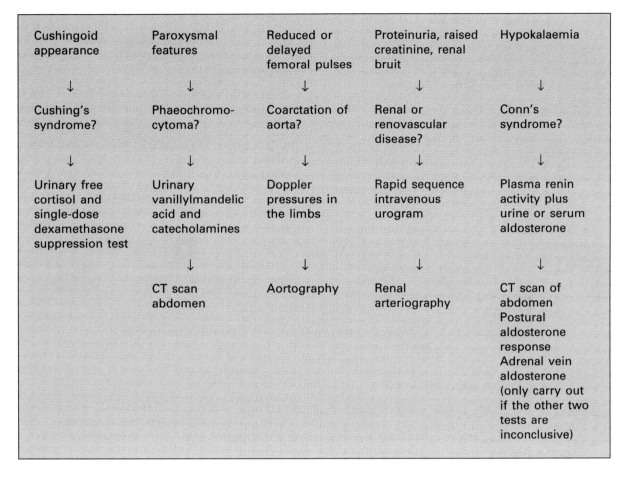

Cushingoid appearance	Paroxysmal features	Reduced or delayed femoral pulses	Proteinuria, raised creatinine, renal bruit	Hypokalaemia
↓	↓	↓	↓	↓
Cushing's syndrome?	Phaeochromo-cytoma?	Coarctation of aorta?	Renal or renovascular disease?	Conn's syndrome?
↓	↓	↓	↓	↓
Urinary free cortisol and single-dose dexamethasone suppression test	Urinary vanillylmandelic acid and catecholamines	Doppler pressures in the limbs	Rapid sequence intravenous urogram	Plasma renin activity plus urine or serum aldosterone
	↓	↓	↓	↓
	CT scan abdomen	Aortography	Renal arteriography	CT scan of abdomen Postural aldosterone response Adrenal vein aldosterone (only carry out if the other two tests are inconclusive)

Table 7.6
Summary of investigation plans for different causes of secondary hypertension.

purpose screening test, capable of detecting not only renovascular disease but also the many other renal abnormalities that are present in this patient population.[23] The rapid sequence intravenous urogram (IVU) is the only test that meets this criterion and that is generally available. No other single test is suitable for diagnosing renal scarring, obstruction, and renovascular disease – the 3 abnormalities detected most commonly in these patients.

Invasive tests such as renal arteriography are particularly inappropriate as a primary investigation, because about 10% of patients have scarring or obstructive uropathy, conditions that are readily diagnosed by less invasive methods.[23] The rapid sequence IVU is the equal of any other non-invasive screening test for renovascular disease as regards sensitivity and specificity. However, it is an imperfect screening test because approximately 25% of patients with renovascular hypertension will have a normal result. Renal arteriography should therefore be considered despite a normal rapid sequence IVU in patients who have severe resistant hypertension, declining renal function, or pulmonary oedema with no identifiable cardiac cause.

The results of transluminal angioplasty are excellent in patients with fibromuscular disease of the renal arteries, as angioplasty is almost always technically sucessful and hypertension is cured completely in 50% of cases.[49] They are, however, a minority of all those with renovascular disease. Atherosclerotic renovascular disease is much the commoner form, occurring particularly in older patients and men. Unfortunately, atherosclerotic lesions are often not amenable to complete correction by angioplasty for technical reasons, for example because of renal artery thrombosis or very severe aortic involvement. Cure of the hypertension by angioplasty is therefore relatively uncommon. Furthermore, angioplasty has a far higher complication rate in atherosclerotic renovascular disease than in fibromuscular disease.[49] As a rule of thumb, transluminal angioplasty is more likely to be successful in patients under 60 years of age who have normal renal function,[57] and investigation efforts should be directed particularly towards such patients.

The availability of transluminal angioplasty is the main justification for renal investigation of difficult hypertension, because attempts to cure renal hypertension by other means have proved disappointing. Renal revascularization and nephrectomy in patients with renovascular disease that is unsuitable for angioplasty have low rates of cure of hypertension, and a relatively high perioperative morbidity and mortality. In patients with other forms of unilateral renal disease, such as scarring or hydronephrosis, the probability of curing hypertension by nephrectomy or surgical correction is again low. As a rule, we favour conservative management of unilateral renal lesions that would require surgery, except in young patients or in those older patients with hypertension that cannot otherwise be controlled. Of course, some of the unilateral renal lesions discovered, such as hydronephrosis or tuberculosis, need treatment in their own right.

The management of phaeochromocytoma, Conn's syndrome, Cushing's disease, and aortic coarctation can all present difficulties in medical evaluation and preparation, anaesthesia, surgery, and postoperative care, and they are best dealt with by a team experienced in these conditions. It is of interest that hypertension is not cured by surgery in approximately 30% of such patients, regardless of the specific cause of the hypertension.

Treat false tolerance

An increase in diuretic treatment should always be tried in resistant hypertension before resorting to drugs of high potency such as minoxidil. Frusemide should be added to the regimen at an initial dose of 40 mg daily and increased stepwise, aiming for weight reduction of at least 1 kg.[20,52] In some patients, particularly those with renal impairment or those taking potent vasodilators such as minoxidil, the dose may have to be increased to 250–500 mg daily. This form of treatment requires painstaking clinical supervision and frequent monitoring of renal function and serum electrolytes, because complications such as orthostatic hypotension, acute gout, hypokalaemia, and declining renal function are relatively common.[20]

Drugs of high potency

In patients who remain uncontrolled despite a regimen including a loop diuretic, beta-blocker and ACE inhibitor or calcium antagonist, the options include the substitution or addition of alternative drugs of moderate potency, for example alpha-blockers, or the use of drugs of high potency. Minoxidil is by far the most effective antihypertensive drug in general use.[58] It is a potent vasodilator, which acts on the precapillary resistance vessels and has to be prescribed with a beta-blocker (to counteract reflex tachycardia) and with a loop diuretic, usually at high dosage (to combat intense fluid retention). Unfortunately it causes severe hirsutism, which is unacceptable to women, and its use is therefore limited to men. Resistant hypertension in men can almost always be controlled satisfactorily by a regimen of loop diuretic, beta-blocker, and minoxidil. Resistant hypertension in women is more difficult because there is no drug equivalent to minoxidil that is suitable for women. We still occasionally use postganglionic adrenergic blockers such as guanethidine as drugs of last resort for women.

Exclude pseudohypertension

When hypertension remains uncontrolled despite these steps, exclusion of pseudohypertension and cuff inflation hypertension should be considered, particularly when the hypertension is both severe and resistant, when evidence for end-organ damage is less than anticipated, or when there are symptoms suggestive of hypotension despite high blood pressure readings. The diagnosis requires direct measurement of intra-arterial blood pressure, which can be difficult to arrange and which carries a small risk. It is sensible to perform renal arteriography simultaneously if this has not been done before and if no cause for hypertension has been identified previously.

Patient and physician resistance

Frohlich classified resistant hypertension into 'patient resistant' hypertension, 'physician resistant' hypertension and resistant hypertension.[1] In doing so, he correctly drew attention to the fact that many (perhaps most) instances of inadequate blood pressure control are due to failure to apply the knowledge we have, and not to inadequacy of the drugs at our disposal. As discussed above, incomplete compliance is one common and important form of 'patient resistance'. In a confidential inquiry into avoidable factors in deaths related to hypertension, 'patient resistance' was thought to have contributed significantly to 37% of the deaths.[59] These deaths had little to do with drug therapy or medical care in the narrow sense. They were largely a failure of patients to modify personal habits, and particularly to stop smoking. 'Patient resistance' in the form of failure to take treatment or to attend for follow-up contributed to death in only 4% of cases.[59] Another form of 'patient resistance' all too familiar to those who run hypertension clinics is seen in patients who find one antihypertensive drug after another quite intolerable, so that the complete therapeutic armamentarium is eventually exhausted. Some patients are singularly unfortunate and develop side effects that are undoubtedly the real thing with every drug – perhaps nightmares with beta-blockers, gout with thiazide, cough with ACE inhibitors, and gross pedal oedema with nifedipine. More common are patients who develop intolerable side effects with drug after drug – but the side effects are remarkably similar with each drug and seem to bear no relation to the recognized side-effect profiles of the individual drugs. In 1 series,[22] this phenomenon was present in 8% of patients with uncontrolled hypertension. The authors suspected, and so do we, that anxiety and depression may play a prominent role in these patients. The role of psychiatric factors in patients with difficult hypertension who have subjective intolerance to multiple drugs deserves further study.

Of even greater concern is 'physician resistance', by which is meant a failure by doctors to apply adequately the knowledge that is available. In the confidential inquiry into hypertensive deaths,[59] shortcomings on the part of doctors were thought to have contributed to death in 40% of cases. The main errors identified were failure to follow-up or treat patients adequately (35%), failure to treat complications appropriately (4%), and failure to detect hypertension (1%).[59] Note that these errors were thought to have contributed to death.

Departures from predetermined minimum standards of care, which were not particularly rigorous, were even commoner. For example, inadequate follow up occurred at some stage in the management of 69% patients; treatment was not started when it clearly should have been in 6% of cases; renal function and urinalysis were not measured in 37% of patients; and there was no record of smoking habit in 26%.[59] These deficiencies are not due to lack of knowledge, and can really be attributed only to sloppy practice of medicine.

Failure of treatment

What should be done when everything has failed? A small number of hypertensive patients remain resistant to treatment even after the management plan above has been implemented. Complete failure of treatment may be due to very severe hypertension, persistent poor compliance, intolerance to numerous antihypertensive drugs, or not uncommonly to a combination of all these factors. In this situation, the goal of treatment should be modified to accept a level of blood pressure control that would normally be considered suboptimal, for example diastolic pressures averaging 100 mmHg or even higher. The rationale is that partial control of severe hypertension provides substantial protection against vascular complications.[55] It is far better to persist with imperfect treatment than to abandon the effort completely, no matter how frustrating this may be. When a policy of accepting imperfect control is adopted it is important to explain this to the patient, and to communicate it clearly to other doctors involved in the management. If this is not done every new doctor who sees the patient and measures the blood pressure is going to attempt the impossible yet again.

References

1 Frohlich ED. Classification of resistant hypertension. *Hypertension* 1988; **11**(suppl II):II67–II70.

2 Toner JM, Close CF, Ramsay LE. Factors related to treatment resistance in hypertension. *Q J Med* 1990; **283**:1195–204.

3 Ramsay LE, Freestone S. The management of resistant hypertension: a systematic approach. *Practical Cardiology* 1983; **9**:70–83.

4 Isaksson H, Danielsson M, Rosenhamer G, Konarski-Svensson JC, Ostergren J. Characteristics of patients resistant to antihypertensive drug therapy. *J Intern Med* 1991; **229**:421–6.

5 Mejia AD, Egan BM, Schork NJ, Zweifler AJ. Artefacts in measurement of blood pressure and lack of target organ involvement in the assessment of patients with treatment-resistant hypertension. *Ann Intern Med* 1990; **112**:270–7.

6 Swales JD, Heagerty A, Russell GI, Bing RF, Pohl JEF, Thurston H. Treatment of refractory hypertension. *Lancet* 1982; **i**:894–6.

7 Gifford RW. An algorithm for the management of resistant hypertension. *Hypertension* 1988; **11**(suppl II): II101–II105.

8 Neusy AJ, Valeri A, Lowenstein J. Refractory hypertension: definition, prevalence, pathophysiology, and management. *Semin Nephrol* 1990; **10**:546–51.

9 Sever P, Beevers G, Bulpitt C et al. Management guidelines in essential hypertension: report of the second working party of the British Hypertension Society. *Br Med J* 1993; **306**:983–7.

10 Setaro JF, Black HR. Refractory hypertension. *N Engl J Med* 1992; **327**:543–7.

11 Neaton JD, Grimm RH, Prineas RJ et al, for the Treatment of Mild Hypertension Study Reasearch Group. Treatment of Mild Hypertension Study. Final results. *JAMA* 1993; **270**:713–24.

12 Materson BJ, Reda DJ, Cushman WC et al. Single drug therapy for hypertension in men. A comparison of six antihypertensive agents with placebo. *N Engl J Med* 1993;**328**:914–21.

13 Andersson O, Berglund G, Hansson L et al. Organisation and efficiency of an out-patient hypertension clinic. *Acta Med Scand* 1978, **203**:391–8.

14 Beilin LJ, Bulpitt CJ, Coles EC et al. Long-term antihypertensive drug treatment and blood pressure control in three hospital hypertension clinics. *Br Heart J* 1980; **43**:74–9.

15 Gifford RW, Tarazi RC. Resistant hypertension: diagnosis and management. *Ann Intern Med* 1978; **88**:661–5.

16 Swales JD. Refractory hypertension. *Hospital Update* 1983; **9**:793–800.

17 Australian National Blood Pressure Study Management Committee. The Australian therapeutic trial in mild hypertension. *Lancet* 1980; **1**:1261–7.

18 Australian National Blood Pressure Study Management Committee. The Australian therapeutic trial in mild hypertension. Prognostic factors in the treatment of mild hypertension. *Circulation* 1984; **69**:668–76.

19 Anonymous. Refractory hypertension. *Lancet* 1973; **2**:486–7 [editorial].

20 Freestone S, Ramsay LE. Frusemide and spironolactone in resistant hypertension: a controlled trial. *J Hypertens* 1983; **1**(suppl 2):326–8.

21 Isaksson H, Konarski K, Theorell T. The psychological and social condition of hypertensives resistant to pharmacological treatment. *Soc Sci Med* 1992; **35**:869–75.

22 Yakovlevitch M, Black HR. Resistant hypertension in a tertiary care clinic. *Arch Intern Med* 1991; **151**:1786–92.

23 Cameron HA, Close CF, Yeo WW, Jackson PR, Ramsay LE. Investigation of selected patients with hypertension by rapid sequence intravenous urogram. *Lancet* 1992; **339**:658–61.

24 Degoulet P, Menard J, Vu H-A et al. Factors predictive of attendance at clinic and blood

pressure control in hypertensive patients. *Br Med J* 1983; **287**:88–93.

25 Henningsen NC, Ohlsson O, Mattiassen I, Trell E, Kristensson H, Hood B. Hypertension, levels of serum gamma glutamyl transpeptidase and degree of blood pressure control in middle-aged males. *Acta Med Scand* 1980; **207**:245–52.

26 Tuomilehto J, Enlund H, Salonen JG, Nissinen A. Alcohol, patient compliance and blood pressure control in hypertensive patients. *Scand J Soc Med* 1984; **12**:177–81.

27 Isles C, Brown JJ, Cumming AMM et al. Excess smoking in malignant-phase hypertension. *Br Med J* 1979; **1**:579–81.

28 Bloxham CA, Beevers DG, Walker JM. Malignant hypertension and cigarette smoking. *Br Med J* 1979; **1**:581–3.

29 Tuomilehto J, Elo J, Nissinen A. Smoking among patients with malignant hypertension. *Br Med J* 1982; **284**:1086.

30 MacKay A, Brown JJ, Cumming AMM, Isles C, Lever AF, Robertson JIS. Smoking and renal artery stenosis. *Br Med J* 1979; **2**:770.

31 Nicholson JP, Teichman SL, Alderman MH, Sos TA, Pickering TG, Laragh JH. Cigarette smoking and renovascular hypertension. *Lancet* 1983; **2**:765–6.

32 Freestone S, Ramsay LE. Effect of coffee and cigarette smoking on the blood pressure of untreated and diuretic-treated hypertensive patients. *Am J Med* 1982; **73**:348–53.

33 Lip GYH, Beevers M, Churchill D, Beevers DG. Hormone replacement therapy and blood pressure in hypertensive women. *J Hum Hypertens* 1994; **8**:491–4.

34 Johnson AG, Simons LA, Simons J, Friedlander Y, McCallum J. Non-steroidal anti-inflammatory drugs and hypertension in the elderly: a community-based cross-sectional study. *Br J Clin Pharmacol* 1993; **35**:455–9.

35 Lewis RV, Toner JM, Jackson PR, Ramsay LE. Effects of indomethacin and sulindac on blood pressure of hypertensive patients. *Br Med J* 1986; **292**:934–5.

36 Pullar T, Kumar S, Peaker S, Feely M. Patterns of compliance in hypertension. *Br J Clin Pharmacol* 1990; **30**: 318P.

37 Littler WA, Honour J, Pugsley DJ, Sleight P. Continuous recording of direct arterial pressure in unrestricted patients; its role in the diagnosis and management of high blood pressure. *Circulation* 1975; **51**:1101–6.

38 Thibonnier M. Ambulatory blood pressure monitoring: When is it warranted? *Postgrad Med* 1992; **91**:263–74.

39 Pickering TG. Clinical applications of ambulatory blood pressure monitoring: the white coat syndrome. *Clin Invest Med* 1991; **14**:212–17.

40 O'Brien E, Cox J, O'Malley K. The role of twenty-four-hour ambulatory blood pressure measurement in clinical practice. *J Hypertens* 1991, **9**(suppl 8):S63–S65.

41 Mallion JM, Maitre A, de Gaudemaris R, Siche JP, Tremel F. Use of ambulatory blood pressure monitoring in the management of antihypertensive therapy. *Drugs* 1992; **44**:12–16.

42 Grin JM, McCabe EJ, White WB. Management of hypertension after ambulatory blood pressure monitoring. *Ann Intern Med* 1993; **118**:833–7.

43 Kuwajima I, Hoh E, Suzuki Y, Matsushita S, Kuramoto K. Pseudohypertension in the elderly. *J Hypertens* 1990; **8**:429–32.

44 Weisser B, Velling P, Geller C et al. Pseudohypertension in hypertensive patients on multiple drug therapy. *J Hypertens* 1990; **8**(suppl 4):S79–S81.

45 Sweifler AJ, Shahab ST. Pseudohypertension: a new assessment. *J Hypertens* 1993; **11**:1–6.

46 Hla KM, Samsa GP, Stoneking HT, Feussner JR. Observer variability of Osler's maneuver in detection of pseudohypertension. *J Clin Epidemiol* 1991; **44**:513–18.

47 Oliner CM, Elliott WJ, Gretler DD, Murphy MB. Low predictive value of positive Osler manoeuvre for diagnosing pseudohypertension. *J Hum Hypertens* 1993; **7**:65–70.

48 Tsapatsaris NP, Napolitna GT, Rothchild J. Osler's maneuver in an outpatient clinic setting. *Arch Intern Med* 1991; **151**:2209–11.

49 Ramsay LE, Waller PC. Blood pressure response to percutaneous transluminal angioplasty for renovascular hypertension: an overview of published series. *Br Med J* 1990; **300**:569–72.

50 Dustan HP, Tarazi RD, Bravo EL. Dependence of arterial pressure on intravascular volume in treated hypertensive patients. *N Engl J Med* 1972; **286**:861–6.

51 Finnerty FA, Davidov M, Mroczek WJ, Gavrilovich L. Influence of extra-cellular fluid volume on response to antihypertensive drugs. *Circ Res* 1970; **26–7**(suppl 1):71–80.

52 Ramsay LE, Silas JH, Freestone S. Diuretic treatment of resistant hypertension. *Br Med J* 1980, **281**:1101–3.

53 Kincaid-Smith P, Fang P, Laver MC. A new look at the treatment of severe hypertension. *Clin Sci Mol Med* 1973; **45**: 75s–87s.

54 Wright EC. Non-compliance – how many aunts has Matilda? *Lancet* 1993; **342**:909–13.

55 Taguchi J, Freis ED. Partial reduction of blood pressure and prevention of complications in hypertension. *N Engl J Med* 1974; **291**:329–31.

56 O'Brien E, Petrie J, Littler W et al. The British Hypertension Society Protocol for the evaluation of automated and semi-automated blood pressure measuring devices with special reference to ambulatory systems. *J Hypertens* 1990; **8**:607–19.

57 Brawn LA, Ramsay LE. Is 'improvement' real with percutanous transluminal angioplasty in the management of renovascular hypertension? *Lancet* 1987; **2**:1313–16.

58 McAreavey D, Ramsay LE, Latham L et al. Third drug trial: comparative study of antihypertensive agents added to treatment when blood pressure remains uncontrolled by a beta-blocker plus thiazide diuretic. *Br Med J* 1984; **288**:106–11.

59 Payne JN, Milner PC, Saul C, Bownes IR, Hannay DR, Ramsay LE. Local confidential inquiry into avoidable factors in deaths from stroke and hypertensive disease. *Br Med J* 1993; **307**:1027–30.

8

Isolated systolic hypertension

Norman M Kaplan

Most hypertension found in people over age 65 is purely systolic, i.e. isolated systolic hypertension (ISH). This is defined as a systolic pressure of 160 mmHg or higher and a diastolic pressure below either 90 or 95 mmHg. Among the participants of the Framingham Heart Study aged 65 to 89 who were hypertensive, 57.4% of the men and 65.1% of the women had ISH.[1] When multiple large populations are surveyed, the prevalence of ISH progressively increases from 0.8% at age 50 to 5.0% at 60, 12.6% at 70, and 23.6% at 80 (Fig. 8.1).[2]

In the Framingham study, an additional 18% of the population aged over 65 had borderline ISH, defined as a systolic pressure of 140–159 mmHg and a diastolic below 90.[3] During 20 years of follow-up, 80% of those with borderline ISH progressed to definite hypertension.

Problems with the prevalence data

Almost all of the prevalence data described in Fig. 8.1 are based upon a few blood pressure measurements taken at a clinic. When such readings are compared with those taken by an automatic ambulatory recorder at multiple times throughout the day, marked differences have been observed similar to those noted in younger subjects.[4] Cox et al[4] obtained ambulatory recordings on 318 patients with ISH based on office readings; the mean daytime ambulatory systolic blood pressure was 27 mmHg lower than that recorded in the clinic.

Assuming that the out-of-the office readings are more representative of patients' usual blood pressure, the prevalence of ISH shown in Fig. 8.1 is obviously somewhat inflated – as are all prevalence data, in young and old, based on only a few clinic measurements. The problem of blood pressure readings being higher in the clinic than out of the office can be minimized, but not entirely corrected, by the simple step of taking at least 3 readings on each visit and using the lowest of these.[5]

In addition, a relatively small percentage of elderly people may be incorrectly diagnosed as hypertensive when they are in fact normotensive, a pattern called 'pseudohypertension'. This refers to normal intra-arterial pressure but elevated pressure readings obtained by routine cuff sphygmomanometry because of rigid, calcified arteries that cannot be compressed and collapsed by the pressure in the balloon.[6] Unfortunately, such patients cannot be reliably identified by the presence of a palpable, though pulseless, radial artery when the cuff is inflated above the systolic pressure (the Osler maneuver).[7] Therefore, pseudohypertension cannot be easily recognized and it probably contributes further to exaggerated prevalence figures for all forms of hypertension in the elderly.

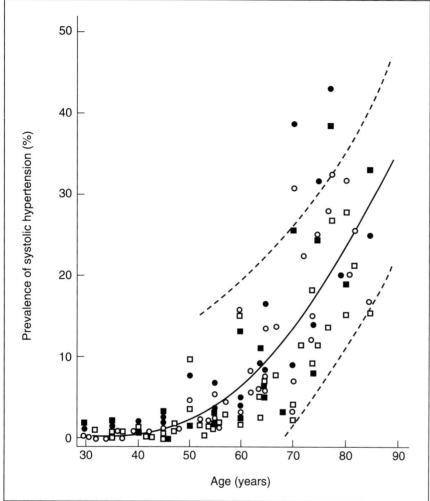

Figure 8.1
Prevalence of isolated systolic hypertension by the mid-point of the age classes reported in various studies. As shown by the regression line (unweighted), the prevalence of systolic hypertension rises curvilinearly with age. The 95% confidence interval for the prediction of individual points is presented for the age range 50–90 years. (From Staessen et al.[2])

□ *white males*
■ *black males*
○ *white females*
● *black females*

Risks of ISH

Even though its prevalence may be somewhat less than claimed, ISH is common in the elderly and, since the population is growing increasingly older, more and more ISH will be seen. Without question, the presence of ISH is a risk factor for cardiovascular disease – particularly stroke – and, as will be reviewed subsequently, the reduction of ISH will protect against these risks.

The epidemiological evidence for an increased risk from ISH, as summarized by Silagy and McNeil,[8] is shown in Table 8.1. The data are remarkably consistent: ISH is associated with increased mortality, with about a 1% increase in all-cause mortality with every millimeter rise in systolic pressure.

Study	Follow-up (yrs)	No of subjects	Definitions		Mortality ratios			
			ISH BP (mmHg)	Normo-tensive BP (mmHg)	All cause	Total cardio-vascular	Stroke	Myo-cardial infarct
Multiple Risk Factor Intervention Trial	6	317 871	≥160 75–79 ≥160 80–84	110–119 75–79 110–119 80–84	2.6 2.4	nc nc	nc nc	nc nc
Hypertension Detection and Follow-Up Program	8	2 376	≥160 < 90	≤160 < 90	2.3	nc	nc	nc
Rancho Bernado	6.4	2 636	≥160 <90	≤160 < 90	1.5	1.3	2.2	0.6*
Leisure World	6	3 245	≥160 > 90	≤160 < 90	1.6	6.9	3.0	2.2
Chicago Stroke Study	3	2 772	≥180 < 95	≥180 > 95	1.6	2.0	2.5	1.7
Chicago People's Gas Company	15	976	≥140 < 90	≥140 < 90	1.7	1.9	nc	2.0
Framingham Study	30	2 470	≥160 < 95	≥140 < 95	1.9† 1.9‡	2.1† 3.1‡	nc nc	nc nc
Dutch Civil Servants	15 25	2 063	≥160 < 90 ≥160 < 90	≥135 < 90 ≥135 < 90	2.4† 3.7‡ 3.2† 1.7‡	nc nc	nc nc	nc nc

*Among patients not taking medication
†Men
‡Women
BP: blood pressure; ISH: isolated systolic hypertension; nc: not calculated

Table 8.1
Mortality ratios for elevated systolic blood pressure compared with normotensive subjects – data from prospective studies. (From Silagy and McNeil.[8])

The only possible exception to the progressive risks of every increment in systolic pressure may be seen in the very old: people aged over 85. In a 3-year follow-up in Finland of 724 non-institutionalized people aged 84–88, the lowest mortality rates were noted in those with systolic pressures in the range of 140–169 mmHg compared to those with either higher or lower levels.[9] Nonetheless, mortality was lower in those whose systolic pressure had decreased from high to middle levels (140–169 mmHg) than in those with consistently high systolic pressures.

Mechanisms for ISH

The systolic pressure rises progressively with age in all acculturated societies but not in primitive people who do not follow our diet and lifestyle.[10] As noted in the Framingham study, ISH is associated with increasing age, female sex, increased weight in women, and higher levels of systolic and diastolic pressure, but not to serum cholesterol, cigarette smoking, glucose intolerance, hematocrit, or uric acid.[1]

It is surprising that these later risk factors for atherosclerosis were not found to be associated with the development of ISH in the Framingham cohort since, in an even larger cross-sectional analysis of people over age 65, ISH was associated with an increased left ventricular mass, electrocardiographic evidence of myocardial infarction, and increased thickness of the intima and media of the carotid artery on sonography.[11]

The associations with these manifestations of atherosclerosis are in keeping with the basic mechanism for the progressive rise in systolic pressure with age: the loss of distensibility and elasticity of the large capacitance vessels, a process nicely demonstrated over 50 years ago

(Fig. 8.2).[12] These curves demonstrate the higher pressures that develop in the aortas of older people compared to those of younger people when they are distended with fluid. This finding reflects the loss of distensibility from atherosclerotic rigidity.

Hemodynamic findings

ISH is characterized by elevated static (peripheral vascular resistance) and dynamic (characteristic impedance and wave reflection) components of left ventricular external load (aortic input impedance) as determined during cardiac catheterization using measures of pulsatile blood pressure and flow.[13] Compared to normotensives, the patients with ISH had 44% higher peripheral vascular resistance, 107% higher characteristic impedance (an index of aortic stiffness), and a 57% higher first harmonic of impedance moduli (an index of wave reflection).[13]

These changes reflect a decrease in the cross-sectional area of the peripheral vascular bed and stiffness of the aorta and large arteries, producing, as Nichols et al[13] wrote, 'an increased pulse wave velocity and an early return of pulse wall reflection in systole'. The authors characterize these effects thus: 'The marked increase in arterial stiffness in ISH offsets the increase in diastolic blood pressure that would have been expected from an increase in peripheral vascular resistance alone, and early return of the reflected pressure wave augmented aortic pressure throughout systole and accounted for the large increase observed in systolic and pulse pressure in the aorta'.[13]

Cardiac findings
Echocardiography in patients with ISH demonstrates left ventricular hypertrophy with well-preserved systolic function but abnormal diastolic filling as determined by reduced

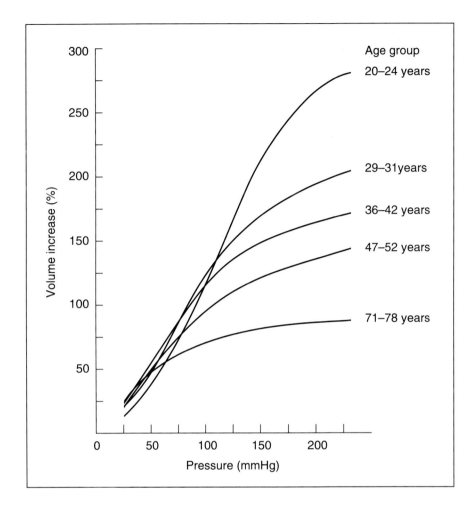

Figure 8.2
These curves show the relation of percentage increase in volume to increase in pressure for 5 different age groups and were constructed from the mean values obtained from a number of aortas excised at autopsy. (From Halloch and Benson.[12])

Doppler-derived pre-ejection period/ejection time ratio.[14] The pattern of transmitral diastolic flow shows greater deceleration time and a lower ratio of early to late peak flow velocities.[15]

The coexistence of postural hypotension

Aging is associated with various changes that may lead to postural hypotension (Table 8.2).

The cardiac output falls with age and, in the elderly with hypertension, it is even lower. When elderly subjects are put under passive postural stress (60° upright tilt), their stroke volume and cardiac index fall further because of an inability to reduce end-systolic volume.[16] Blood pressure is maintained through an increase in peripheral resistance. These 'normal' changes obviously predispose the elderly to postural hypotension from any process that further reduces fluid volume or vascular integrity.

Decreases baroreceptor responsiveness
Autonomic dysfunction
Increased stiffness of heart and large
   arteries
Reduced cardiac output and intravascular
   volume
Defective cerebral autoregulation
Venous pooling
Postprandial hypotension
Reduced renin–angiotensin reactivity
Systolic hypertension

Table 8.2
Age-related changes leading to postural
hypotension.

As systolic blood pressure rises from atherosclerosis, baroreceptor sensitivity and vascular compliance are further reduced, so that the high systolic pressures persist but, at the same time, the fall in pressure that accompanies standing is not immediately countered. This leads to increasing postural hypotension with higher levels of basal supine systolic hypertension (Fig. 8.3).[17] Moreover, chronic hypertension shifts the threshold for cerebral autoregulation so that a small fall in systemic blood pressure may precipitate a fall in cerebral blood flow.[18]

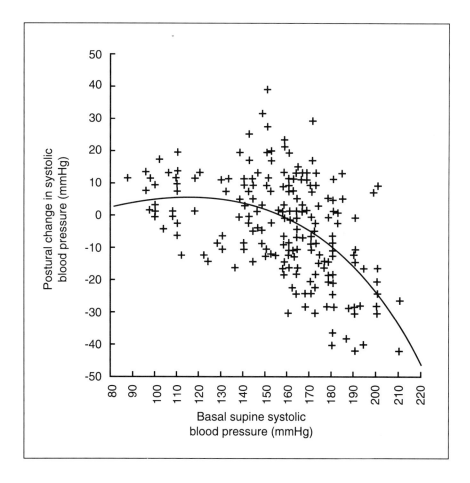

Figure 8.3
Relationship between basal supine systolic blood pressure and postural change in systolic blood pressure for aggregate data from elderly subjects. (From Lipsitz et al.[17])

The prevalence of postural hypotension

Among healthy normotensive elderly people, fewer than 7% will have a 20 mmHg or greater fall in systolic pressure after 1 minute of quiet standing (the usual definition of postural hypotension).[19] Among those seen as outpatients, about 20% over 65 years of age and 30% over 75 will have such a postural fall. Moreover, a marked postprandial fall in pressure with inadequate heart rate responses are often seen in well elderly persons.[20]

The recognition of postural hypotension

Blood pressure and pulse should be measured after the patient has been supine for 5 minutes, and immediately after standing up and after at least 2 minutes of standing. Support may be provided to those who are unstable, but the patient should bear his or her own weight. If, despite a postural fall of 20 mmHg in systolic pressure, the pulse increases by less than 10 beats per minute, baroreceptor reflex impairment is likely. If tachycardia above 100 beats per minute is noted, either volume depletion or progressive autonomic failure with postsynaptic denervation supersensitivity are probably present.[21]

Management

Before systolic hypertension is treated, attempts must be made to overcome postural hypotension if it is present. The physical measures listed in Table 8.3 often are helpful but, if they fail, a number of drugs may be tried.[22,23]

Non-drug treatment of ISH

Strong evidence is now available for a protective effect of antihypertensive therapy in elderly patients with ISH.[24,25] However, before starting

---

Correct precipitating factors and withdraw offending drugs
  (diuretics, vasodilators, tranquillizers, and sedatives)
Physical measures
  Sleep with the head of the bed elevated by 15–20°
  Get up slowly, in stages, from supine to seated to standing
  Dorsiflex the feet, or perform handgrip isometric or mental
    exercise before standing. Leg-crossing and squatting may help
  Eat small meals and drink coffee only in the early morning
  Wear fitted (jobst) stockings and pressure suits
Drugs[22]
  Fludrocortisone ± non-steroidal anti-inflammatory drugs
  For 'pure' autonomic dysfunction: pindolol
  For CNS dysfunction: desmopressin
  If the above fail: ergotamine, yohimbine,
    alpha-sympathomimetics, dopamine antagonists
  Octreotide (a somatostatin analogue) has been helpful in patients
    with autonomic neuropathy[23]

Table 8.3
Management of postural hypotension.

Table 8.4
Life-style modifications for treatment of hypertension.

Stop smoking
Of proven value:
  Lose weight, particularly for upper body obesity
  Reduce sodium intake to 110 mmol per day (2.4 g sodium or 6 g
    of sodium chloride)
  Reduce alcohol intake to no more than 2 standard portions
    per day
  Exercise (isotonic) regularly
  Increase potassium intake from fresh fruits and vegetables
Of unproven value:
  Relax and relieve stress
  Eat less saturated fat, more fish oils
  Maintain adequate calcium and magnesium intake

antihypertensive drugs, non-drug therapies, (better referred to as lifestyle modifications) should be encouraged (Table 8.4). Although the rigid large arteries that are responsible for ISH might be expected not to respond to these maneuvers, the fact that they do respond to the same antihypertensive agents as well as or better than the more compliant arteries in the non-elderly with combined systolic–diastolic hypertension suggests that they will also respond to the various modifications in life-style. Fewer trials on these life-style modifications have been done on the elderly, but enough data are available to document their efficacy.[26]

Dietary changes

Moderate sodium restriction

The effectiveness of a more restrictive diet than usually recommended was shown by Niarchos et al,[27] whose 32 patients with ISH reduced their average daily urine sodium excretion to 48 mmol from a baseline of 143 mmol. Those with initially low or normal levels of plasma renin activity achieved a marked fall in systolic pressure, whereas the few with a high plasma renin activity changed little (Fig. 8.4). These results were similar to what was noted with diuretic therapy.

The antihypertensive efficacy of sodium restriction progressively increases with age.[28] Therefore, moderate sodium restriction (to 100–120 mmol per day) should be advised for all elderly hypertensives. However, they may have at least two additional hurdles to overcome in achieving this goal: first, their taste sensitivity may be less so they may ingest more sodium to compensate for this; and second, they may depend more upon processed and prepackaged foods, which are high in sodium rather than eating fresh foods that are low in sodium.

Moderation of alcohol intake

Excessive alcohol consumption is responsible for 5–10% of the hypertension found among men, including the elderly who often are alcohol abusers.[29] About half of all published data show the pressor effect only when

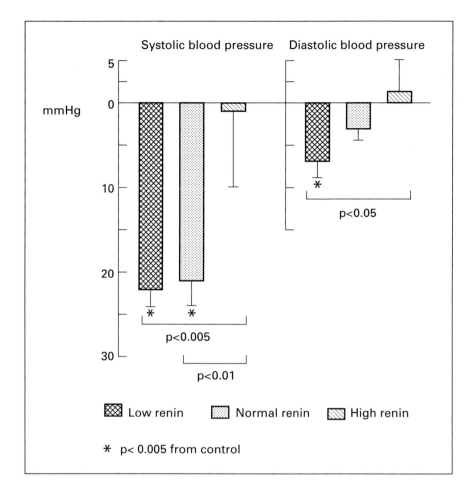

Figure 8.4
Comparison of the effects of low sodium intake on systolic and diastolic blood pressure in low-renin, normal-renin, and high-renin ISH. (From Niarchos et al.[27])

average daily consumption is greater than 2 drinks, the equivalent of one ounce of ethanol.[30] Therefore, alcohol consumption should be restricted to no more than 2 standard portions per day but there is no need to advise abstinence unless there are over-riding health reasons. Such moderation of alcohol consumption is likely to prevent a considerable amount of hypertension while, at the same time, providing the protection from coronary disease that comes from moderate drinking.

Physical activity

Aerobic or dynamic physical activity will lower the blood pressure in most but not all hyper-tensives, including the elderly. Elderly women who perform more physical activity tend to have lower blood pressures, a benefit that is independent of changes in body weight and plasma insulin.[31] The manner by which repeti-tive aerobic exercise lowers blood pressure probably involves a dampening of sympathetic nervous system activity.

In those who are taking antihypertensive medication, problems may be noted either with the ability to perform exercise or with the ability to reach a training effect. Thus, diuretic-induced hypokalemia may reduce muscle blood flow and beta-blockers may reduce performance by limiting the needed rise in cardiac output.

Drug treatment of ISH

Results from trials

Even though considerable confusion about the criteria used for the diagnosis and treatment of hypertension in the elderly by practitioners in England and elsewhere was noted a few years ago,[32] the situation seems to be changing toward a more aggressive approach to the use of antihypertensive medications to lower elevated systolic pressures.[33] With increasing awareness of the results of recently published trials in both ISH[24,25] and combined systolic–diastolic hypertension in the elderly,[34] therapy will almost certainly continue to be increasingly provided to the steadily growing population of elderly hypertensives. The potential to prevent about 24 000 strokes and 44 000 major cardiovascular events in the USA each year just in those with ISH has led to a clear call for immediate application of the results of these trials to the large population of patients with ISH.[35]

SHEP data
The Systolic Hypertension in the Elderly Program (SHEP) was the first study to address the treatment of ISH.[24] To obtain the desired number of subjects, 450 000 people were screened (Table 8.5). The relatively healthy state of those who were enrolled (as indicated by the fact that 95% had no limitation of activities of daily living) brings up the issue of the applicability of these data to the larger population of elderly hypertensives who are less fit.

The treatment protocol started with low doses of the long-acting diuretic chlorthalidone (Table 8.6). If that was not enough, a low dose of a beta-blocker was added. By the end of the trial, about one third were on both medications. In addition, almost half of the placebo group had to be switched to drug therapy because of a rise in blood pressure beyond the acceptable upper limit. This admixture probably dilutes the strength of the protection found by the end of the study. Nonetheless, those on drugs had considerably less morbidity and mortality than those on placebo (even though almost half of the original placebo group were taking drugs) (Table 7).

Side effects were increased in those on drugs and they were characterized as 'intolerable' in 28.1% of those on drug therapy, compared to 20.8% of those on placebo. However, medication had to be stopped because of side effects in only 13% of those on drug therapy compared to 7% of those on placebo.

MRC Trial in the Elderly
Of the 4396 subjects aged 65–74 enrolled in this trial, 43% had ISH.[25] They were not analyzed separately, but the report states that 'there was no evidence that systolic or diastolic blood pressure at entry . . . influenced response to treatment'. Therefore, it is likely that the 43% with ISH responded in a similar manner to the 57% with combined systolic and diastolic hypertension.

The subjects were randomly allocated in equal numbers to either hydrochlorothiazide 25 mg plus amiloride 2.5 mg or matching placebo or to atenolol 50 mg or matching placebo. Depending on how high the pressures were initially, the goal of therapy was to reach

After screening 450 000 persons, enrolled 4736 subjects (43% male, 57% female; 14% black)
3161 not previously on antihypertensive therapy
Average age: 71.6 (60–80+)
Average blood pressure: 170/77 mmHg
No limitation of activities of daily living – 95%
Baseline ECG abnormalities – 61%

Table 8.5
Systolic Hypertension in the Elderly Program[24]

Random assignment to placebo or drug; once allocated to drug, the doses could be progressive raised:
1. Chlorthalidone   12.5 mg (morning)
2. Chlorthalidone   25 mg (morning)
3. plus Atenolol   25 mg (morning)
   or Reserpine   0.05 mg (morning)
4. plus Atenolol   50 mg (morning)
Placebo-treated subjects were switched to active treatment if BP > 240/115 mmHg on 1 occasion or 220/90 mmHg on a sustained basis
After 1 year, 90% allocated to drug, 19% allocated to placebo were on drug
After 5 years, 90% allocated to drug, 44% allocated to placebo were on drug

Table 8.6
Therapeutic regimen of the Systolic Hypertension in the Elderly Program. (Data extracted from SHEP Cooperative Research Group.[24])

	Active	Placebo
Number of patients	2365	2371
Mean BP at 5 years (mmHg)	144/68	155/71
Fall from baseline	27/9	16/6
Number of events (relative risk in parentheses)		
Strokes	96	149 (0.63)
Deaths from stroke	10	14 (0.71)
Myocardial infarction	50	74 (0.67)
Deaths from coronary artery disease	59	73 (0.80)
Left ventricular failure	48	102 (0.46)
Non-cardiovascular deaths	109	103 (1.05)

Table 8.7
Results of the Systolic Hypertension in the Elderly Program. (Data extracted from SHEP Cooperative Research Group.[24])

a systolic level of either 150 or 160 mmHg. This could be accomplished by doubling the dose of initial drug, adding the other trial drug, or starting nifedipine and other supplementary drugs. Follow-up averaged 5.8 years.

The systolic and diastolic pressures fell rapidly, with a greater immediate reduction in systolic levels in those on the diuretic. To achieve the goal blood pressure, 52% of those on beta-blocker and 38% of those on diuretics had to be given supplementary drugs by the 5th year.

By the end of the study, about 25% of the subjects had been lost to follow-up and even more had stopped taking their randomized treatment, so that more than half of the study population were not on their prescribed therapy. Despite these dropouts and withdrawals, there was a significant 25% decrease in fatal and non-fatal strokes and an almost significant 19% reduction in coronary events. Although deaths from cardiovascular causes were slightly fewer in the treated group than the placebo group (161 versus 180), all-cause mortality was similar, in large part because of more cancer deaths in those given beta-blocker. Analysis of the two treatment groups separately showed significantly fewer coronary events and cardiovascular events and deaths in those given diuretic than in those given beta-blocker.

The high rates of dropout and withdrawal, although probably inherent in the nature of this study design, are of concern. Similarly, the high rate of admixture of drugs to achieve the goals of therapy cloud the purity of the data. Nonetheless, the striking differences between the diuretic and beta-blocker group must be significant, not just statistically but clinically as well.

Recommendations for management

This conclusion was reached by the 6 British hypertension experts whose analysis of the 6 published randomized trials of the treatment of hypertension in elderly patients follows the report of the MRC trial.[36] The authors make a number of recommendations on the basis of these data, including:

- treatment should be considered for patients up to age 80 with systolic pressure above 160 mmHg;
- the goal of therapy should be a blood pressure below 160/90 mmHg;
- non-pharmacological measures should be utilized, particularly a modest reduction in salt intake and a higher intake of dietary potassium;
- the choice of antihypertensive therapy should be based upon the presence of concomitant conditions (Table 8.8), and therapy should be individualized rather than based on the stepped care approach;
- first-line therapy for those with uncomplicated hypertension should be low doses of a diuretic, e.g. 12.5 mg per day of hydrochlorothiazide, probably with a potassium-sparing agent;
- beta-blockers 'cannot now be considered the treatment of choice in elderly hypertensive patients', although they may be used in those with angina or a prior myocardial infarction;
- even though the newer agents (ACE inhibitors, calcium entry blockers, alpha-blockers) have not been subjected to controlled trials, 'such drugs may be favoured on a number of theoretical and practical grounds, particularly when diuretics or beta-blockers are contraindicated. They may have a major role in managing patients with coexistent disease, such as heart failure, chronic lung disease, and diabetes' (see Table 8.8).

This succinct summary offers strong support for the treatment of hypertension in most elderly

Coexisting disease	Diuretic	Beta-blocker	Calcium blocker	ACE inhibitor
None	++	+	+	+
Heart failure	++	–	–	++
Angina	+	++	++	+
Asthma or chronic obstructive airways disease	++	–	+	+
Peripheral vascular disease	+	–	++	–*
Gout	–	+	+	+
Diabetes	–	–	+	++

++: first-line drug; +: suitable alternative drug; –: usually contraindicated; *A high proportion of patients with peripheral vascular disease will have occult renovascular disease

Table 8.8
Selection of antihypertensive drug treatment according to coexisting disease in elderly patients. (From Beard et al.[36])

patients, unless they have serious other diseases that 'dominate the clinical picture'. Such therapy has been shown to provide benefits that are 'considerably greater than those conferred by treating younger patients'. These recommendations, including the use of small doses of drugs with gradual reduction of pressure and avoidance of postural hypotension, seem to be excellent guidelines for all to follow in treating this rapidly expanding population of elderly patients at increased risk from hypertension.

At least one other large clinical trial on the treatment of ISH is in progress, the SYST-EUR study.[37] Unless those results provide strong data that support other modalities of therapy, the results of the SHEP trial and the MRC in the elderly trial will serve as strong support for the appropriate treatment of ISH.

References

1 Wilking SVB, Belanger A, Kannel WB, D'Agostino RB. Determinants of isolated systolic hypertension. *JAMA* 1988; **260**:3451–5.

2 Staessen J, Amery A, Fagard R. Isolated systolic hypertension in the elderly. *J Hypertens* 1990; **8**:393–405.

3 Sagie A, Larson MG, Levy D. The natural history of borderline isolated systolic hypertension. *N Engl J Med* 1993; **329**:1912–17.

4 Cox JP, O'Brien E, O'Malley K. Ambulatory blood pressure measurement in the elderly. *J Hypertens* 1991; **9**(suppl 3):S73–S77.

5 Fotherby MD, Potter JF. Variation of within visit blood pressure readings at a single visit in the elderly and their relationship to ambulatory measurements. *J Hum Hypertens* 1994; **8**:107–11.

6 Spence JD, Sibbald WJ, Cape RD. Pseudohypertension in the elderly. *Clin Sci Mol Med* 1978; **55**:399s–402s.

7 Oliner CM, Elliott WJ, Gretler DD, Murphy MB. Low predictive value of positive Osler manoeuvre for diagnosing pseudohypertension. *J Hum Hypertens* 1993; **7**: 65–70.

8 Silagy CA, McNeil JJ. Epidemiologic aspects of isolated systolic hypertension and implications for future research. *Am J Cardiol* 1992; **69**:213–18.

9 Heikinheimo RJ, Haavisto MV, Kaarela RH, Kanto AJ, Koivunen MJ, Rajala SA. Blood pressure in the very old. *J Hypertension* 1990; **8**:361–7.

10 Intersalt Cooperative Research Group. Intersalt: an international study of electrolyte excretion and blood pressure. Results for 24 hour urinary sodium and potassium excretion. *Br Med J* 1988; **297**:319–28.

11 Psaty BM, Furberg CD, Kuller LH et al. Isolated systolic hypertension and subclinical cardiovascular disease in the elderly. Initial findings from the Cardiovascular Health Study. *JAMA* 1992; **268**:1287–91.

12 Hallock P, Benson IC. Studies on the elastic properties of human isolated aorta. *J Clin Invest* 1937; **16**:595–602.

13 Nichols WW, Nicolini FA, Pepine CJ. Determinants of isolated systolic hypertension in the elderly. *J Hum Hypertens* 1992; **10**(Suppl 6):S73–S77.

14 Pearson AC, Gudipati C, Nagelhout D et al. Echocardiographic evaluation of cardiac structure and function in elderly subjects with isolated systolic hypertension. *J Am Coll Cardiol* 1991; **17**:422–30.

15 Dart A, Silagy C, Dewar E, Jennings G, McNeil J. Aortic distensibility and left ventricular structure and function in isolated systolic hypertension. *Eur Heart J* 1993; **14**:1465–70.

16 Shannon RP, Maher KA, Santinga JT, Royal HD, Wei JY. Comparison of differences in the hemodynamic response to passive postural stress in healthy subjects > 70 years and < 30 years of age. *Am J Cardiol* 1991; **67**:1110–16.

17 Lipsitz LA, Storch HA, Minaker KL, Rowe JW. Intra-individual variability in postural blood pressure in the elderly. *Clin Sci* 1985; **69**: 337–41.

18 Wollner L, McCarthy ST, Soper NDW, Macy DJ. Failure of cerebral autoregulation as a cause of brain dysfunction in the elderly. *Br Med J* 1979; **1**:1117–18.

19 Lipsitz LA. Orthostatic hypotension in the elderly. *N Engl J Med* 1989; **321**:952–6.

20 Peitzman SJ, Berger SR. Postprandial blood pressure decrease in well elderly persons. *Arch Intern Med* 1989; **149**:286–8.

21 Wieling W, ten Harkel ADJ, van Lieshout JJ. Spectrum of orthostatic disorders: Classification based on an analysis of the short-term circulatory response upon standing. *Clin Sci* 1991; **81**:241–8.

22 Ahmad RAS, Watson RDS. Treatment of postural hypotension. A review. *Drugs* 1990; **39**:74–85.

23 Hoeldtke RD, Davis KM. The orthostatic tachycardia syndrome: Evaluation of autonomic function and treatment with octreotide and ergot alkaloids. *J Clin Endocrinol Metab* 1991; **73**:132–9.

24 SHEP Cooperative Research Group. Prevention of stroke by antihypertensive drug treatment in older persons with isolated systolic hypertension. Final results of the Systolic Hypertension in the Elderly Program (SHEP). *JAMA* 1991; **265**:3255–64.

25 MRC Working Party. Medical Research Council trial of treatment of hypertension in older adults: Principal results. *Br Med J* 1992; **304**:405–12.

26 Applegate WB, Miller ST, Elam JT et al. Nonpharmacologic intervention to reduce blood pressure in older patients with mild hypertension. *Arch Intern Med* 1992; **152**:1162–6.

27 Niarchos AP, Weinstein DL, Laragh JH. Comparison of the effects of diuretic therapy and low sodium intake in isolated systolic hypertension. *Am J Med* 1984; **77**:1061–88.

28 Weinberger MH, Fineberg NS. Sodium and volume sensitivity of blood pressure. Age and pressure change over time. *Hypertension* 1991; **18**:67–71.

29 Hurt RD, Finlayson RE, Morse RM, Davis LJ Jr. Alcoholism in elderly persons: Medical aspects and prognosis of 216 inpatients. *Mayo Clin Proc* 1988; **63**:753–60.

30 World Hypertension League. Alcohol and hypertension – implications for management. *J Hum Hypertens* 1991; **5**:227–32.

31 Reaven PD, Barrett-Connor E, Edelstein S. Relation between leisure-time physical activity and blood pressure in older women. *Circulation* 1991; **83**:559–65.

32 Fotherby MD, Harper GD, Potter JF. General practitioners' management of hypertension in elderly patients. *Br Med J* 1992; **305**:750–2.

33 Glynn RJ, Field TS, Satterfield S et al. Modification of increasing systolic blood pressure in the elderly during the 1980s. *Am J Epidemiol* 1993; **138**:365–79.

34 Dahlof B, Lindholm LH, Hansson L, Schersten B, Ekbom T, Wester PO. Morbidity and mortality in the Swedish Trial in Old Patients with Hypertension (STOP-Hypertension). *Lancet* 1991; **338**:1281–5.

35 Stamler J, Berge KG, Davis BR, Hadley E, Pressel S, Probsfield J. Prevention of stroke in older persons with isolated systolic hypertension. *JAMA* 1991; **266**:2829–30 [reply to letter to the editor].

36 Beard K, Bulpitt C, Mascie-Taylor H, O'Malley K, Sever P, Webb S. Management of elderly patients with sustained hypertension. *Br Med J* 1992; **304**:412–16.

37 Staessen J, Bert P, Bulpitt C et al. Nitrendipine in older patients with isolated systolic hypertension: second progress report on the SYST-EUR trial. *J Hypertens* 1993; **7**:265–71.

SECTION III

THE SETTING

9

The management of hypertension in the diabetic patient

Simon RJ Maxwell and Anthony H Barnett

Diabetes mellitus is associated with a greatly increased risk of premature vascular disease.[1] This may occur in the form of macrovascular disease (typical large vessel atherosclerosis) or microvascular disease, a unique pathology of small vessels leading to complications such as nephropathy and retinopathy. A variety of factors contribute to the excess risk of cardiovascular disease in diabetes.[2]

Amongst these factors, arterial hypertension deserves special attention. Epidemiological surveys show a striking association between non-insulin dependent (type 2) diabetes and hypertension. Hypertension occurs twice as frequently in diabetic patients as in non-diabetic subjects[3] and up to 50% of diabetic patients eventually develop hypertension.[4,5] Hypertension represents an important risk factor for the development of both macrovascular and microvascular complications.[6] Patients in whom both diabetes and hypertension are present are at particular risk of coronary artery disease,[7] the major cause of premature death in the UK.

These facts emphasize the potential impact that hypertension might have on the life expectancy of diabetic patients and the importance of adequate blood pressure control. This task is hindered by the fact that tolerance to the side effects of common antihypertensive drugs is reduced in the presence of diabetic complications such as autonomic neuropathy, renal disease, and peripheral vascular disease.

Furthermore, the recent suggestion that type 2 diabetes and hypertension may be linked pathophysiologically by the presence of insulin resistance and hyperinsulinaemia has important implications for the choice of antihypertensive drug therapy.

Association of hypertension and diabetes: is hypertension an insulin-resistant state?

The first suggestion of an association between hypertension and insulin resistance was made by Welborn et al who found that hyperinsulinaemia was common in hypertensive patients.[8] Subsequent epidemiological studies have consistently shown a high prevalence of hypertension amongst patients with type 2 diabetes when compared to non-diabetic cohorts.[3] Hypertension may be present in as many as half of all diabetics.[1,4,9] Among patients with type 2 diabetes who were recruited to the UK Prospective Diabetes Study, 40% were found to be hypertensive at entry.[10] Similarly, patients who are initially diagnosed with hypertension are prone to develop type 2 diabetes.[11] This striking association is independent of both age and obesity, two factors strongly associated with each condition.

Reaven and Modan[12] suggested that insulin resistance and hyperinsulinaemia may form the

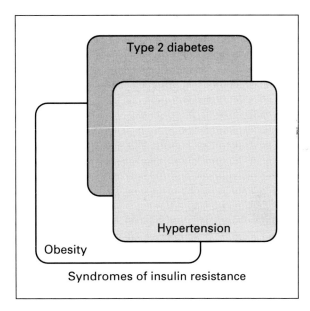

Figure 9.1
The association of hypertension, diabetes, obesity and insulin resistance.

link between hypertension, diabetes, and obesity (Fig. 9.1). When hypertensive patients, whether obese or of normal weight, are compared with matched normotensive control subjects, an increased plasma insulin response to a glucose challenge is consistently observed.[13,14] Using the insulin glucose clamp technique, it has been possible to demonstrate that the major site of insulin resistance in hypertensive patients is glycogen synthesis in skeletal muscle.[15] Importantly, glucose intolerance, hyperinsulinaemia and insulin resistace persist even after hypertension has been successfully controlled.[16]

The evidence that non-diabetic hypertensives have abnormal insulin responses to a standard glucose tolerance test and are therefore insulin resistant and hyperinsulinaemic (but not overtly diabetic) has two important implications. First, hyperinsulinaemia itself may be an important factor in the development of hypertension. Second, hyperinsulinaemia might make a substantial contribution to the risk of vascular disease in hypertensive patients even in the absence of hyperglycaemia and overt diabetes. The hypothetical relationship of insulin resistance, diabetes, hypertension and vascular risk is shown in Fig. 9.2.

Hyperinsulinaemia as a cause of hypertension

If hyperinsulinaemia does promote hypertension, then evidence of glucose intolerance would be expected to antedate the development of hypertension. Men with a high 1-hour plasma glucose in a standard glucose tolerance test have an increased chance of subsequently developing hypertension.[17] The high rates of precipitation of type 2 diabetes amongst patients being treated for hypertension with thiazides or beta-blockers can also be considered as indirect evidence for the pre-existence of an insulin-resistant state.[18–20] Infusions of pharmacological doses of insulin cause an increase in blood pressure in normal healthy volunteers.[21]

Several putative mechanisms by which hyperinsulinaemia may lead to hypertension have been put forward (Table 9.1).[15,22–24]

Sodium retention
Sympathetic nervous system activation
Disturbed membrane ion transport
Proliferation of vascular smooth muscle cells
Altered prostaglandin metabolism

Table 9.1
Factors linking hyperinsulinaemia to the development of hypertension.

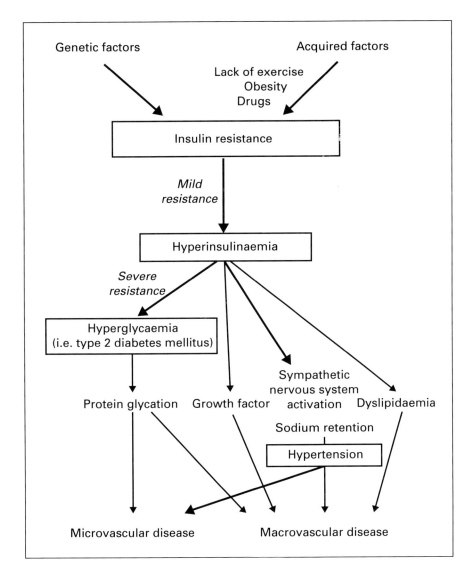

Figure 9.2
The relationship between insulin resistance and the development of diabetes, hypertension and vascular disease.

Hyperinsulinaemia and insulin therapy are both known to activate the sympathetic nervous system and increase the reactivity of the cardiovascular system to noradrenaline; these actions are independent of changes in blood glucose.[25-27] These changes favour an increase in peripheral vascular resistance and cardiac output, resulting in elevation of blood pressure. Insulin also promotes sodium and water retention by its effects on the renal tubule; this leads in turn to increases in intravascular volume and therefore in blood pressure.[28] Increases in total body exchangeable sodium have been noted in patients with both type 1 and type 2 diabetes, and this imbalance may play a central role in diabetic hypertension.[29] In addition to the direct effect of insulin,[28] enhanced glomerular filtration of glucose by promoting sodium–glucose cotransport in the proximal convoluted tubule and decreasing tubular responses to atrial natriuretic factor, may contribute to sodium retention in diabetes.[30]

Insulin-induced defects in ion transport systems such as sodium–potassium ATPase and sodium–hydrogen countertransport (which is linked to calcium exchange) may induce arteriolar muscular contraction, resulting in increased total peripheral resistance. Cytosolic calcium is increased and pH is decreased in erythrocytes of hypertensive type 2 diabetic patients, and this would be expected to promote vasoconstriction in smooth muscle cells.[31] The increased sodium load may also contribute to vascular hyperreactivity to pressor hormones such as noradrenaline and angiotensin II.[32,33]

A more recent suggestion involves the possible interaction of insulin and prostaglandins PGI_2 and PGE_2, which modulate blood pressure. Insulin may cause changes in vascular resistance and blood pressure by decreasing the production and secretion of these vasoactive prostaglandins. Insulin infusion and insulin-resistant states with hyperinsulinaemia are known to decrease the rate of production of these prostaglandins.[23] Insulin may also act as a growth factor that stimulates proliferation of arterial smooth muscle cells.[34] The resulting vascular hyperplasia would favour an increase in total peripheral resistance and in blood pressure.

Hyperinsulinaemia as a risk factor for coronary artery disease

Since hypertension is an insulin-resistant state, many of its associated complications may be related to hyperinsulinaemia rather than to the haemodynamic effects of blood pressure itself. The relative ineffectiveness of simple blood pressure control to prevent complications such as coronary artery disease in non-diabetic populations supports the concept that another independent factor (such as hyperinsulinaemia) may be involved in the coronary risk.[35–37] Results from large populations studies in several countries support the concept that relatively minor degrees of hyperinsulinaemia are associated with increased risk for coronary artery disease.[38,39]

Pathogenesis

Hyperinsulinaemia and insulin resistance may promote atherogenesis and coronary artery disease in a number of ways (Table 9.2). Both defects are central to the well-recognized abnormalities in lipoprotein metabolism in diabetes. The secretion rate of triglyceride-rich very-low-density lipoproteins (VLDL) from the liver is significantly correlated with insulin resistance and hyperinsulinaemia.[40] This explains the frequent occurence of hypertriglyceridaemia in diabetes. If insulin resistance is reduced by

Dyslipidaemia
    VLDL and triglycerides increased
    LDL more dense
    HDL reduced
Insulin as a growth factor
    smooth muscle cells
Hyperglycaemia
    protein glycation/oxidation

Table 9.2
Factors linking insulin resistance and hyperinsulinaemia to the development of coronary artery disease.

weight reduction then plasma insulin and triglycerides also fall.[41] Insulin resistance and hypertriglyceridaemia are also associated with two further important changes. First, there is an inverse relationship of both insulin resistance and triglyceride levels with high-density lipoprotein (HDL) concentration, a protective lipoprotein fraction, which may explain much of the coronary artery disease risk associated with hypertriglyceridaemia in epidemiological surveys.[42] Second, insulin resistance and hypertriglyceridaemia are also associated with abnormalities in the size and density of low-density lipoprotein (LDL) particles. When compared to controls, type 2 diabetics have an excess of smaller LDL particles which are more readily taken up by the vascular wall.[43]

Hyperinsulinaemia may also have direct effects on the arterial wall. Migration of and morphological changes in smooth muscle cells are important features of atherogenesis. Insulin in physiological concentrations can stimulate the proliferation of human arterial smooth muscle cells,[34] and it may also enhance the action of other growth factors such as PDGF.[44] These effects might enhance atherogenesis at the cellular level, but they depend on the growth regulatory functions remaining unimpaired despite the limitation of insulin-stimulated glucose uptake. The failure of the beta-cells to compensate for resistance to the effects of insulin on the peripheral disposal of glucose leads to hyperglycaemia and heralds the onset of type 2 diabetes (see Fig. 9.2). Prolonged periods of hyperglycaemia predispose to glycation of plasma proteins, including lipoproteins. This non-enzymatic reaction forms an unstable product that can undergo further reactions with the potential to oxidize and damage the protein structure. These changes have been strongly implicated in the pathogenesis of macrovascular and microvascular diabetic complications.[2,45]

Complications of hypertension in diabetes

Vascular complications

Hypertension represents a significant risk factor for the development of both macrovascular[46] and microvascular[47] diabetic complications. Among the 3648 newly diagnosed type 2 diabetic patients recruited into the UK Prospective Diabetic Study, 40% were hypertensive at entry (blood pressure greater than or equal to 160/90 mmHg).[48] During a median 4.6 years follow-up, the hypertensive patients had an increased risk of death from diabetes-related events (mainly cardiovascular: odds ratio 1.82) or death combined with major cardiovascular morbidity such as myocardial infarction, angina, stroke, or amputation (odds ratio 1.56). The presence of hypertension seems to be particularly important in accelerating the risk of atherosclerosis of the coronary arteries.[7]

Hypertension is also a risk factor for the progression of microvascular disease, which affects all vessels but is most apparent in the eyes (retinopathy) and kidneys (nephropathy). Diabetic retinopathy is still the commonest cause of blindness in the UK and hypertension is a risk factor for its progression. One study examined the incidence of exudates over a 5-year period and found that patients with a systolic blood pressure of over 145 mmHg had more than twice the number of retinal exudates compared with those with blood pressures below this level.[49] Cross-sectional data also supports a role for hypertension in the development of retinopathy.[50] The mechanisms that contribute to retinopathy are unknown but enhanced capillary leakage may be a factor.[51]

Renal complications

Diabetic nephropathy accounts for approximately 20% of deaths in diabetics below the age of 50 years,[52–54] and is also associated with a significantly increased risk of cardiovascular disease.[55] Hypertension is also a significant risk factor for the development of diabetic nephropathy and appears to accelerate its progression.[56] Recent data suggest that the genetic predisposition to hypertension, as evidenced by parental hypertension and altered sodium–lithium transport in red blood cells is a risk factor for nephropathy, even in the presence of a normal blood pressure.[57,58] These factors also increase the risk of developing hypertension itself.[59] A recent study of factors associated with the presence of microvascular complications in 157 patients with type 1 diabetes concluded that hypertension was associated with the development of nephropathy and retinopathy.[47]

Is treating hypertension worthwhile in diabetic patients?

Although many large prospective trials have examined the benefits of treating hypertension in the general population, similar trials are yet to be undertaken in diabetic patients. Since the accelerated development of atherosclerosis and its complications in diabetes seems to be governed by the same pathophysiological processes as in non-diabetic patients, we can reasonably extrapolate from existing trials. These show significant reduction of risk of stroke and congestive cardiac failure but have been disappointing from the point of view of coronary artery disease.[35–37,60] Possible reasons for this include inadequate length and efficacy of treatment, blood pressure reductions that are too great, and inadequate control of other risk factors. Particular emphasis has also been given to the contention that conventional therapy (diuretics and beta-blockers) actually aggravates risk factors, including insulin resistance and dyslipidaemia. Advocates of this hypothesis argue that antihypertensive therapy should not only lower blood pressures but also have an impact on these risk factors for coronary artery disease.

The data supporting the benefits of antihypertensive therapy in patients with diabetic nephropathy are particularly convincing. Adequate control of even mild hypertension significantly reduces albumin excretion rate and slows the decline in renal function in established nephropathy.[61–63] However, blood pressure control does not reverse the process – once it is established, eventual progression to end stage renal failure is inevitable. In patients with diabetic nephropathy, the earliest clinical manifestation of renal disease is an elevated urinary albumin excretion rate of 20–200 µg/min, known as microalbuminuria. Its presence has an 80% predictive capacity for those who will go on to develop overt nephropathy, which is characterized by proteinuria and hypertension. A very important question is whether the progression from incipient disease with microalbuminuria to overt nephropathy can be arrested by antihypertensive therapy. Recent trials give some cause for optimism (see below). Adequate blood pressure control in patients with retinopathy also appears to reduce disease progression as judged by the incidence of retinal exudates.[49]

Treating hypertension in the diabetic patient

Conservative measures

The treatment of hypertension in the diabetic patient involves conservative and pharmacological measures as for the rest of the population. In the case of diabetes, the benefits of the non-pharmacological measures are particularly evident and should be considered as the initial step in tackling hypertension and as an important adjunct to drug treatment.[64] Dietary sodium restriction has, in general, been relatively unhelpful as a means of controlling blood pressure, but it may be useful in cases of dietary excess. Diabetic patients, in particular, have increased exchangeable body sodium and are likely to benefit from reduced dietary intake.[29] Obesity is a major co-existent problem in elderly patients with insulin resistance, and it undoubtedly contributes to hypertension and reduces the chances of successful pharmacological treatment. For this reason, many patients will also benefit from a low-fat, high-fibre, calorie-restricted diet. Not only is this approach successful in leading to weight reduction, but it may also improve glycaemic control, plasma insulin levels and plasma lipids.[64,65] High alcohol intake should not be forgotten as a contributory factor to hypertension, obesity, and dyslipidaemia.

There is currently much interest in the role of exercise in the prevention of cardiovascular disease. Not only does increased exercise help to relieve obesity, but it may also reduce blood pressure and improve other risk factors such as dyslipidaemia.[66–68] Exercise may also reduce postprandial hyperinsulinaemia by increasing insulin sensitivity and glucose disposal.[66,68]

These changes may be fundamental in improving cardiovascular risk in the insulin-resistant patient, apart from any direct benefits they may have on blood pressure for the reasons previously discussed. Suitable aerobic exercise programmes of appropriate intensity can be found for most patients.

Drug therapy

When choosing antihypertensive drug therapy in the diabetic patient, a number of factors should be taken into account. Some drugs have the potential to interfere with diabetic control by exacerbating insulin resistance, a fundamental abnormality in type 2 diabetes. Other drugs may impair the response to hypoglycaemia, which would be a disadvantage for patients concurrently treated with insulin or oral hypoglycaemics. Some drugs may exacerbate co-existent risk factors such as hyperinsulineamia, hyperglycaemia, and dyslipidaemia. Drugs that have a potential impact on the underlying vascular disease process or retard the development of complications would be advantageous. Table 3

Effective in lowering blood pressure
Should not impair (ideally should improve) sensitivity to insulin
  • should reduce hyperinsulinaemia
  • should not worsen hyperglycaemia
Should not impair the ability to recognize or react to hypoglycaemia
Impact on the pathogenesis of diabetic complications
  • Macrovascular disease
      Lipids
      glycation/oxidative damage
  • Microvascular disease
      nephropathy
Should not exacerbate common diabetic complications
  • Postural hypotension
  • Impotence
  • Decreased peripheral blood flow
  • Decrease renal function

Table 9.3
Characteristics of an 'ideal' antihypertensive drug for the diabetic patient.

outlines a number of qualities that would be expected in an ideal antihypertensive agent for diabetic patients.

Diuretics

The potential for thiazide diuretics to induce hyperglycaemia was recognized soon after their introduction in the 1950s.[69] This effect was originally believed to be restricted to patients with underlying diabetes, but it is now known to occur during long-term thiazide treatment in non-diabetic patients.[18,70] The hyperglycaemic effect is reversible on withdrawal of the thiazide.[70] The deterioration in glucose tolerance has been attributed to diuretic-induced potassium depletion, and this is supported by studies showing that the effect can be offset by regular potassium supplementation.[71] In subjects with established glucose intolerance, thiazide treatment further impairs tolerance and causes a deterioration in glycaemic control.[72,73] Many of the earlier studies, however, employed higher doses than would now be considered optimal, so offering little extra hypotensive effect at the expense of more side effects.

High plasma levels of total cholesterol or LDL cholesterol and low levels of HDL cholesterol predispose to coronary artery disease. Drug-induced reductions in plasma cholesterol reduce the risk of developing coronary artery disease.[74] Therefore, the impact of antihypertensive drugs on plasma lipoproteins may make an important contribution to overall coronary risk. Short-term treatment of non-diabetics with high doses of hydrochlorothiazide (50–100 mg) caused rises of total cholesterol (+6.5%), LDL cholesterol (+15%), triglyceride (+23%) and VLDL (+28%).[75] If these rises were sustained over a long period then the risk of coronary artery disease might be substantially increased.[76]

Although longer studies, lasting for over a year, have suggested that these adverse changes are only transitory,[77,78] it is generally accepted that thiazides aggravate diabetic dyslipidaemia.[79,80] Their adverse effect on the lipid profile probably results from the increase in insulin resistance,[81] emphasizing its central importance in influencing cardiovascular risk. Neurohumoral activation in response to diuretic-induced volume contraction, including increased levels of catecholamines, may also contribute to the disturbance in lipid and carbohydrate metabolism.[82]

Thiazide diuretics are unlikely to impair renal function or worsen peripheral vascular disease at normal therapeutic dosage. This class of drug is notable for causing impotence in non-diabetics,[83] and this may be a particular problem in diabetic populations where the prevalence of impotence may already be as high as 50%.[84] The potential for thiazide diuretics to induce hypokalaemia has also been the subject of considerable attention.

The treatment of essential hypertension in the non-diabetic population reduces mortality from stroke and heart failure.[60,85] Though treating essential hypertension reduces overall mortality,[86] the effects on coronary artery disease mortality have been conflicting and less impressive.[37,87,88] The reasons for these unimpressive results might include disturbance of insulin sensitivity and of electrolytes. Further worries were raised by the MRFIT trial, in which a subgroup of men with electrocardiogram abnormalities had an increased risk of sudden death following diuretic therapy.[37] A subsequent critical analysis of the evidence suggested that these worries are unfounded.[89]

No prospective trials have assessed the impact of antihypertensive therapy on mortality in diabetic patients. Two retrospective analyses, however, have suggested that diuretic therapy may be associated with excess mortality.[90,91] The study of Warram et al[90] was based on observations in 759 diabetic outpatients

	Insulin resistance	Glucose	Lipids	Potassium	Urate
Diuretics	↑	↑	↑	↓	↑
Beta-blockers	↑	<-->↑	↑	<-->	<-->
Calcium antagonists	<-->	<-->	<-->	<-->	<-->
ACE Inhibitors	↓	<-->↓	↓	<-->(↑)	<-->

Table 9.4
The therapeutic characteristics of anti-hypertensive drug therapy in diabetes mellitus. [↑ = increase or deterioration, ↓ = decrease or improvement and <--> = neutral effect.]

with severe retinopathy. It found that cardio-vascular mortality was increased 3.8 times in patients treated with diuretics alone compared with those with untreated hypertension. When combined, these data suggest that the side effects associated with chronic diuretic therapy have an adverse effect on cardiovascular risk.

In summary, thiazides are effective antihypertensive agents but have adverse effects on glycaemic profile and are associated with electrolyte imbalances, a deterioration in lipid profile, and increased insulin resistance.[92] They are also a common cause of impotence, which already has a prevalence of 50% in male diabetics. Indapamide is a non-thiazide diuretic that does not seem to have the same deleterious effects on diabetic control and serum lipids.[93,94] Table 9.4 summarizes the important characteristics of thiazide diuretics and other antihypertensive drugs with regard to the diabetic patient.

Beta-blockers

Beta-blockers have been considered as first-line agents in the treatment of hypertension since the 1960s. Propranolol, the first drug in this class, effectively lowered blood pressure, owing primarily to blockade of beta$_1$-receptors in the heart. However, because propranolol also blocked beta$_2$-receptors, which are responsible for bronchodilatation, vasodilatation in peripheral vessels, and metabolic activities such as lipolysis and glycogenolysis, it had a variety of unwanted side effects and contraindications. Beta-blocking drugs, such as atenolol and metoprolol, which are relatively selective for beta$_1$-receptors, have since been developed in an attempt to overcome these problems. Newer beta-blockers, such as celiprolol, even have some beta$_2$-agonist properties, which allows the cardiac effects to be supplemented with peripheral vasodilatation.

Glucose tolerance is reduced in patients on beta-blockers.[95] Following beta-blockade, peak plasma glucose concentrations are higher after an oral glucose tolerance test,[96] although this effect may be less marked with beta$_1$-selective agents.[97] Beta-adrenergic stimulation by circulating catecholamines makes a major contribution to recovery from insulin-induced hypoglycaemia by mobilizing glucose from the liver (glycogenolysis).[98] Recovery is significantly impaired in patients on non-selective beta-blockers, although this appears to be less of a problem with metoprolol and atenolol.[99] Beta-blockers also modify haemodynamic responses to insulin-induced hypoglycaemia and may therefore prevent early recognition of such events.[100] Despite these observations, a long-term study of diabetic patients on beta-blockers found that hypoglycaemic reactions were not common on treatment, and there was no evidence that they were less likely to occur with selective agents.[101]

A number of studies of the effects of beta-blockers on serum lipids have been conducted; these have been reviewed elsewhere.[102] The findings of these studies are not entirely consistent, but a reasonably clear pattern emerges if we consider only those trials in which blood pressure has been successfully lowered, in which treatment lasted for more than a month, and in which a sufficiently large number of patients were studied. Selective and non-selective drugs increase triglycerides and lower HDL, although the effect on HDL is less marked that selective agents. Drugs that have intrinsic sympathomimetic activity, such as pindolol and acebutolol, do not adversely effect lipids and may even improve them.

Like thiazides, beta-blockers have the potential to exacerbate pre-existing diabetic complications. All beta-blockers reduce cardiac output and limb perfusion pressure and may exacerbate peripheral vascular insufficiency. Selective agents may have some advantage in not harming beta$_2$-mediated vasodilatation, but they are not free from such problems.[96] In non-diabetic subjects, the potential for beta-blockers to cause impotence is less than for diuretics.[83] Beta-blockers do not cause postural hypotension.

A major advantage of beta-blocking drugs in hypertensive patients is their potential to reduce the risk of developing fatal complications of coronary artery disease,[103] the major cause of premature mortality in diabetes mellitus. These complications include myocardial infarction and sudden cardiac death, often due to ventricular arrhythmias, which itself accounts for approximately one half of all cardiac deaths.[104] The beneficial or 'cardioprotective' effects include decreased myocardial contractility and heart work (and therefore reduced oxygen consumption), increased coronary flow due to increased diastolic time, and reduced platelet aggregability.[105] During ischaemic events in animals, pretreatment with beta-blockers may limit infarct size.[106] Beta-blockers also have a well-documented anti-arrhythmic effect.[107] In primary prevention studies that have examined the treatment of hypertension, sudden cardiac death and myocardial infarction have been found to be significantly reduced with beta-blockers compared with thiazide diuretics or placebo.[60,108–110] The beneficial effects of beta-blockers on the secondary prevention of cardiac mortality after myocardial infarction are also evident,[111–113] partly as a result of their impact on ventricular tachyarrhythmias.[114] Since the pathophysiology and presentation of coronary disease is similar, it is assumed that diabetic patients will also benefit from beta-blockade.[103] Indeed, beta-blockers have been used without problems in diabetic patients after myocardial infarction.[115,116]

In summary, beta-blockers are not ideal antihypertensive drugs for the diabetic patient. The potential to impair glucose tolerance and reduce peripheral perfusion may be seen as particularly disadvantageous side effects. However, their proven benefits in preventing morbidity make them worth consideration in patients with established coronary artery disease. Beta-blockers do not have specific effects on the rate of development of complications. Indeed, the disturbances of carbohydrate and lipid metabolism may have adverse effects (see Table 9.4). Selective beta-blockers should be used in preference to the non-selective agents.

Calcium antagonists

Calcium antagonists have become increasingly popular antihypertensive agents, but they are associated with a relatively high incidence of side effects.[117] It was anticipated that calcium antagonists would interfere with glucose homoeostasis because both glucose-induced insulin secretion and glycogenolysis are calcium-dependent processes.[118,119] Indeed, a small open trial on healthy volunteers did suggest that nifedipine had a significant hyperglycaemic effect.[120] Larger trials conducted over longer periods, however, do not suggest that nifedipine is diabetogenic.[121-123] Nifedipine therapy had no effect on insulin release and fasting blood sugar levels in non-diabetic hypertensives.[121] When compared with controls in a crossover trial lasting for one year, nifedipine and verapamil did not impair long-term glucose control (HbA1$_C$) in hypertensive patients with type 2 diabetes.[123] It can be concluded that despite trials of short-term high-dose treatment suggesting otherwise,[124] nifedipine does not appear to be diabetogenic in normal subjects nor does it significantly affect glucose tolerance in diabetic patients. When nifedipine was used to treat insulin-requiring diabetics, there was no evidence of increased insulin requirements.[125]

Verapamil is a non-dihydropyridine calcium antagonist less frequently used as an antihypertensive agent in the UK. The majority of studies suggest that verapamil has no effect on glucose tolerance or insulin secretion in non-diabetics[126-128] or type 2 diabetic patients.[123] Diltiazem was found to have no effect on the response to an oral glucose tolerance test in healthy volunteers.[129] Similarly, no adverse effects on glucose homoeostasis have been found with the newer calcium antagonists, including isradipine,[130] felodipine,[131] nicardipine,[132] nitrendipine,[133] or nilvadipine.[134] Evidence for the metabolic neutrality of calcium antagonists with respect to carbohydrate metabolism has been reviewed recently.[135]

Calcium antagonists appear to be free of recognized adverse effects upon serum electrolytes and deleterious effects on lipid metabolism.[136] This can be seen as a distinct advantage over the thiazides and beta-blockers. As vasodilators they tend to improve blood flow to the limbs and have no effect on impotence. Although calcium antagonists have vasodilating effects, they tend not to trigger the renal compensatory mechanisms that lead to fluid and electrolyte retention.[137] Their effects on renal blood flow and tubular transport of fluid and electrolytes culminate to produce a mild natriuresis and diuresis that tends to counteract the effects of fluid and salt retention seen with other vasodilators.[138] Furthermore, renal disease tends not to interfere with the pharmacokinetics of calcium antagonists, which are metabolized by the liver.

Troublesome side effects of dihydropyridine calcium antagonists include peripheral oedema, flushing, and tachycardia. Constipation is common with verapamil.

Calcium antagonists may have some beneficial effects on the development of the vascular complications of systemic hypertension. In animal models of atherosclerosis, nifedipine suppresses the development of atherosclerotic plaques.[139] This effect is achieved without reductions in plasma lipids and may involve alterations in lipid metabolism in the vascular wall. These laboratory results are partially supported by the findings of a study that showed that diltiazem may reduce the chances of myocardial infarction in patients with established coronary artery disease.[140]

Another interesting property of calcium antagonists is their effect upon hypertrophy of the left ventricle in hypertension. Regression of the structural changes has been demonstrated in many animal models, and there is some evidence that similar effects are seen in humans.[141]

The lack of adverse effects of calcium antagonists on glucose tolerance and their proven efficacy mean that these drugs can be considered as first-choice antihypertensive agents for diabetic patients (see Table 9.4). Their tendency to improve peripheral blood flow and renal function and their potential impact on structural damage to the cardiovascular system may be important additional benefits.

ACE inhibitors

The angiotensin-converting enzyme (ACE) inhibitors are now well-established antihypertensive agents following the introduction of captopril and then enalapril. All drugs in this class tend to reduce insulin resistance and therefore increase insulin sensitivity.[142,143] Studies in both normotensive and hypertensive type 2 diabetic patients have confirmed that hepatic and peripheral sensitivity to insulin is increased after ACE inhibition.[144-147] Meta-analysis of trials involving the long-term treatment of type 2 diabetic patients with ACE inhibitors showed that there was an average reduction in blood glucose of 15% and in glycosylated haemoglobin of 8%.[148] This effect is a major advantage in diabetes, in which hyperglycaemia and insulin resistance are probably central factors in the development of vascular complications. ACE inhibitors do not appear to have adverse effects on serum lipids, and they may even increase the HDL:total cholesterol ratio.[146,149]

ACE inhibitors may have an important role in preventing the development of diabetic renal disease, which is a major cause of premature mortality in both type 1 and type 2 diabetic patients (see below). This beneficial effect may relate to their relatively specific effect on renal haemodynamics.

Left ventricular hypertrophy is an important risk factor for ventricular arrhythmias and sudden death in hypertensive patients.[150,151] Hypertensive diabetics are at particular risk of developing left ventricular hypertrophy.[152] There is not much data available about the effects of individual antihypertensive drugs on LVH in diabetics. In non-diabetic hypertensives, however, the potential to regress structural changes in the myocardium seems to rest with ACE inhibitors, calcium antagonists, and perhaps beta-blockers.[153] Whether clinically relevant regression of structural changes in resistance vessels is possible remains to be clarified.

The benefits in diabetic nephropathy and the favourable metabolic effects are becoming increasingly persuasive arguments for choosing ACE inhibitors as first-line antihypertensive agents in the diabetic patient. Furthermore, this class is unlikely to exacerbate pre-existing problems such as peripheral vascular insufficiency or impotence.

Caution should be exercised in the presence of renal impairment. In some cases, most notably renal artery stenosis, renal perfusion is preserved by activation of the renin–angiotensin system. Treatment with an ACE inhibitor may precipitate a rapid decline in renal function. This rare complication may be a problem in diabetic populations, in whom occult disease of the renal artery is more common. Therefore, vigilance is required when treating patients with established renal insufficiency since any decline in renal function is usually reversed on discontinuation of the drug.

Another problem encountered at initiation of ACE inhibitors is first-dose hypotension.[154] This is particularly likely in those previously treated with diuretics or in those with renovascular hypertension, but it is also a problem in elderly patients with reduced autonomic function.[155] Problems can be avoided if treatment is initiated with a low dose at night (and preferably under medical supervision) if hypotension is anticipated.

Other antihypertensive drugs

Other drugs with proven antihypertensive efficacy in diabetes include alpha-blockers, methyldopa, and the serotonin-2-receptor antagonist ketanserin.[156–158]

Alpha-blockers, such as prazosin and doxazosin, tend to improve the cardiovascular risk profile by lowering total and LDL cholesterol and improving the LDL:HDL ratio.[159] There is also considerable evidence to suggest that alpha-blockers increase sensitivity to insulin,[135,160] and so improve glucose control in type 2 diabetic patients.[161] Although they share many of the desirable properties of calcium antagonists and ACE inhibitors, alpha-blockers tend to cause orthostatic hypotension, and this makes them unacceptable to many diabetic patients. Ketanserin is a serotonin-2 receptor antagonist that combines metabolic neutrality with effective blood pressure control.[158] It may also have specific benefits in patients who have established peripheral vascular disease.

Diabetic nephropathy

About 30–40% of all diabetics develop diabetic nephropathy with persistent albuminuria, a decline in glomerular filtration rate, and raised blood pressure. Nephropathy accounts for 20% of deaths in diabetics under the age of 50,[52–57] and for 25% of all patients in the UK with end-stage renal failure. Patients destined to develop nephropathy can be detected with reasonable accuracy by screening for microalbuminuria, the earliest manifestation of a glomerular abnormality.

A variety of factors are involved in pathogenesis and progression of diabetic nephropathy (Fig. 9.3). Although the duration of diabetes and glycaemic control are important, it is haemodynamic rather than metabolic factors that appear to have the greatest influence upon glomerular damage and loss of function. Of these, glomerular hypertension and hyperfiltration are particularly damaging to the kidney and are consistently found in patients with newly diagnosed type 1 diabetes.[162,163] This is the result of concomitant elevation of glomerular plasma flow and of mean glomerular transcapillary hydrostatic pressure difference.

The role of the renin–angiotensin system in this state is unknown, but such patients are known to have high levels of renin.[164] Blocking the renin–angiotensin system leads to increased renal plasma flow but causes no change in glomerular filtration rate. This suggests a reduction in filtration fraction due to reduced glomerular filtration pressure. This reduction seems to result from a preferential relaxing effect on the efferent rather than the afferent arteriole.[165,166] Although proteinuria forms a convenient method of screening for nephropathy, it may also be involved in disease progression. Increased macromolecular traffic across the glomerular basement membrane has been implicated as a factor in glomerular injury.[167] This implies that, ideally, drug therapy should effectively reduce proteinuria as well as reducing glomerular pressures.

Once nephropathy is established, arterial hypertension is the most important influence on the rate of progression of the renal damage. Indeed, adequate control of hypertension is critical in preserving renal function in the presence of nephropathy.[63,168,169] Therefore, all diabetic patients, and especially those with

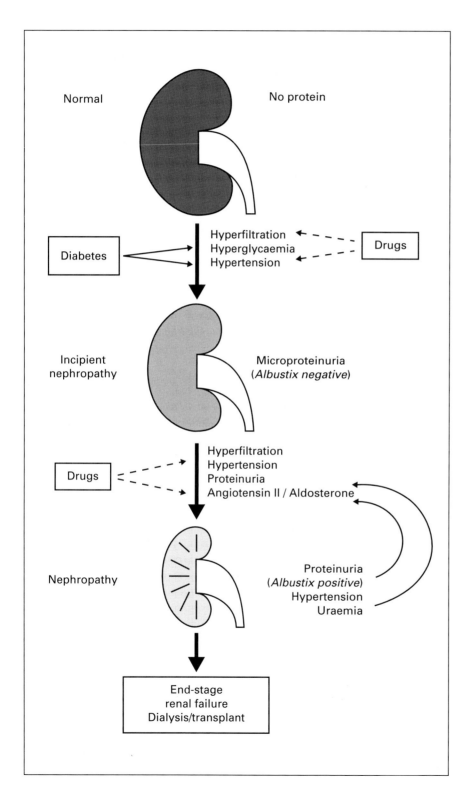

Figure 9.3
The pathogenesis of diabetic nephropathy.

incipient and overt renal disease, must be screened for hypertension and effectively treated if hypertension is present. The factors involved in progression were examined in a longitudinal study of a cohort of 131 diabetic patients with nephropathy.[170] This identified not only hypertension but also plasma levels of angiotensin II and aldosterone as independent risk factors for progression of nephropathy. These findings further supported the rationale of using drugs that block the renin–angiotensin system and raised concern about the use of agents (such as diuretics) that might make these changes in angiotensin II and aldosterone levels worse.

Most trials of antihypertensive drugs in diabetic nephropathy have shown that blood pressure control reduces the rate of decline of renal function in those with established nephropathy, irrespective of the class of agent used.[61–63,170–172] This confirms that pressure reduction alone is effective in protecting the kidney. However, the potential of ACE inhibitors to produce local pressure reduction at a glomerular level may be beneficial in diabetic nephropathy over and above any antihypertensive effect on the systemic circulation.[30,173–177] The concept of a class-specific effect on the kidney is supported by a study of captopril treatment in nephropathic patients which showed that the rate of deterioration of glomerular filtration rate was reduced and that this was not correlated with its efficacy on blood pressure reduction in individual patients.[175] A recent placebo-controlled trial of ACE inhibition in 409 patients with insulin-dependent diabetes (urinary protein excretion > 500 mg per day and serum creatinine > 221 μmol/l) found a 50% reduction in combined end-points (death, dialysis, or transplantation) in the treatment group despite near parity in blood pressure between the two groups.[178] Several studies have also reported significant

renal protective effects of ACE inhibitors in non-hypertensive microproteinuric diabetics.[179,180]

ACE inhibition may also produce a significant reduction of approximately 50% in urinary albumin excretion.[148,168,181–183] This effect is not restricted to treatment with ACE inhibitors and can also be seen to a lesser extent with calcium antagonists.[168,184] A notable exception is nifedipine which appears to exacerbate albuminuria.[30] This effect is once again related to reductions of intraglomerular pressure as a result of efferent arteriolar dilatation.[185] The effects of individual drugs differs in this respect – nifedipine dilates both afferent and efferent arterioles and is therefore less effective.

Captopril was compared with conventional therapy (hydrochlorothiazide and metoprolol) in 74 hypertensive type 2 diabetics, of whom 21 had microalbuminuria.[186] Albuminuria was reduced in the patients treated with captopril, but it rose in the majority of those on conventional therapy. The effects on proteinuria of 12 months' treatment with enalapril (40 mg per day) and 12 months' treatment with nifedipine (40 mg per day) were compared in 30 type 2 diabetics. Although blood pressure reduction and preservation of creatinine clearance were the same in both groups, proteinuria was markedly reduced only by enalapril.[181] In contrast, the calcium antagonists nitrendipine and diltiazem appear to be effective in reducing albuminuria.[184] Some studies have suggested that an ACE inhibitor and calcium antagonist in combination are best at limiting albuminuria and decline in renal function, with fewer side effects than either agent alone.[168]

A meta-analysis of published studies of diabetic patients with microalbuminuria or clinical proteinuria who were treated for more than 4 weeks with antihypertensive drugs related changes in urinary protein excretion to reduction in blood pressure.[30] This showed that for conventional therapy (diuretics ± beta-blocker) there was a direct correlation in the two parameters. The same was also true for ACE inhibitors, but even with no change in blood pressure there was a 30% fall in protein excretion. This emphasizes the specific benefits of using this class of drug.

Who to treat and with which drug?

When the results of large prospective trials carried out in the non-diabetic hypertensive population are extrapolated to the higher-risk diabetic population, we can conclude that patients with diastolic pressure ≥ 90 mmHg and systolic pressure ≥ 160 mmHg are likely to benefit from intervention.[88,187] In addition, diabetic patients with borderline blood pressure elevation (intermittent measurements above and below 140/90 mmHg) and a strong family history of hypertension and cardiovascular disease may also benefit from early treatment.[188] Patients with incipient or overt diabetic nephropathy even in the presence of normal blood pressures are likely to benefit from treatment with ACE inhibitors. Those with a strong family history of hypertension are particularly prone to develop nephropathy and require close monitoring for proteinuria and rises in blood pressure.

The conservative measures outlined above are probably appropriate advice for most diabetic patients irrespective of blood pressure, but are particularly important if pharmacological measures are also being considered. ACE inhibitors are to be preferred as initial therapy for hypertension in most patients. For diabetic patients with incipient nephropathy, even those with normal blood pressure, ACE inhibitors can reduce proteinuria without affecting blood pressure. Alternative first-line agents are the calcium antagonists which are also free from metabolic effects and interactions with diabetic complications. Nifedipine may have some disadvantages compared with other drugs in this class because of its tendency to exacerbate proteinuria. ACE inhibitors and calcium antagonists can also be used satisfactorily in combination. Beta-blocking drugs are relatively contraindicated in diabetes, but beta$_1$-selective drugs may cause little interference and are better tolerated than other beta-blockers. Beta-blockers may be considered advantageous in patients with established coronary disease where, at least in the non-diabetic population, they undoubtedly reduce coronary mortality. If a diuretic drug is required, indapamide has advantages over the thiazides. Given the current concerns about their effect on mortality, thiazide diuretics are best avoided.

Conclusion

Hypertension and diabetes often coexist, and the reasons for this are much debated. Hypertension is a major risk factor for macrovascular and microvascular disease in diabetes and its treatment is worthwhile in preventing both kinds of complication. The threshold for treatment is debated but it should be lower for younger patients and for those with overt nephropathy. Non-pharmacological measures, including dietary modification and increase in exercise, are of utmost importance.

Based on their efficacy and side effects, the ACE inhibitors and calcium antagonists have established themselves as first-line agents for the management of hypertension in diabetes. The theoretical advantages of the ACE inhibitors are particularly clear – they improve insulin sensitivity and may have an impact on the development of complications. In diabetic patients with nephropathy, effective antihypertensive therapy can reduce proteinuria and slow the progression of nephropathy. ACE inhibitors may reduce proteinuria even in the absence of a change in blood pressure. Whether they actually prolong life or reduce morbidity over a prolonged period compared to the other antihypertensives remains to be clarified in prospective trials. In the absence of another indication, diuretics are best avoided for the management of hypertension in diabetes.

References

1 Panzram G. Mortality and survival in type 2 (non-insulin-dependent) diabetes mellitus. *Diabetologia* 1987; **30**:123–31.

2 Bierman EL. Atherogenesis in diabetes. *Arteriosclerosis Thrombosis* 1992; **12**:647–56.

3 Teuscher A, Egger M, Herman JB. Diabetes and nephropathy: blood pressure in clinical diabetic patients and control population. *Arch Int Med* 1989; **149**:1942–5.

4 Turner RC. United Kingdom prospective diabetes study III. Prevalence of hypotension and antihypertensive therapy in patients with newly diagnosed diabetes. A Multicentre Study. *Hypertension* 1985; 7(suppl II):8–13.

5 Reaven GM. Role of insulin resistance in human disease. *Diabetes* 1988; **37**:1595–607.

6 Barnett AH. Hypertension as a risk factor for diabetic complications. In: Barnett AH, Dodson PM eds. *Hypertension and Diabetes*. London: Science Press, 1990:2.1–2.18.

7 Kannel WB, McGee DL. Diabetes and cardiovascular disease. *JAMA* 1979; **241**:2035–8.

8 Welborn TA, Breckenridge A, Rubinstein HT et al. Serum insulin in essential hypertension and in peripheral vascular disease. *Lancet* 1966; **i** : 1336–7.

9 Pell S, D'Alonzo CA. Some aspects of hypertension in diabetes mellitus. *JAMA* 1967; **202**:10–16.

10 Hypertension in Diabetes Study (HDS). I. Prevalence of hypertension in newly presenting type 2 diabetic patients and the prevalence of risk factors for cardiovascular and diabetic complications. *J Hypertens* 1993; **11**:309–17.

11 Epstein M, Sowers JR. Diabetes mellitus and hypertension. *Hypertension* 1992; **19**:403–18.

12 Modan M, Halkin H, Almog et al. Hyperinsulinaemia: a link between hypertension, obesity and glucose intolerance. *J Clin Invest* 1985; **75**:809–17.

13 Ferrannini E, Buzzigoli G, Bonadona R et al. Insulin resistance in essential hypertension. *N Engl J Med* 1987; **317**:350–7.

14 Stamler J, Rhomberg P, Schoenberg JA et al. Multivariate analysis of the relationship between seven variables to blood pressure: findings of the Chicago Heart Association detection project in industry 1967–1972. *J Chronic Dis* 1975; **28**:527–48.

15 Passa P. Hyperinsulinemia, insulin resistance and systemic hypertension. *Horm Res* 1992; **36**:33–6.

16 Swislocki ALM, Hoffman BB, Reaven GM. Insulin resistance, glucose intolerance and hyperinsulinaemia in patients with hypertension. *Am J Hypertension* 1989; **2**:419–23.

17 Salomaa VV, Strandberg TE, Vanhansen H et al. Glucose tolerance and blood pressure. Long term follow-up study in middle-aged men. *Br Med J* 1991; **303**:493–6.

18 Bengtsson C, Blohme G, Lapidus L et al. Do antihypertensive drugs precipitate diabetes? *Br Med J* 1984; **289**:1495–7.

19 Skarfors ET, Lithel HO, Selinus I et al. Do antihypertensive drugs precipitate diabetes in predisposed men? *Br Med J* 1989; **298**:1147–52.

20 Skarfors ET, Selinus I, Lithel HO. Risk factors for developing non-insulin dependent diabetes: a ten year follow-up of men in Uppsala. *Br Med J* 1991; **303**:755–60.

21 Gans ROB, van der Toorn L, Bilo HJG, Nauta JJP, Heine RJ, Donker AJM. Renal and cardiovascular effects of insulin in healthy volunteers. *Clin Sci* 1991; **80**:219–25.

22 Axelrod L. Insulin, prostaglandins and the pathogenesis of hypertension. *Diabetes* 1991; **40**:1223–7.

23 Dodson PM. Hypertension and insulin resistance: mechanisms and implications for treatment. *J Human Hypertens* 1991; **5**:349–54.

24 Pritchard BN, Smith CC, Sen S, Betteridge DJ. Hypertension and insulin resistance. *J Cardiovasc Pharmacol* 1992; **20**(suppl 11):577–84.

25 Rooney DP, Edgar DJ, Sheridan B, Atkinson AB, Bell PM. The effect of low dose insulin infusions on the renin–angiotensin and sympathetic nervous systems in normal man. *Eur J Clin Invest* 1991; **21**:430–5.

26 Rowe JW, Young JB, Minaker KL, Stevens AL, Palotta J, Landsberg L. Effect of insulin and glucose infusions on sympathetic nervous system activity in normal man. *Diabetes* 1981; **30**:219–25.

27 Gans ROB, Bilo HJG, van Maarschalkerweerd WWA, Heine RJ, Nauta JJP, Donker AJM. Exogenous insulin augments in healthy volunteers the cardiovascular reactivity to noradrenaline but not to angiotensin II. *J Clin Invest* 1991; **88**:512–17.

28 DeFronzo RA. The effect of insulin on renal sodium metabolism. *Diabetologia* 1981; **21**:165–71.

29 Feldt-Rasmussen B, Mathiesen ER, Deckert T et al. Central role for sodium in the pathogenesis of blood pressure independent of angiotensin, aldosterone and catecholamines in type 1 (insulin-dependent) diabetes mellitus. *Diabetologia* 1987; **30**:610–17.

30 Weidmann P, Boehlen LM, de Courten M. Pathogenesis and treatment of hypertension associated with diabetes mellitus. *Am Heart J* 1993; **125**:1498–1513.

31 Resnick LM, Gupta RK, Bhargava KK, Gruenspan H, Alderman MH, Laragh JH. Cellular ions in hypertension, diabetes and obesity: a nuclear magnetic spectroscopic study. *Hypertension* 1991; **17**:951–7.

32 Wiedmann P, Beretta-Piccoli C, Keusch G et al. Sodium–volume factor, cardiovascular reactivity and hypotensive mechanisms of diuretic therapy in hypertension associated with diabetes mellitus. *Am J Med* 1979; **67**:779–84.

33 Drury PL, Smith GM, Ferriss JB. Increased vasopressor responsiveness to angiotensin II in uncomplicated type I (insulin-dependent) diabetes. *Diabetologia* 1984; **27**:174–9.

34 Pfeifle B, Ditshuneit H. Effect of insulin on the growth of cultured human arterial smooth muscle cells. *Diabetologia* 1981; **20**:155–8.

35 Veterans' Administration Cooperative Study Group on Antihypertensive Agents. Effects of treatment on morbidity in hypertension. II. Results in patients with diastolic blood pressure averaging 90 through 114 mmHg. *JAMA* 1970; **213**:1143–52.

36 Korner PI, Bauer GE, Doyle AE et al. Untreated mild hypertension: a report by the management committee of the Australian therapeutic trial in mild hypertension. *Lancet* 1982; **1**:185–91.

37 Multiple Risk Factor Intervention Trial Research Group. Multiple Risk Factor Intervention Trial: risk factor changes and mortality results. *JAMA* 1982; **248**:1465–77.

38 Pyörälä K, Savolainen E, Kaukola S, Haapakoski J. Plasma insulin as coronary heart disease risk factor: Relationship to other risk factors and predictive capacity during 9½ year follow-up on the Helsinki Policemen Study Population. *Acta Med Scand Suppl* 1985; **701**:38–52.

39 Fontbonne A, Charles MA, Thibult N et al. Hyperinsulinaemia as a predictor of coronary heart disease mortality in a healthy population: The Paris Prospective Study, 15 year follow up. *Diabetologia* 1991; **34**:356–61.

40 Reaven GM, Lerner RL, Stern MP, Farquar JW. Role of insulin in endogenous hypertriglyceridaemia. *J Clin Invest* 1967; **46**:1756–67.

41 Olefsky JM, Reaven JM, Farquar JW. Effects of weight reduction in obesity: studies of carbohydrate and lipid metabolism. *J Clin Invest* 1974; **53**:64–76.

42 Castelli WP. The triglyceride issue: a view from Framingham. *Am Heart J* 1986; **112**:432–40.

43 Stewart MW, Laker MF, Dyer RG et al. Lipoprotein compositional abnormalities and insulin resistance in type II diabetic patients with mild hyperlipidemia. *Arteriosclerosis Thrombosis* 1993; **13**:1046–52.

44 Connell JM, McLellan AR. Hypertension, insulin and atherogenesis. *J Cardiovasc Pharmacol* 1991; **18**(suppl 2):S45–S50.

45 Brownlee M, Cerami A, Vlassara H. Advanced glycosylation end-products in tissue and the biochemical basis of diabetic complications. *N Engl J Med* 1988; **318**:1315–21.

46 Janka HU. Five year incidence of macrovascular complications in diabetes mellitus. *Horm Metab Res Supp* 1985; **15**:15–19.

47 Billault BM, Passa PL. Factors associated with diabetic microangiopathy: a study of 157 type I (insulin-dependent) diabetic patients. *J Diabet Complications* 1991; 5:238–43.

48 Hypertension in Diabetes Study (HDS). II. Increased risk of cardiovascular complications in hypertensive type 2 diabetic patients. *J Hypertens* 1993; **11**:319–25.

49 Knowler WC, Bennett PH, Balintine EJ. Increased incidence of retinopathy in diabetics with elevated blood pressure. *N Engl J Med* 1980; 301:645–50.

50 Barnett AH, Britton JR, Leatherdale BA. Study of possible risk factors for severe retinopathy in non-insulin dependent diabetes. *Br Med J* 1983; 287:529.

51 Waltman SR, Krupin T, Singer P, Becker B. Effects of therapy on vitreous fluorimetry in diabetes mellitus. *Trans Ophthalmol Soc UK* 1979; 99:8–9.

52 White P. Natural course and prognosis of juvenile diabetes. *Diabetes* 1956; 5 :445–50.

53 Deckert T, Poulsen JE, Larsen M. Prognosis of diabetics and diabetes onset before the age of thirty-one. *Diabetologia* 1978; **14**:363–70.

54 Tunbridge WMG. Factors contributing to the deaths of diabetics under fifty years of age. *Lancet* 1981; ii:569–72.

55 O'Donnell MJ. Hypertension and nephropathy in diabetes mellitus. In: Barnett AH, Dodson PM, eds. *Hypertension and Diabetes*. London: Science Press, 1990:3.1–3.18.

56 Drury PL. Diabetes and arterial hypertension. *Diabetologia* 1983; **24**:1–9.

57 Krolewski AJB, Canessa M, Warram JH, Laffel LM, Christlieb AR, Knowler WC, Rand LI. Predisposition to hypertension and susceptibility to renal disease in insulin-dependent diabetes mellitus. *N Engl J Med* 1988; 318:140–5.

58 Walker JD, Tariq T, Viberti G. Sodium lithium countertransport activity in red cells of patients with insulin dependent diabetes and nephropathy and their parents. *Br Med J* 1990; 302635–8.

59 Facchini F, Ida Chen YD, Reaven GM. Insulin resistance, hyperinsulinemia and dyslipidemia in non-obese individuals with a family history of hypertension. *Am J Hypertens* 1993; 5:694–9.

60 Medical Research Council Working Party. MRC trial of treatment of mild hypertension: principal results. *Br Med J* 1985; **291**:97–104.

61 Mogensen CE. Progression of nephropathy in long-term diabetics with proteinuria and effect of initial antihypertensive treatment. *Scand Clin Lab Invest* 1976; 36:383–8.

62 Mogensen CE. Long-term antihypertensive treatment inhibiting progression of diabetic nephropathy. *Br Med J* 1982; **285**:685–8.

63 Parving HH, Andersen AR, Smidt UM, Svendsen PA. Early aggressive antihypertensive treatment reduces rate of decline in kidney function in diabetic nephropathy. *Lancet* 1983; i:1175–8.

64 O'Donnell MJ, Dodson PM. The non-drug treatment of hypertension in the diabetic patient. *J Hum Hypertens* 1991; 5:287–94.

65 Fagerberg B, Berglund A, Andersson OK, Berglund G. Weight reduction versus antihypertensive drug therapy in obese men with high blood pressure: effects upon plasma insulin levels and association with changes in blood pressure and serum lipids. *J Hypertens* 1992; **10**:1053–61.

66 Dodson PM, Pacy PJ, Bal P, Kubicki AJ, Fletcher RF, Taylor KG. A controlled trial of a high fibre, low fat and low sodium diet for mild hypertension in type 2 (non-insulin-dependent) diabetic patients. *Diabetologia* 1984; **27**:522–6.

67 Jennings G, Nelson L, Nestel P et al. The effect of changes in physical activity on major cardiovascular risk factors, haemodynamics, sympathetic function and glucose utilization in man: a controlled study of four levels of activity. *Circulation* 1986; **73**:30–40.

68 Uusitupa M. Hypertension in diabetic patients – use of exercise in treatment. *Ann Med* 1991; **23**:335–8.

69 Wilkins RW. New drugs for the treatment of hypertension. *Ann Inter Med* 1959; **50**:1-10.

70 Murphy MB, Lewis PJ, Kohner E, Schumer B, Dollery CT. Glucose intolerance in hypertensive patients treated with diuretics. A fourteen year follow-up. *Lancet* 1982; ii:1293–5.

71 Helderman JH, Elahi D, Andersen DK et al. Prevention of glucose intolerance of thiazide diuretics by maintainance of body potassium. *Diabetes* 1983; **32**:106–11.

72 Strathers AD, Murphy MB, Dollery CT. Glucose tolerance during antihypertensive therapy in patients with diabetes mellitus. *Hypertension* 1985; **7(suppl 2)**:95–101.

73 Pacy PJ, Dodson PM, Kubicki AJ, Fletcher RF, Taylor KG. Comparison of the hypotensive and metabolic effects of bendrofluazide therapy and a high fibre, low fat, low sodium diet in diabetic subjects with mild hypertension. *J Hypertens* 1984; **2**:215–20.

74 Thompson GR. Evidence that lowering serum lipids favourably influences coronary artery disease. *Q J Med* 1987; **62**:87–95.

75 Ames RA. The effects of antihypertensive drugs on serum lipids and lipoproteins. I. Diuretics. *Drugs* 1986; **32**:260–78.

76 Kannel WB, Castelli WP, Gordon T. Cholesterol in the prediction of atherosclerotic disease. *Ann Intern Med* 1979; **90**:85–91.

77 Greenberg G, Brennan PJ, Miall WE. Effects of diuretic and beta blocker therapy in the Medical Research Council Trial. *Am J Med* 1984; **76**:45–51.

78 Helgeland A, Hjermann I, Leren P, Enger S, Holme I. High-density lipoprotein cholesterol and antihypertensive drugs: the Oslo Study. *Br Med J* 1978; **2**:403.

79 Ferrari P, Rosman J, Weidmann P. Antihypertensive agents, serum lipoproteins and glucose metabolism. *Am J Cardiol* 1991; **67**:26B–35B.

80 Weidmann P, De Courten M, Ferrari P. Effect of diuretics on plasma lipid profile. *Eur Heart J* 1992; **13**(suppl 6):61–7.

81 Ames RA, Hill P. Antihypertensive therapy and the risk of coronary artery disease. *J Cardiovasc Pharmacol* 1982; **4**(suppl II): S206–S212.

82 Weinberger MH. Mechanisms of diuretic effects carbohydrate tolerance, insulin sensitivity, and lipid levels. *Eur Heart J* 1992; **13**(suppl. 6):5–9.

83 Medical Research Council Working Party. MRC Trial: Report of Medical Research Council Working Party on mild to moderate hypertension. Adverse reaction to bendrofluazide and propranolol for the treatment of mild hypertension. *Lancet* 1981; **ii**:539–42.

84 Barnett DM, Desantels RE. Sexual function in diabetes. In: Marble A, Bradley RF, Christlieb AR, Soeldner SS, eds. *Joslin's Diabetes Mellitus* 12th Ed. Philadelphia: Lea and Febiger, 1985:686–97.

85 Veteran' Administration Cooperative Study Group on Antihypertensive Agents. Effects of treatment on morbity in hypertension. I. Results in patients with diastolic blood pressure averaging 115 mmHg through 129 mmHg. *JAMA* 1967; **202**:1028–34.

86 Hypertension Detection and Follow-Up Program (HDFP) Cooperative Group. Five year findings of the Hypertension Detection and Follow-Up Program I. Reduction in mortality of persons with high blood pressure including mild hypertension. *JAMA* 1979; **242**:2562–71.

87 Amery A, Birkenhager W, Brixko P et al. Mortality and morbidity results from the European Working Party on High Blood Pressure in the Elderly Trial. *Lancet* 1985; **i**:1349–54.

88 Collins R, Peto R, MacMahon S et al. Blood pressure, stroke and coronary heart disease. Part 2: short-term reduction of blood pressure: overview of randomized drug trials in their epidemiological context. *Lancet* 1990; **i**:827–38.

89 Papadremetriou V. Diuretics, hypokalaemia and cardiac arrhythmias: a critical analysis. *Am Heart J* 1986; **III**:1217–24.

90 Warram JH, Laffel LM, Valsania P, Christlieb AR, Krolewski AS. Excess mortality associated with diuretic therapy in diabetes mellitus. *Arch Int Med* 1991; **151**:1350–56.

91 Klein R, Moss SE, Klein BEK, DeMets DL. Relation of ocular and systemic factors to survival in diabetes. *Arch Int Med* 1989; **149**:266–72.

92 Kendall MJ, Lewis H, Griffiths M, Barnett AH. Drug treatment of the hypertensive diabetic. *J Hum Hypertens* 1988; **1**:249–58.

93 Gerber A, Weidmann P, Bianchetti MG et al. Serum lipoproteins during treatment with the antihypertensive agent indapamide. *Hypertension* 1985; **7**:164–9.

94 Gambardella S, Frontoni S, Grazia-Felici M et al. Efficacy of antihypertensive treatment with indapamide in patients with non-insulin-dependent diabetes and persistent microalbuminuria. *Am J Cardiol* 1990; **65**:46H–50H.

95 Pollare T, Lithell H, Selinus I, Berne C. Sensitivity to insulin during treatment with atenolol and metoprolol: a randomised double-blind study of effects on carbohydrate and lipoprotein metabolism in hypertensive patients. *Br Med J* 1989; **298**:1152–7.

96 Kendall MJ. Are selective beta-adrenoreceptor blocking drugs an advantage? *J R Coll Physicians Lond* 1981; **15**:33–40.

97 Wright AD, Barber SG, Kendall MJ, Poole PH. Beta-adrenoreceptor blocking drugs and blood sugar control in diabetes mellitus. *Br Med J* 1979; **1**:159–61.

98 Garber AJ, Cryer PE, Santiago JV, Haymond MW, Pagliara AS, Kipnis DM. The role of adrenergic mechanisms in the substrate and hormonal response to insulin-induced hypoglycaemia in man. *J Clin Invest* 1976; **58**:7–15.

99 Deacon SP, Barnett D. Comparison of atenolol and propranolol during insulin-induced hypoglycaemia. *Br Med J* 1976; **2**:272–3.

100 Lloyd-Mostyn RH, Oram S. Modification by propranolol of cardiovascular effects of induced hypoglycaemia. *Lancet* 1975; **i**:1213–15.

101 Barnett AH, Leslie RDG, Watkins PG. Can insulin-dependent diabetics be given beta-adrenergic blocking drugs? *Br Med J* 1980; **280**:976–8.

102 Ames RA. The effects of antihypertensive drugs on serum lipids and lipoproteins. II Non-diuretic drugs. *Drugs* 1986; **32**:335–57.

103 Tse WY, Kendall MJ. Is there a role for beta-blockers in hypertensive diabetic patients? *Diabetic Med* 1994; **11**:137–44.

104 Surawicz B. Prevention of sudden cardiac death: three promising approaches. *Rhythmology* 1987; **11**:3–10.

105 Campbell WB, Johnson AR, Callahan KS, Graham RM. Antiplatelet activity of beta-adrenergic antagonists. *Lancet* 1981; **ii**:1382–4.

106 Hearse DJ, Yellon DM, Downey JM. Can beta-blockers limit myocardial infarct size? *Eur Heart J* 1986; **7**:925–30.

107 Murray DP, Murray RG, Littler WA. The effects of metoprolol given early in acute myocardial infarction on ventricular arrhythmias. *Eur Heart J* 1986; **7**:217–22.

108 Wikstrand J, Warnold I, Tuomilehto J, Olsson G, Elmfeldt D, Berglund G. On behalf of the advisory committee. Metoprolol versus thiazide diuretics in hypertension. Morbidity results from the MAPHY study. *Hypertension* 1991; **17**:570–88.

109 Olsson G, Tuomilehto J, Berglund G et al. Primary prevention of sudden cardiac cardiovascular death in hypertensive patients: Mortality results from the MAPHY study. *Am J Hypertens* 1991; **4**:151–8.

110 The IPPPSH Collaborative Group. Cardiovascular risk and risk factors in a randomized trial of treatment based on the beta-blocker oxprenolol: The International Prospective Primary Prevention Study in Hypertension (IPPPSH). *J Hypertens* 1985; **3**:379–92.

111 The ISIS Collaborative Group. A randomised trial of intravenous atenolol among 16,027 cases of suspected myocardial infarction. *Lancet* 1986; **ii**:57–66.

112 Beta Blocker Heart Attack Trial Research Group. A randomized trial of propranolol in patients with acute myocardial infarction. 1. Mortality results. *JAMA* 1982; **247**:1707–13.

113 Olsson G, Wikstrand J, Warnold I et al. Metoprolol-induced reduction in post-infarction mortality: Pooled results from five double-blind randomised trials. *Eur Heart J* 1992; **13**:28–32.

114 Ryden L, Ariniego R, Arnman K et al. A double blind trial of metoprolol in acute myocardial infarction: effects on ventricular arrhythmias. *N Engl J Med* 1983; **308**:614–18.

115 Gundersen T, Kjekshus JK. Timolol treatment after myocardial infarction in diabetic patients. *Diabetes Care* 1983; **6**:285–90.

116 Kjekshus J, Gilpin E, Cali G, Blackey AR, Henning H, Ross JR Jr. Diabetic patients and beta-blockers after myocardial infarction. *Eur Heart J* 1990; **11**:43–50.

117 Gill JS, Zezulka AV, Beevers M, Beevers DG. An audit of nifedipine in a hypertension clinic. *J Clin Hosp Pharm* 1986; **11**:107–16.

118 Grodsky G, Bennett LL. Cation requirements for insulin secretion in the isolated perfused pancreas. *Diabetes* 1966; **15**:910–13.

119 Janis RA, Scriabine A. Sites of action of Ca^{2+} channel inhibitors. *Biochem Pharmacol* 1983; **32**:3499–507.

120 Charles S, Ketelslegers JM, Buysschaert M, Lambert A. Hyperglycaemic effects of nifedipine. *Br Med J* 1981; **283**:19–20.

121 Landmark K. Antihypertensive and metabolic effects of long term therapy with nifedipine slow-release tablets. *J Cardiovasc Pharmacol* 1985; **7**:12–17.

122 Collins WCJ, Cullen MJ, Feely J. The effects of therapy with dihydropyridine calcium channel blockers on glucose tolerance in non-insulin-dependent diabetes. *Br J Clin Pharmacol* 1986; **21**:568P.

123 Whitcroft I, Thomas J, Davies IB, Wilkinson N, Rawthorne A. Calcium antagonists do not impair long term glucose control in hypertensive non-insulin dependent diabetic (NIDDs). *Br J Clin Pharmacol* 1986; **22**:208P.

124 Zezulka AV, Gill JS, Beevers DG. Diabetogenic effects of nifedipine. *Br Med J* 1984; **289**:437–8.

125 Donnelly T, Harrower ATB. Effect of nifedipine on glucose tolerance and insulin secretion in diabetic and non-diabetic patients. *Curr Med Res Opin* 1980; **6**:690–3.

126 Rojdmark S, Andersson DEH. Influence of verapamil on glucose tolerance. *Acta Med Scand Suppl* 1984; **681**:37–42.

127 Semple CG, Thomson JA, Beastall GH, Lorimer AR. Oral verapamil does not affect glucose tolerance in non-diabetics. *Br J Clin Pharmacol* 1983; **15**:570–1.

128 Shamoon H, Baylor P, Kambosos D, Charlap S, Plawes S, Frishman W. Influence of oral verapamil on glucoregulatory hormones in man. *J Clin Endocrinol Metab* 1985; **60**:536–41.

129 Segrestaa JM, Caulin C, Dahan R et al. Effect of diltiazem on plasma glucose, insulin and glucagon during an oral glucose tolerance test in healthy volunteers. *Eur J Clin Pharmacol* 1984; **26**:481–3.

130 Parreira JM, Correia LG, Pereira E, Duarte RS, Pape E. Antihypertensive efficacy, safety, and tolerability of isradipine in hypertensive patients with diabetes. *Am J Hypertens* 1993; **6**:104S–106S.

131 Gradman AH. Treatment of hypertension with felodipine in patients with concomitant diseases. *Clin Cardiol* 1993; **16**:294–301.

132 Giugliano D, Saccomanno F, Paolisso G et al. Nicardipine does not cause deterioration in glucose homeostasis in man: a placebo controlled study in elderly hypertensives with and without diabetes mellitus. *Eur J Clin Pharmacol* 1992; **43**:39–45.

133 Giuntoli F, Galeoli F, Natali A, Gabani S, Saba P. Antihypertensive and metabolic effects of nitrendipine in non-insulin-dependent diabetes mellitus with hypertension. *J Cardiovasc Pharmacol* 1992; **19**(suppl 2):S39–S40.

134 Kawai K, Suzuki S, Murayama Y, Watanabe Y, Yamashita K. Comparison of the effects of nilvadipine and captopril on glucose and lipid metabolism in NIDDM patients with hypertension. *Diabetes Res Clin Pract* 1992; **16**:137–43.

135 Ramsay LE, Yeo WW, Jackson PR. Influence of diuretics, calcium antagonists, and alpha-blockers on insulin sensitivity and glucose tolerance in hypertensive patients. *J Cardiovasc Pharmacol* 1992; **20**(suppl 11):S49–S53.

136 Faergeman O, Meinertz H, Hansen JF. Serum lipoproteins after treatment with verapamil for six months. *Acta Med Scand Suppl* 1984; **681**:49–51.

137 Bauer JH, Reams G. Short- and long-term effects of calcium entry blockers on the kidney. *Am J Cardiol* 1987; **59**:66A–71A.

138 Chellingsworth M, Kendall MJ. Calcium antagonists and the kidney. *J Hum Hypertens* 1987; **1**:3–8.

139 Bernini F, Catapano AL, Corsini A, Fumagalli R, Paoletti R. Effects of calcium antagonists on lipids and atherosclerosis. *Am J Cardiol* 1989; **64**:129I–134I.

140 Gibson RS, Boden WE, Theroux P et al. Diltiazem and reinfarction in patients with non-Q-wave myocardial infarction. *New Engl J Med* 1986; **315**:423–7.

141 Agabibi-Rosei E, Muiesan ML, Romanelli G, Beschi M, Castellano M, Muiesan G. Reversal of cardiac hypertrophy by long-term treatment with calcium antagonists in hypertensive patients. *J Cardiovasc Pharmacol* 1988; **12**(suppl 6):S75–S78.

142 Pollare T, Lithell H, Berne C. A comparison of the effects of hydrochlorothiazide and captopril on glucose and lipid metabolism in patients with hypertension. *N Engl J Med* 1989; **321**:868–73.

143 Paolisso G, Gambardella A, Verza M, D'Amore A, Sgambaro S, Varricchio M. ACE inhibition improves insulin-sensitivity in aged insulin-resistant hypertensive patients. *J Hum Hypertens* 1992; **6**:175–9.

144 Jauch KW, Hartl W, Guenther B, Wicklmayr M, Rett K, Dietze G. Captopril enhances insulin responsiveness of forearm muscle tissue in non-insulin-dependent diabetes mellitus. *Eur J Clin Invest* 1987; **17**:448–54.

145 Torlone E, Rambotti AM, Perriello G et al. ACE-inhibition increases hepatic and extra-hepatic sensitivity to insulin in patients with type 2 (non-insulin-dependent) diabetes mellitus and arterial hypertension. *Diabetologia* 1991; **34**:119–25.

146 Bak JF, Gerdes LU, Sorensen NS, Pedersen O. Effects of perindopril on insulin sensitivity and plasma lipid profile in hypertensive non-insulin-dependent diabetic patients. *Am J Med* 1992; **92**(suppl 4B):69S–72S.

147 De Feo P, Torlone E, Perriello G et al. Short-term metabolic effects of the ACE inhibitor benazepril in type 2 diabetes mellitus associated with arterial hypertension. *Diabete Metab* 1992; **18**:283–6.

148 Bergemann R, Wohler D, Weidmann P, Betzin J, Nawrath T. Improved glucose regulation and microalbuminuria/proteinuria in diabetic patients treated with ACE inhibitors. A meta-analysis of published studies of 1985–1990. *Schweiz Med Wochenschr* 1992; **122**:1369–76.

149 Jandrain B, Herbaut C, Depoorter JC, Voorde KV. Long-term (1 year) acceptability of perindopril in type II diabetic patients with hypertension. *Am J Med* 1992; **92**:91S–94S.

150 McLenachan JM, Henderson E, Morris KI, Dargie HJ. Ventricular arrhythmias in patients with hypertensive left ventricular hypertrophy. *N Engl J Med* 1987; **317**:787–92.

151 Koren MJ, Deveraux RB, Casale PN, Savage GG, Laragh JH. Relation of left ventricular mass and geometry to morbidity and mortality in uncomplicated essential hypertension. *Ann Int Med* 1991; **114**:345–52.

152 Sampson MJ, Drury PL. Hypertension and the heart in insulin-dependent diabetes. *J Hum Hypertens* 1991; **5**:273–6.

153 Cruickshank JM, Lewis J, Moore V, Dodd C. Reversibility of left ventricular hypertrophy by differing types of antihypertensive therapy. *J Hum Hypertens* 1992; **6**:85–90.

154 Cleland JGF, Dargie HG, McAlpine H, Ball SG, Morton JJ et al. Severe hypotension after the first dose of enalapril in heart failure. *Br Med J* 1985; **291**:1309–12.

155 Reid JL. Angiotensin converting enzyme inhibitors in the elderly. *Br Med J* 1987; **295**:943–4.

156 Feher MD, Henderson AD, Wadsworth J et al. Alpha-blocker therapy, a possible advance in the treatment of diabetic hypertension – results of a cross-over study of doxazosin and atenolol monotherapy in hypertensive non-insulin-dependent diabetic subjects. *J Hum Hypertens* 1990; **4**:571–7.

157 Trost BN, Weidmann P. Antihypertensive therapy in diabetic patients. *Hypertension* 1985; **7**(suppl II):II-102–II-108.

158 Janssens M, Symoens J, Robertson MP. Ketanserin in the treatment of peripheral vascular disease or hypertension in patients with diabetes mellitus: a review. *J Cardiovasc Pharmacol* 1991; **17**(suppl 5):S54–S66.

159 Feher MD. Doxazosin therapy in the treatment of diabetic hypertension. *Am Heart J* 1991; **121**:1294–301.

160 Pollare T, Lithell H, Selinus I, Berne C. Application of prazosin is associated with an increase in insulin sensitivity in obese patients with hypertension. *Diabetologia* 1988; **31**:415–20.

161 Taylor SH. Efficacy of doxazosin in specific hypertensive patient groups. *Am Heart J* 1991; **121**:286–92.

162 Mogensen CE. Glomerular filtration rate and renal plasma flow in short-term and long-term juvenile diabetes mellitus. *Scand J Lab Clin Invest* 1971; **28**:91–100.

163 Christiansen JS, Gammelgaard S, Tronier B, Svendsen PA, Parving HH. Kidney function and size in diabetics before and during

initial insulin treatment. *Kidney Int* 1982; **21**:683–8.

164 Wiseman MJ, Drury PL, Keen H, Viberti GC. Plasma renin activity in insulin-dependent diabetics with raised glomerular filtration rate. *Clin Endocrinol (Oxf)* 1984; **21**:409–14.

165 Steffes MW, Brown DM, Mauer SM. Diabetic glomerulopathy following unilateral nephrectomy in the rat. *Diabetes* 1978; **27**:35–41.

166 Keane WF, Anderson S, Aurell M, de Zeuw D, Narins RG, Povar G. Angiotensin converting enzyme inhibitors and progressive renal insufficiency. *Ann Int Med* 1989; **111**:503–16.

167 Mogensen CE, Hansen KW, Osterby R, Damsgaard EM. Blood pressure elevation versus abnormal albuminuria in the genesis and prediction of renal disease in diabetes. *Diabetes Care* 1992; **15**:1192–204.

168 Bakris GL. Hypertension in diabetic patients. An overview of interventional studies to preserve renal function. *Am J Hypertens* 1993; **6**:140S–147S.

169 Neuringer JR, Brenner BM. Hemodynamic theory of progressive renal disease: a ten year update in brief review. *Am J Kidney Dis* 1993; **22**:98–104.

170 Walker WG. Hypertension-related renal injury: a major contributor to end-stage renal disease. *Am J Kidney Dis* 1993; **22**:164–73.

171 Parving HH, Hommel E. Prognosis in diabetic nephropathy. *Br Med J* 1989; **299**:230–3.

172 Christiansen CK, Mogensen CE. Effect of antihypertensive treatment on progression of incipient diabetic nephropathy. *Hypertension* 1985; **7**(suppl 2):109–13.

173 Taguma Y, Kitamoto Y, Futaki G et al. Effect of captopril on proteinuria in azotemic diabetics. *N Engl J Med* 1985; **313**:1616–20.

174 Hommel E, Parving HH, Mathiesen E, Edsberg B, Nielsen MD, Giese J. Effect of captopril on kidney function in insulin-dependent diabetic patients with nephropathy. *Br Med J* 1986; **293**:467–70.

175 Bjorck S, Nyberg C, Mulec H, Granerus G, Herlitz H, Aurell M. Beneficial effects of angiotensin converting enzyme inhibition on renal function in patients with diabetic nephropathy. *Br Med J* 1986; **293**:471–4.

176 Parving HH, Hommel E, Smidt UM. Protection of kidney function and decrease in albuminuria by captopril in insulin dependent diabetics with nephropathy. *Br Med J* 1988; **297**:1086–91.

177 Kasiske BL, Kalil RSN, Ma JZ, Liao M, Keane WF. Effect of antihypertensive therapy on the kidney in patients with diabetes: a meta-regression analysis. *Ann Int Med* 1993; **118**:129–38.

178 Lewis EJ, Hunsicker LG, Bain RP, Rohde RD for the Collaborative Study Group. The effect of angiotensin-converting enzyme inhibition on diabetic nephropathy. *N Engl J Med* 1993; **329**:1456–62.

179 Parving HH, Hommel E, Damkjaer Nielsen M, Giese J. Effect of captopril on blood pressure and kidney function in normotensive insulin dependent diabetics with nephropathy. *Br Med J* 1989; **299**:533–6.

180 Marre M, Chantellier G, Leblanc H, Guyene TT, Menard J, Passa P. Prevention of diabetic nephropathy with enalapril in normotensive diabetics with microalbuminuria. *Br Med J* 1988; **297**:1092–5.

181 Ferder L, Daccordi H, Martello M, Panzalis M, Inserra F. Angiotensin converting enzyme inhibitors versus calcium antagonists in the treatment of diabetic hypertensive patients. *Hypertension* 1992; **19**(suppl II):II-237–II-242.

182 Ferrier C, Ferrari P, Weidmann P, Keller U, Beretta-Piccoli C, Riesen WF. Swiss hypertension treatment programme with verapamil and/or enalapril in diabetic patients. *Drugs* 1992; **44**(suppl 1):74–84.

183 O'Donnell MJ, Rowe BR, Lawson N et al. A placebo-controlled trial of lisinopril in diabetic patients with incipient nephropathy. *J Hum Hypertens* 1993; **7**:327–32.

184 Jungmann E, Usadel KH. Renal long-term effects of calcium antagonist treatment in patients with diabetes mellitus. *Clin Investig Med* 1992; **70**:942–8.

185 Murray KM. Calcium channel blockers for the treatment of diabetic nephropathy. *Clin Pharm* 1991; **10**:862–5.

186 Lacourciere Y, Nadeau A, Poirier L, Tancrede G. Captopril or conventional therapy in hypertensive type II diabetics. Three year analysis. *Hypertension* 1993; **21**:786–94.

187 SHEP Cooperative Research Group. Prevention of stroke by antihypertensive drug treatment in older persons with isolated systolic hypertension. *JAMA* 1991; **285**:3255–64.

188 Earle K, Walker J, Hill C, Viberti G. Familial clustering of cardiovascular disease in patients with insulin-dependent diabetes and nephropathy. *N Engl J Med* 1992; **326**:673–7.

10

Renal Disease and Hypertension

Wai Y Tse and Dwomoa Adu

The occurrence of hypertension in renal diseases and the impact of hypertension on the progression of renal insufficiency have long been topics of importance to physicians. The kidney plays a crucial role in the pathogenesis of essential hypertension, and primary parenchymal renal disease and renal vascular disease can result in secondary hypertension.[1] In addition, many experimental studies have shown that systemic hypertension can cause a decline in renal function, and malignant hypertension rapidly leads to irreversible loss of renal function.[2,3]

Between 80% and 90% of patients with end-stage renal failure that requires dialysis have hypertension. Treatment of hypertension and correction of other cardiovascular risk factors are important in these patients, as they have an unacceptably high prevalence of cardiovascular disease and more than half die from a cardiac or vascular event.[4] Moreover, there is evidence that treatment of hypertension can reduce the rate of decline of renal function in patients with renal insufficiency and primary hypertension.[5]

Essential hypertension as the cause of renal failure

In the early stages of essential hypertension, the kidney is histologically normal. However, in long-standing benign hypertension, the kidney becomes contracted and granular. There is patchy ischaemic atrophy and sclerosis of the glomeruli, together with fibrosis due to hyaline arteriosclerosis. However, despite the presence of histological abnormalities, it is rare for benign hypertension to lead to renal failure,[6] although a number of studies have shown that hypertension can adversely affect renal function.[2,3,7] In the Hypertension Detection and Follow-up Program (HDFP), the group with the highest blood pressure at entry had the highest serum creatinine, suggesting that the rate of decline of renal function amongst hypertensive patients before entry into the study was related to blood pressure at entry.[2] The Modification of Diet in Renal Disease Study has also shown that subjects with mean diastolic blood pressure levels of 100 mmHg or more exhibited a significantly greater decline in renal function than subjects with blood pressures below this level.[7] In another retrospective study of 86 patients on dialysis, 50% of whom were black, Brazy et al found a positive correlation between mean diastolic blood pressure and rate of decline in renal function.[3]

Indirect evidence of the harmful role of hypertension is also provided by the observation that renal damage can be prevented or improved by antihypertensive drugs.[8] Brazy and Fitzwilliam were able to show that the slope of the reciprocal of serum creatinine against time was reduced by approximately

40% when diastolic arterial blood pressure was maintained below 90 mmHg.[9] Similarly, Lindeman et al showed, in a cohort of 446 subjects, that the decline of renal function was greatest in those with blood pressure of 140/90 mmHg or greater compared to those who were either normotensive or hypertensive with adequately controlled blood pressure.[10]

Identification of prognostic indicators of progressive renal failure is obviously desirable, as it would allow clinicians to identify those patients requiring closer monitoring of blood pressure control. In the HDFP study, blacks, older subjects (over 60 years), and patients with the highest diastolic blood pressure at entry were shown to be the most likely to develop renal impairment.[2]

For reasons that remain unclear, hypertensive renal failure is more prevalent in black patients. Essential hypertension now accounts for 28% of all end-stage renal disease in the USA and is the commonest cause of end-stage renal disease in blacks.[11] There is some evidence to suggest that the fundamental mechanisms responsible for hypertension may be different in blacks and whites. Compared to whites, black hypertensive patients have a more expanded intravascular volume, lower plasma renin activity, and reduced natriuretic response to a sodium load.[12] Black patients typically respond well to diuretics, calcium channel blockers, alpha-blockers and central alpha-blockers, but not so well to ACE inhibitors, and poorly to beta-blockers.

Despite increased treatment of patients with hypertension, the number of patients with end-stage renal diseases is increasing. It has been suggested that this is the result of the high prevalence of hypertension among black patients and among patients with diabetes mellitus. Other contributory factors may include inadequate treatment, poor patient compliance with the treatment program, and delayed diagnosis of the hypertensive state. Moreover, at present there are no studies that quantitatively correlate the severity of renal blood flow and glomerular filtration rate reduction with the degree of elevated blood pressure levels, with the histologic changes of nephrosclerosis, or with progressive renal failure.

Hypertension in primary renal diseases

The prevalence of hypertension is increased in all types of parenchymal disease, although the proportion of patients affected varies in the different parenchymal disorders. Glomerulonephritis is more likely than chronic interstitial nephritis to cause hypertension.[13] Even within the category of glomerulonephritis, the prevalence of hypertension varies. Hypertension is more commonly found in lupus nephritis, IgA nephropathy, membranoproliferative glomerulonephritis and focal sclerosis, but less frequently found in membranous nephropathy or minimal change disease.[14,15]

Apart from the type of renal disease, the prevalence of hypertension also depends on the duration of disease. Thus, in children with chronic pyelonephritis, approximately 10% are hypertensive, whereas in adults 33% have hypertension at presentation, and by the time end-stage renal failure is reached approximately 80% are hypertensive.[16]

It has been postulated that when renal mass is reduced, glomerular hyperfiltration occurs as the result of compensatory dilatation of the afferent arteriole.[17] Superimposed systemic hypertension will further increase the transcapillary hydrostatic pressure difference, leading to a more severe proteinuria and glomerulosclerosis.[18] In addition, hypertension itself can directly lead to hyaline arteriosclerosis of the afferent arteriole, which can result in further renal injury via an ischaemic mechanism.

The deleterious effect of superimposed hypertension was confirmed in several experimental models of glomerulonephritis involving rats.[19,20] It was found that rats with superimposed hypertension had an accelerated deterioration of renal function and more proteinuria than those rats with the same model of renal disease but without hypertension. In man, there is also evidence that hypertension can accelerate the decline of renal function in subjects with parenchymal renal diseases. In patients with chronic glomerulonephritis, chronic pyelonephritis, and adult polycystic kidney disease, hypertension was found to be the most prominent adverse factor causing a deterioration in renal function.[21-23]

Maschio et al also found a negative role for hypertension in the course of non-diabetic chronic renal disease.[24] They were able to show that, at comparable levels of serum creatinine upon entry to the study, normotensive patients had a greater likelihood of maintaining renal function than hypertensive patients. In a separate series of 174 patients with advanced chronic renal failure (plasma creatinine > 900 µmol/l) due to well-defined primary renal diseases (including glomerulonephritis, interstitial nephritis, polycystic kidneys disease, hypertensive nephrosclerosis and Alport's syndrome), it was again demonstrated that decline in renal function was faster in those who were hypertensive than in those subjects with normal blood pressure.[25] Indirect evidence of the harmful effect of hypertension is also provided by the observation that treatment of hypertension in patients with renal disease can retard the progression of renal failure.[3,21,26]

Malignant hypertension

Malignant hypertension is a distinct clinical and pathological entity characterized by:

- a marked elevation of blood pressure (diastolic pressure often > 120–130 mmHg), and hypertensive retinopathy, consisting of flame-shaped haemorrhages, cotton-wool exudates, and (in the later stages) papilloedema.
- Untreated malignant hypertension rapidly causes renal failure, often with heart failure and intracerebral haemorrhage with or without hypertensive encephalopathy. Fortunately, hypertensive crises are uncommon, but untreated hypertensive crises have a significant morbidity and carry a 90% mortality rate at 2 years.

Renal failure used to be the predominant cause of death, responsible for 68% of deaths in the Hammersmith series,[27] but dialysis facilities have now improved outcome dramatically. Nonetheless, the initial serum creatinine remains a good prognostic indicator of patient survival. Men have a higher incidence than women of both primary hypertension and hypertensive crisis, and blacks have a higher incidence than whites. Malignant hypertension usually occurs in patients with preexisting benign hypertension, although *de novo* cases have been described. It should be noted that isolated raised blood pressure of the same magnitude as malignant hypertension can occur in subjects with hypertension but without evidence of acute end-organ damage or retinopathy. This entity of severe 'uncomplicated' hypertension should be differentiated from malignant hypertension, as the prognosis differs greatly between the two conditions.

The precise mechanisms responsible for the transition from the benign to the malignant phase of hypertension are not altogether clear, but several mechanisms have been proposed. Vascular reactivity is often increased as the result of increased release of vasoconstrictor substances such as noradrenaline, angiotensin II, and antidiuretic hormone. In addition, vasoconstriction of the renal efferent arterioles leads to increased glomerular capillary pressure and to diuresis and volume depletion. Hypovolaemia leads to a reflex increase in the release of vasoconstrictor substances, which in turn induces further endothelial damage and narrowing of the renal arteries, thus setting up a vicious circle.[28] More recently, the vascular endothelium has been implicated as having a crucial role in the regulation of vascular tone through the release of mediators such as endothelium-derived relaxing factor (nitric oxide) and endothelin-1, a potent vasoconstricting agent.[29] Theoretically, an imbalance in the release of these agents could lead to uncontrolled hypertension.

Patients with evidence of end-organ damage secondary to hypertensive emergencies should be hospitalized. Normally initial treatment should be by mouth with a beta-blocker or a calcium antagonist but virtually any antihypertensive agents can be used, provided the blood pressure is not reduced too quickly. Very rapid falls in blood pressure can adversely affect perfusion to vital organs and in particular, can lead to cerebral infarction, blindness, azotaemia and myocardial ischaemia. In patients with malignant hypertension and left ventricular failure, intravenous nitroprusside may be used to reduce the blood pressure. It has the advantages of a rapid onset of action and a short duration of action, thus providing minute-to-minute control. Effective alternatives include intravenous bolus administration of labetolol. In practice, however, intravenous agents are rarely used. The initial goal of therapy should be to reduce diastolic blood pressure by approximately 25%, but not below 100–110 mmHg. Blood pressure should be maintained at this target level for the first 24 hours, and then reduced to normotensive level over the course of the next few days using a combination of beta-blockers, calcium antagonists, diuretics, vasodilators or angiotensin converting enzyme inhibitors.

Renovascular hypertension

Renovascular disease is the commonest cause of secondary hypertension, accounting for 1–5% of unselected hypertensives and 10–30% of patients presenting with malignant phase hypertension.[30] Atherosclerosis or fibromuscular dysplasia are responsible for almost all cases of renal artery stenosis. Fibromuscular dysplasia of the arterial wall is commonest among younger people (those under 40 years)

Age of onset of hypertension: aged under 30 years or aged over 50 years of age
Acute onset of hypertension
Hypertension refractory to drug treatment
Well-controlled hypertension that suddenly worsens
Accelerated (malignant) hypertension
Presence of abdominal or flank bruits
Symptoms of vascular disease elsewhere
Azotaemia following the use of angiotensin converting enzyme inhibitors
Unexplained hypokalaemia
Unexplained pulmonary oedema

Table 10.1
Features that should prompt investigation for underlying renovascular disease in a hypertensive patient.

and is commoner in women, whereas atherosclerotic disease predominate in older people. Although there are no clinical characteristics that absolutely distinguish the patient with renovascular hypertension from the patient with essential hypertension, some clinical features do warrant further screening for renovascular hypertension (Table 10.1).

Methods of screening

Plasma renin activity, rapid sequence intravenous urography, and isotope dynamic renography have traditionally been used as screening methods for renovascular disease, but these techniques lack adequate sensitivity and specificity.[31] Intravenous digital angiography is expensive and fails to visualize the renal artery in up to 20% of cases.[32] Duplex ultrasonography has been used, but this is often operator dependent and, again in up to 20% of cases, the renal artery cannot be localized.[33] The administration of a single dose of captopril before performing isotope renogram has resulted in improved diagnostic accuracy, with an average sensitivity and specificity rates of 90%.[34] In patients with significant renal artery stenosis, captopril will lead to a marked fall in glomerular filtration rate, resulting from the loss of the efferent arteriolar vasoconstriction mediated by angiotensin II. Arteriography remains the definitive screening test, but it has the disadvantage of being an invasive test with all the risks attendant to an arterial puncture.

Treatment

Patients with renovascular hypertension are typically resistant to conventional antihypertensive drugs. Given that the underlying mechanism responsible for renovascular hypertension is the increased activation of the renin–angiotensin–aldosterone system, ACE inhibitors would be the obvious drug of choice in this clinical setting. Indeed, ACE inhibitors have exhibited great efficacy in controlling blood pressure in animals[35,36] and in patients with renovascular hypertension.[37,38] In 1 study, captopril alone or combined with diuretics successfully controlled the blood pressure of 90% of 160 patients with renovascular hypertension.[37] The efficacy of ACE inhibitors in controlling the blood pressure in subjects with renovascular hypertension was confirmed in another study that used enalapril.[39] In this study, a combination of enalapril and thiazide diuretic controlled more patients than the combination of a thiazide with a beta-blocker and hydralazine. ACE inhibitors can be used to control the blood pressure in patients who have unilateral renal artery stenosis, but they should be avoided in patients with bilateral renal artery stenosis and in patients with stenosis in the artery to a solitary functioning kidney. In patients with significant renal artery stenosis, angiotensin II is required to exert a pressor effect on the efferent arteriole and maintain filtration pressure. Administration of ACE inhibitors in such patients can, by preventing the formation of angiotensin II, abolish efferent arteriolar constriction, thereby causing a reduction in glomerular filtration rate, and hence lead to renal failure. Therefore, ACE inhibitors should be used only in these patients after screening tests have excluded critical renal artery stenosis.

Control of blood pressure is clearly important, but many patients with renovascular hypertension have progressive arterial disease that is likely to cause progressive narrowing of the arteries. Therefore, when possible, patients with significant renal artery stenosis should be considered for angioplasty or operative treatment. If angioplasty or surgery is not a possible option, satisfactory blood pressure control is mandatory to retard the potential decline of renal function and to prevent the cardiovascular complications associated with hypertension.

Role of hypertension in diabetic nephropathy

Diabetic nephropathy develops in 30–50% of patients with insulin dependent diabetes mellitus.[40] Much less is known about susceptibility to diabetic nephropathy in non-insulin-dependent diabetes mellitus. Renal failure is uncommon in white patients with non-insulin-dependent diabetes mellitus, occurring in only 5–10%. However, in populations with an increased prevalence of non-insulin-dependent diabetes mellitus, such as native Americans, Hispanics, and blacks, the frequency of end-stage renal disease due to diabetic nephropathy approaches (or may exceed) that in insulin-dependent diabetes mellitus.[41]

Following a variable period of glomerular hyperfiltration, patients develop microalbuminuria (urinary albumin excretion rate of 30–300 mg/24 hours). This is associated with the development of hypertension, left ventricular hypertrophy, a twenty-fold increased risk of developing renal insufficiency and a hundredfold increase in mortality.[42] Treatment of hypertension at the microalbuminuric stage appears to arrest progression of renal disease completely, whereas treatment at the stage of clinical proteinuria only slows the rate of deterioration.[43] Currently, in the UK, there are an estimated 600 cases per year of end-stage renal failure as a consequence of diabetes mellitus.[44]

Prolonged tight glycaemic control may prevent the development of diabetic nephropathy but there is no evidence of benefit in renal disease that is already established. Hypertension is a characteristic feature of diabetic nephropathy and is the single most important factor in exacerbating the progression of renal failure in diabetic patients.[45,46] In a study of patients with renal insufficiency from diabetic nephropathy, hypertension control was associated with a 33% reduction in the rate of decline in the glomerular filtration rate.[45]

Treatment

Metabolic side effects such as hypokalaemia, hyperuricaemia, glucose intolerance, hyperinsulinaemia, and decreased insulin sensitivity have caused concern over the use of diuretics. Likewise, non-selective beta-blockers have a negative impact on glycaemic control, but this can be minimized by the use of selective $beta_1$-blockers.[47] Beta-blockers have an established cardioprotective role, particularly in the post-infarct period,[48,49] and since cardiovascular disease is prevalent in diabetics, the use of selective $beta_1$-blockers remains a logical choice of antihypertensive agent in diabetic patients with ischaemic heart disease. Calcium antagonists are also useful agents in diabetics with ischaemic heart disease, and they have the advantage of being metabolically neutral with little adverse effect on glucose and lipid levels.

There is a growing body of evidence from clinical studies that ACE inhibitors are particularly effective in the treatment of hypertension in patients with diabetic nephropathy. A number of studies have found that ACE inhibitors may be more beneficial than other agents such as beta-blockers and diuretics, because, despite similar reduction in blood pressure, ACE inhibitor therapy results in a greater reduction in proteinuria and in the rate of decline in glomerular filtration rate.[43,50]

However, not all studies in diabetics have shown a superior effect with ACE inhibitors. Zuchelli et al reported that the same deceleration in renal function was obtained with an ACE inhibitor and with a calcium antagonist in a 4-year study in 142 patients.[51] Similarly, O'Donnnell et al, comparing lisinopril and nifedipine, also failed to show any significant differences in proteinuria or renal haemodynamics.[52]

Nonetheless, from a metabolic standpoint, ACE inhibitors represent an excellent choice for antihypertensive therapy in diabetics since there is no adverse effect on lipid or glucose metabolism. Recently, Kasiske et al conducted a meta-analysis of 100 controlled and uncontrolled studies in diabetic patients and concluded that ACE inhibitors decrease proteinuria and preserve glomerular filtration rate in patients with diabetes mellitus, independent of their effect in lowering blood pressure.[53] The finding that ACE inhibitors can decrease albuminuria even in normotensive diabetics with microalbuminuria supports this hypothesis.[43] It should be noted that patients with diabetic nephropathy often have accelerated atherosclerosis that diffusely involves the arterial system. An unexpected increase in the serum creatinine after ACE inhibitor therapy has been initiated should prompt consideration of renovascular disease.

In summary, it appears that lowering the blood pressure, regardless of the type of antihypertensive medication used, will slow the rate of progression of diabetic nephropathy. At present, an ACE inhibitor should probably be included in the antihypertensive regime unless there are specific contraindications.

Hypertension in renal transplants

Hypertension is observed frequently in patients with renal transplants, and a number of mechanisms may be responsible. The hypertension may be related to:

- the donor kidneys (genetic predisposition to hypertension);
- graft kidney pathology (immunological rejection, renal artery stenosis, or occurrence of original disease);
- immunosuppressive drugs;
- the development of primary or secondary hypertension in the recipient; or
- the presence of pre-existing hypertension in the recipient.

Post-transplantation hypertension is often multifactorial, resulting from one or more of these factors. High blood pressure is thought to contribute to the accelerated vascular disease observed in patients who have received a renal transplant, and it is associated with decreased graft survival. Thus, hypertension in renal transplant patients should be treated aggressively.

Genetically determined alterations to the donor kidney

In humans, a genetically determined tendency to the development of post-transplantation hypertension in the donor kidney may be involved in the pathogenesis of hypertension. In a study involving 50 recipients of a cadaver kidney, it was found that those patients whose donor came from a hypertensive family had higher mean blood pressure and required significantly more antihypertensive treatment than those patients whose donor came from a normotensive family.[54]

However, interpretation of such data in humans is confounded by other factors, including immunosuppressive and antihypertensive drug treatment and the presence of graft rejection. Animal studies supporting a genetic predisposition of the donor to hypertension are much more convincing.[55,56]

Conversely, patients with primary hypertension as the cause of end-stage renal failure may become normotensive after bilateral nephrectomy and successful transplantation of a kidney from a normotensive donor.[57] In long-term survivors (over 7 years), hypertension is present in 65% of patients with native kidneys, but only in 50% of bilaterally nephrectomized patients, an observation suggesting that native kidneys cause hypertension in 15% of transplanted patients.[58]

Graft kidney pathology

Renal artery stenosis

Renal artery stenosis as a complication of renal transplantation causing hypertension occurs in 10–12% of recipients and should be ruled out as the cause of post-transplant hypertension. Atherosclerosis or local factors (such as technical faults, cannula-induced injury, and reaction to suture material) have all been implicated in its pathogenesis. Rejection has also been considered as a causal factor, and the rate of stenosis is indeed greater in cadaver than in living donor kidney recipients.[57] Graft-artery stenosis should be suspected if a bruit can be heard over the graft or if the hypertension is refractory to medical treatment. Transplant renal artery stenosis should also be suspected if the introduction of an ACE inhibitor leads to impaired renal function. Treatment decisions which should be made individually for each patient include ureteric stenting and surgical reimplantation of the artery.

Rejection

Hypertension often occurs in acute rejection crisis and usually resolves with anti-rejection therapy. In this setting, hypertension appears renin-dependent. West et al showed that plasma renin levels increased with the onset of allograft rejection and decreased with the return of renal function,[59] and a significant correlation was found between diastolic blood pressure and plasma renin in acute rejection episodes.[60]

Chronic rejection may also result in hypertension and a number of studies have shown a correlation between blood pressure and serum creatinine.[61,62] In chronic rejection, reduced renal blood flow and cortical ischaemia can lead to increased renin secretion and this may be the explanation for the hypertension.[63]

Drugs

Steroids

A positive correlation between blood pressure and prednisolone dosage has been described, but the evidence is restricted to the first 2 months after transplantation, when steroid dose is greatest and only in those with good graft function.[62] In studies including less selected patients, maintenance steroid dose is not greater in hypertensive than in normotensive patients.[61] Multivariate analysis suggests that blood pressure after renal transplantation is correlated with the cumulative prednisolone dosage but not with the maintenance prednisolone dosage, and that it is independent of graft tolerance and function.[64] There is some data to suggest that an alternate day steroid dose regime can lead to a fall in the blood pressure.[65]

Cyclosporin

Cyclosporin was introduced in the late 1970s and is now a valuable adjunct in the field of organ transplantation. Studies have shown that cyclosporin can improve renal graft survival by some 20% at 1 year.[66] However, decreases in renal blood flow and glomerular filtration rate have been demonstrated with high blood levels of cyclosporin, and renal dysfunction in association with structural damage has been described.[67] In addition, the use of cyclosporin is associated with a higher prevalence of hypertension in transplant patients.[68] The hypertension observed in patients treated with cyclosporin is characterized by sodium dependency, enhanced sympathetic nervous system activity, marked intrarenal vasoconstriction (predominantly at the afferent level), and lower renin values compared to patients on conventional immunosuppressive drugs. As the result of impaired sodium handling and increased vascular resistance, extracellular volume is often expanded. Cyclosporin may also induce hypertension by altering eicosanoid metabolism, and there is evidence to suggest that the response to endogenous vasoconstrictor agents is enhanced.[68]

Management

Treatment of hypertension in renal-transplant patients is important, as hypertension can directly damage the renal transplant. Moreover, renal-transplant patients with previous renal failure, often have advanced atherosclerosis, and poorly controlled hypertension will further accelerate the atherosclerotic process. The cause of hypertension should be identified and appropriate treatment instigated. In the case of transplant renal artery stenosis, ureteric stenting or surgical correction of the stenosis should be offered if possible. During acute rejection episodes, effective antirejection therapy will lead to a reduction both in plasma renin levels and arterial blood pressure. Sodium restriction, diuretic administration, and conventional antihypertensive medication are effective therapy in most hypertensive transplant recipients in whom no remediable cause for the hypertension can be identified. There is as yet no convincing evidence in favour of the use of a particular antihypertensive agent in renal transplant recipients with hypertension. In post-transplant hypertension that is resistant to medical therapy, removal of the diseased host kidneys may be indicated, particularly when they are a source of increased renin secretion.

Hypertension associated with erythropoietin

Human erythropoietin is effective in the management of anaemia in patients with chronic renal failure. There are, however, a number of adverse side-effects, including thrombosis of fistulae and haemodialysis lines, the development of epileptic seizures and hypertension.[69,70] Approximately one third of the patients treated with recombinant human erythropoietin will experience an aggravation of pre-existing hypertension or will develop *de novo* hypertension.[77] Cases of malignant hypertension induced by erythropoietin have also been described in the literature.[72]

In the vast majority of cases, hypertension develops during the first few months of treatment in association with the rise in haematocrit and haemoglobin. The mechanism of worsening hypertension is unclear but it is probably related to changes in blood viscosity and peripheral resistance.[73] Peripheral resistance rises because the compensatory vasodilatation induced by renal anaemia is relieved.[74] It has also been suggested that alterations in the renin–angiotensin–aldosterone system during erythropoietin treatment may contribute to the hypertension.[75] Not all patients who became hypertensive soon after the introduction of erythropoietin therapy remain hypertensive, and presumably autoregulation occurs.

Treatment

Erythropoietin remains an important asset to the management of chronic renal failure and the benefits far outweigh the side effects. Apart from the obvious reduced need for blood transfusion with its inherent risks, there are beneficial effects on the heart, including a reduction in heart size in those with cardiomegaly, reduced myocardial oxygen consumption, and a reduction in cardiac output. This leads to improved exercise tolerance and better cognitive function, and there is evidence that it leads to an overall improved quality of life.[76] The current accepted practice is to intensify the antihypertensive treatment, but phlebotomy has been used successfully in erythropoietin-induced malignant hypertension.[77]

Hypertension in dialysis patients

It is estimated that 80–90% of all patients with end-stage renal failure have hypertension. In the vast majority of these, blood pressure is volume dependent and the hypertension usually indicates either inadequate removal of salt and water during dialysis or excessive intake between dialysis. Strict volume control is mandatory in treating hypertension in dialysis patients. Patients whose hypertension does not respond to sodium and fluid restriction tend to have inappropriately high plasma renin activity.[78] In such patients, ACE inhibitors are the logical choice of antihypertensive agent, and indeed they have been found to be effective.[79]

However, renin is by no means the sole substance responsible for dialysis-refractory hypertension. Zuchelli et al have found that renin values of normotensive and hypertensive patients overlapped widely and failed to find a correlation between plasma renin activity and blood pressure.[80] Often, satisfactory control of blood pressure can be achieved only by using a combination of antihypertensive drugs and strict volume control. Antihypertensive medication is usually omitted before haemodialysis, to reduce the risk of intradialysis hypotension.

Management of hypertension in renal failure

Nonpharmacological treatment

Non-pharmacological treatment should be tried before commencing antihypertensive drugs unless the hypertension is severe. Other risk factors for cardiovascular morbidity should be aggressively corrected; these include obesity, high alcohol intake, smoking, and hyperlipidaemia. In patients with advanced renal disease, hypertension is often salt-dependent and so a sodium-restricted diet is a useful initial step in the management of hypertension.

There is still considerable controversy surrounding the usefulness of protein restriction. In animals, a high protein diet is associated with a greater degree of proteinuria and the accelerated development of glomerular sclerosis.[81,82] In humans, the evidence is inconclusive. Nonetheless, protein restriction is usually recommended in those with advanced renal impairment, as this alleviates the symptoms of uraemia.

Pharmacological treatment of hypertension

Diuretics
The antihypertensive efficacy of thiazide diuretics is sharply diminished in patients with renal impairment and is lost when the glomerular filtration rate is below 25 ml/min. In contrast, loop diuretics such as frusemide can still produce an adequate diuresis when little renal function remains. Potassium-sparing diuretics should be avoided in advanced renal impairment because of the danger of hyperkalaemia.

Other adverse effects include hyperuricaemia, glucose intolerance, hyperinsulinaemia, and decreased insulin sensitivity. As these are all risk factors for cardiovascular disease, this has led to some concern over the use of diuretics. However, in spite of the adverse metabolic effects, thiazide diuretics are effective in reducing cardiovascular mortality.[83,84] Fluid overload is a frequently encountered problem in subjects with renal impairment, and loop diuretics have an important role in the overall management of these patients.

ACE inhibitors

The intrarenal renin–angiotensin system may play a pivotal role in the pathogenesis of progressive renal injury, and the inappropriately high renin–angiotensin activity that is usually found in chronic renal insufficiency provides a rationale for the use of ACE inhibitors in patients with renal insufficiency and hypertension. Angiotensin raises glomerular capillary pressure, affects mesangial traffic of macromolecules, and influences mesangial cell mitogenesis.[85,86]

In many rat models of systemic and glomerular hypertension, ACE inhibitors normalize glomerular capillary hydraulic pressure and limit the development of structural injury.[87] Mann et al compared the effects of a conventional antihypertensive therapy with the effects of captopril or enalapril in patients with similarly elevated pretherapy creatinine and blood pressure levels.[88] After 1 year, blood pressure levels were controlled comparably in both groups but serum creatinine levels had stabilized in the group treated with ACE inhibitors while they had risen steadily in the other group. Similarly, Rodicio et al observed the effects of captopril in a group of patients whose renal function had deteriorated during a 12–24 month period despite satisfactory control of hypertension by hydralazine, propanolol,

and frusemide: the progression of renal failure was arrested by captopril over a 3-year period.[89]

However, a recent review of both short-term (less than 12 months) and long-term (more than 12 months) studies of ACE inhibition in non-diabetic renal disease concluded that the majority of studies in humans had not been adequately randomized and had been of too short a duration or confounded by design difficulties to allow any conclusions concerning the effect of ACE inhibitors on the progression of renal disease.[90]

The beneficial effects of ACE inhibitors in retarding the progression of diabetic nephropathy is more convincing and has already been discussed.[43,50,53] Apart from a possible renal-protective effect, ACE inhibitors are of proven benefit in patients with left ventricular dysfunction and lead to reduced cardiovascular morbidity and mortality.[91,92] Improved outcome was also seen in post-infarct patients with left ventricular dysfunction.[93,94]

Reversible acute renal failure is an important hazard of ACE inhibitor therapy, and its presence strongly suggests bilateral renal artery stenosis or an arterial stenosis of a solitary kidney. However, renal failure can occur after ACE inhibitor therapy in patients who have no demonstrable stenosis of the renal arteries. In such patients, sodium depletion is almost invariably present. ACE inhibitors and diuretics should be used with caution, particularly in elderly, atheromatous, and diabetic patients and in patients with diffuse small vessel disease. Renal function should be closely monitored when initiating therapy and a rise in serum creatinine should lead one to suspect renovascular disease.

Since nearly all ACE inhibitors are excreted by the kidneys, dose adjustment is necessary in patients with severely impaired renal function. For some ACE inhibitors, such as captopril, enalapril, lisinopril, and perinopril, the high elimination fraction by haemodialysis necessitates a supplemental dose after dialysis. As glomerular filtration rate falls in patients with renal disease, serum potassium tends to rise. Inhibition of aldosterone production by administration of ACE inhibitors further reduces potassium excretion and may precipitate life-threatening hyperkalaemia, especially when combined with potassium supplements or potassium-sparing diuretics. Serum potassium should be checked several days after the start of therapy in order to exclude hyperkalaemia, particularly in diabetics and in patients already on beta-blockers or non-steroidal anti-inflammatory agents.

It is still debatable whether ACE inhibitors are better than other antihypertensive drugs in retarding the decline of renal function, and if so to what extent this is due to better blood pressure control and to what extent it is due to another, specific effect. Patients with renal failure are more susceptible to cardiovascular disease and so the beneficial effects, particularly in patients with reduced left ventricular function, make ACE inhibitors a valuable asset in the management of hypertension. Furthermore, they have the added advantage of being metabolically neutral, and they do not affect either lipids or glycaemic control.

Calcium antagonists

Calcium antagonists reverse afferent arteriolar vasoconstriction but have little effect on the efferent arteriole. In contrast to direct-acting vasodilators, such as hydralazine and minoxidil, calcium antagonists attenuate the expected adaptive changes in peripheral vascular resistance, heart rate, and extracellular fluid volume that eventually counteract the initial reduction in blood pressure. Renal blood flow, glomerular filtration rate, filtration fraction, and urinary sodium excretion are all increased. From the theoretical point of view, calcium

antagonists should not be effective in preventing glomerular injury, because they result in glomerular hypertension. However, in a study involving patients with a variety of chronic renal disease, calcium antagonists were found to slow the decline in renal function.[9] Others have failed to find a beneficial effect of calcium antagonists on proteinuria in hypertensive patients with chronic renal failure.[95] Recently, Zuchelli et al compared the effects of captopril and nifedipine on renal function[51] and no difference was found in the progression rate of renal insufficiency between the groups over a 3-year period. However, this study did show that those with higher blood pressure had a greater rate of decline of renal function, thus confirming again the importance of blood pressure control. Another advantage of using calcium antagonists is that they are metabolically neutral and do not affect either glucose or lipid metabolism

Aside from their role in treating hypertension, it appears that calcium antagonists have a protective role in several models of acute renal insufficiency, including the prevention of acute renal failure and protection against the nephrotoxic effects of cyclosporin.

There is evidence that elevated intracellular calcium plays a role in the pathogenesis of acute renal failure.[96] In animal studies, in renal failure induced by glycerol and certain nephrotoxic antibiotics and in renal failure induced by arterial clamping, administration of calcium antagonists before the manoeuvres that led to renal failure can reduce renal damage.[97,98,99] In humans too, studies have shown that calcium antagonists can protect the kidney against damage from radiographic contrast agents.[100] It is postulated that calcium antagonists attenuate nephrotoxicity by reducing the intracellular calcium load, resulting in less vasoconstriction.

Calcium antagonists appear to be able to protect the kidneys against the nephrotoxic effect of cyclosporin. Several randomized clinical trials have demonstrated that calcium antagonists reverse cyclosporin-mediated renal vasoconstriction, and that they confer renal protection in cadaver kidney transplant recipients.[101,102] Moreover, the prophylactic administration of calcium antagonists to donor kidneys has been shown to ameliorate post-transplantation renal insufficiency.[101,103,104]

Dosage adjustment is not necessary for the dihydropyridine class of calcium antagonists which are predominantly excreted by the liver. Nifedipine is one such agent. In addition, dialysis has little effect on the clearance of these drugs, largely because they are protein-bound and lipophilic, and so supplemental dosing is not needed after dialysis. In summary, calcium antagonists are effective antihypertensive agents. They may also have renal protective effects that favour their use in many clinical situations when renal function is impaired.

Beta-blockers

Beta-blockers may be chosen as initial therapy, particularly in patients with coronary artery disease, as their cardioprotective role, particularly in the post-infarct period, is established beyond doubt.[48,49] They should, however, be used with caution in patients with congestive cardiac failure because of their negative inotropic effect. Both selective and non-selective beta-blockers increase plasma triglyceride concentrations and may lower HDL cholesterol, though it seems that non-selective drugs have a more consistent effect on HDL. However these changes are modest and have to be weighed against the cardioprotective effect of beta-blockers. Moreover, renin secretion is suppressed by beta-blockers, which makes beta-blockers a logical antihypertensive agent in hypertension associated with renal diseases where there is often hyper-reninaemia.

In general, beta-blockers with low lipid solubility are excreted by the kidney, and dose reduction is necessary in renal failure.

Alpha-blockers and direct vasodilators

Alpha-blockers inhibit postjunctional alpha-receptors. Prazosin, doxazosin, terazosin, and indoramin are drugs in this group. They have a favourable effect on lipids, decreasing total cholesterol, triglycerides, LDL cholesterol, and VLDL cholesterol and increasing HDL cholesterol levels. Moreover, alpha-blockers can induce a reduction in left ventricular mass, another risk factor for cardiovascular diseases. However, despite an improvement in the risk factors profile, there is as yet no long-term data that they can reduce mortality from cardiovascular disease. Postural hypotension can occur and may be a particular problem in diabetic patients with renal failure, especially if they have concomitant autonomic neuropathy. Other vasodilators, such as minoxidil and hydralazine, can be used in patients with renal impairment, but fluid retention and tachycardia occur, and these side effects often necessitate the addition of diuretics and beta-blockers.

Role of bilateral nephrectomy

In a small proportion of patients with end-stage renal failure, blood pressure remains elevated despite adequate volume control. These patients often have an inappropriately high levels of renin, and bilateral nephrectomy in these patients sometimes leads to a reduction in blood pressure. However, bilateral nephrectomy is now infrequently performed as, apart from the obvious operative risks, patients who have had the operation have a greater problem with anaemia and renal osteodystrophy. Moreover, with the availability of more antihypertensive drugs, particularly ACE inhibitors, blood pressure can usually be controlled without resorting to nephrectomy. Occasionally, in renal transplant patients whose hypertension is poorly controlled despite being on maximal antihypertensive medication, bilateral nephrectomy is performed in order to preserve the allograft function.

Summary and recommendations

The primary aim of antihypertensive treatment in patients with renal failure is to attenuate the decline in renal function and to reduce the incidence of cardiovascular disease, the most important cause of morbidity and mortality among patients with chronic renal failure. Hypertension, lipid-profile abnormalities, glucose intolerance, and left ventricular hypertrophy are found in most patients with chronic renal failure and are responsible for the increased incidence of atherosclerosis. Four groups of hypertensive patients who are particularly at risk of progressing to end stage renal failure were identified by the Working Group on Hypertension and Chronic Renal Failure:[2] blacks, those with chronic renal failure, diabetics, and the elderly. Apart from these groups of patients, the presence of significant proteinuria might be the marker of the subset of patients with essential hypertension who risk developing progressive renal disease. Recently, an independent association between cardiovascular mortality and proteinuria has been described in patients with type 2 diabetes and in patients with essential hypertension..[42,105]

There is currently no consensus about the target blood pressure that is most beneficial for ameliorating the progression of renal failure. In patients with diabetic nephropathy reduction of blood pressure to values well within the normal range has been shown to slow the decline in renal function, and there is little to suggest the opposite in patients with nephropathy due to other causes. All available information concerning chronic renal failure and hypertension suggests that reduction of severe, moderate, and mild hypertension to less than 140/90 mmHg could reduce the incidence of end-stage renal failure. Cruickshank et al have demonstrated a J-shaped relationship between blood pressure and cardiovascular mortality.[106] Although this concept of excessive lowering of blood pressure resulting in increased cardiovascular risk is not universally accepted, caution should perhaps be exercised when treating hypertension in renal patients with pre-existing coronary heart disease.

A beta-blocker should be the drug of choice for a patient with hypertension and ischaemic heart disease but should be avoided in patients with peripheral vascular disease, heart block, or chronic obstructive airways disease. An ACE inhibitor should be introduced early in patients with left ventricular dysfunction, and there is evidence supporting a potential renal protective role in retarding the progression of renal dysfunction; this evidence is particularly strong in the diabetic subgroup. ACE inhibitors are useful agents in renin-dependent hypertension and are often effective in treating resistant hypertension in dialysis patients. Diuretics are useful in the treatment of fluid retention but their usefulness rapidly diminishes when there is significant renal impairment. Generally speaking, calcium antagonists and alpha-blockers are well-tolerated agents and can be considered for use either as first-line antihypertensive agents or as adjunctive therapeutic agents in the management of hypertension in renal failure.

Treatment should be tailored to the needs of the patients and should be individualized. The drugs prescribed should have the least adverse effects and the ultimate aim is to reduce end-organ damage. Finally, the pharmacokinetics of many drugs change in end-stage renal failure, and this should be borne in mind when antihypertensive drugs are prescribed.

References

1   Luke RG. Essential Hypertension: A renal disease? A review and update of the evidence. *Hypertension* 1993; **21**:380–90.

2   National High Blood Pressure Education Program Working Group Report on hypertension and chronic renal failure. *Arch Intern Med* 1991; **151**:1280–7.

3   Brazy PC, Stead WW, Fitzwilliam JF. Progression of renal insufficiency. Role of blood pressure. *Kidney Int* 1989; **35**:670–4.

4   Disney AP. *Australia and New Zealand Dialysis and Transplant Registry* (ANZDATA), 13th Report, Issue no. 727-3738. Woodville: Queen Elizabeth Hospital, 1990.

5   ter Wee PM, Donker AJM. Clinical strategies for arresting progression of renal disease. *Kidney Int* 1992; **42**(suppl 38):S114–S120.

6   Whelton PK, Klag MJ. Hypertension as a risk factor for renal disease. Review of clinical and epidemiological evidence. *Hypertension* 1989; **13**(suppl I): I-19.

7   Klahr S. The modification of diet in renal disease study. *N Eng J Med* 1989; **320**:864–6.

8   Baldwin DS, Neugarten J. Role of hypertension in the evolution of renal disease. In Maschio G, Campese VM, Valvo E, Oldrizzi L, eds. 1987; **54**:63–76: Hypertension and Renal Disease. *Contrib Nephrol*. Basel: Karger.

9   Brazy PC and Fitzwilliam JF. Progressive renal disease; role of race and antihypertensive medication. *Kidney Int* 1990; **37**:1113–19.

10 Lindeman RD, Tobin JD, Shock NW. Association between blood pressure and the rate of decline in renal function with age. *Kidney Int* 1984; **26**:861–8.

11 Excerpts from United States Renal Data System 1991. Annual Report: III. Causes of end stage renal disease. *Am J Kidney Dis* 1990; **16**(suppl 2):22–8.

12 Frolich ED, Messerli FH, Dunn FG, Oigman W, Ventura HO, Sundgaard-Riise K. Greater renal vascular involvement in the black patient with essential hypertension. A comparision of systemic and renal haemodynamics in black and white patients. *Miner Electrolyte Metab* 1984; **10**:173.

13 Kincaid-Smith P,Whitworth JA. Pathogenesis of hypertension in chronic renal failure. *Semin Nephrol* 1988; **8**:155.

14 Budman DR, Steinberg AD. Hypertension and renal disease in systemic lupus erythematosus. *Arch Intern Med* 1967; **136**:1003.

15 Danielson H, Kornerup HJ, Olsen S, Posborg V. Arterial hypertension in chronic glomerulonephritis. An analysis of 310 cases. *Clin Nephrol* 1983; **19**:284–7.

16 Arze RS, Ramos JM, Owen JP et al. The natural history of chronic pyelonephritis in the adult. *Q J Med* 1982; **51**:396–410.

17 Dworkin LD, Feiner HD. Glomerular injury in uninephrectomised spontaneously hypertensive rats. A consequence of glomerular capillary hypertension. *J Clin Invest* 1986; **77**:797–808.

18 Dworkin LD, Feiner HD, Randazzo J. Glomerular hypertension and injury in deoxycorticosterone-salt rats on antihypertensive therapy. *Kidney Int* 1987; **31**:718–24.

19 Blantz RC, Gabbai F, Gushwa LC, Wilson CB. The influence of concomitant experimental hypertension and glomerulonephritis. *Kidney Int* 1987; **32**:652–3.

20 Neugarten J, Feiner HD, Schacht RG, Gallo GR, Baldwin DS. Aggravation of experimental glomerulonephritis by superimposed clip hypertension. *Kidney Int* 1982; **22**(3):257–63.

21 Arze RS, Ramos JM, Owen JP, Wilkinson R, Kerr DNS. The natural history of chronic pyelonephritis in the adult. *Q J Med* 1982; **210**:396–410.

22 Reubi FC. Hypertension. In: Grantham JJ, Gardner KD, eds. *Problems in Diagnosis and Management of Polycystic Kidney Disease*. Kansas City: PKR Foundation, 1985:121–8.

23 Blythe WB. Natural history of hypertension in renal disease. *Am J Kidney Dis* 1985; **4**:A50–A56.

24 Maschio G, Oldrizzi L, Rugiu C. Role of hypertension on the progression of renal disease in man. *Blood Purif* 1988; **6**:250–7.

25 Hannedouche T, Chauveau P, Kalou F, Albouze G, Lacour B. Factors affecting progression in advanced chronic renal failure. *Clin Nephrol* 1993; **39**:312–20.

26 Pettinger WA, Lee HC, Reisch J, Mitchell HC. Long-term improvement in renal function after short-term strict blood pressure control in hypertensive nephrosclerosis. *Hypertension* 1989; **13**:766–72.

27 Kincaid-Smith P, McMichael J, Murphy EA. Clinical course and pathology of hypertension with papilloedema. *Q J Med* 1958; **37**:117–53.

28 Nolan CR, Linas SL. Accelerated and malignant hypertension. In: Schrier RW, Gottschalk CW, eds. *Diseases of the Kidney*, 4th edition. Boston: Little, Brown, 1988: 1703–824.

29 Vane JR, Anggard EE, and Botting RM. Regulatory functions of the vascular endothelium. *N Engl J Med* 1990; **323**:27.

30 Davis BA, Crook JE, Vestal RE, Oates JA. Prevalence of renovascular hypertension in patients with grade III or IV hypertensive retinopathy. *N Engl J Med* 1979; **301**:1273–6.

31 Carmichael DJS, Mathias CJ, Sneu ME, Peart S. Detection and investigation of renal artery stenosis. *Lancet* 1986; **i**:667–70.

32 Harvey RJ, Krumlovsky F, Deljerco F, Martin HG. Screening for renovascular hypertension. Is renal digital subtraction angiography the preferred non-invasive test? *JAMA* 1985; **254**:388–93.

33 Dresberg AL, Paushter DM, Lammert GK, Hale JC, Troy RB, Novick AC et al. Renal artery stenosis: evaluation with colour flow imaging. *Radiology* 1990; **177**:749–53.

34 Jonker GJ, Huisman RM, de Zeeuw D. Enhancement of screening tests for renovascular hypertension by angiotensin-converting enzyme inhibition. *Nephrol Dial Transplant* 1993; **8**:798–807.

35 Bengis RG, Coleman TG. Antihypertensive effect of prolonged blockade of angiotensin formation in benign and malignant, one and two kidney Goldblatt hypertensive rats. *Clin Sci* 1979; **57**:53–62.

36 Michel JB, Dussaule JC, Choudat L et al. Effects of antihypertensive treatment in one-clip two-kidney hypertension in rats. *Kidney Int* 1985; **29**:1011–20.

37 Hollenberg NK. Medical therapy of renovascular hypertension: efficacy and safety of captopril in 269 patients. *Cardiovasc Rev Rep* 1983; **4**:854–79.

38 Jackson B, Murphy BF, Johnston CI, Kincaid-Smith P, Whitworth JA. Renovascular hypertension: treatment with the oral angiotensin-converting enzyme inhibitor enalapril. *Am J Nephrol* 1986; **6**:182–6.

39 Franklin SS, Smith RD. Comparison of effects of enalapril plus hydrochlorothiazide versus standard triple therapy on renal function in renovascular hypertension. *Am J Med* 1985; **79**(suppl 3C):14–23.

40 Andersen AR, Christiansen JS, Andersen JK, Kreiner S, Deckert T. Diabetic nephropathy in type 1 (insulin-dependent) diabetes: An epidemiological study. *Diabetologia* 1983; **25**:496–501.

41 Cowie CC, Port FK, Wolfe RA, Savage PJ, Mou PP, Hawthorne VM. Disparities in incidence of diabetic end-stage renal disease according to race and type of diabetes. *N Eng J Med* 1989; **16**:1074–9.

42 Viberti GC, Hill RD, Jarrett RJ, Argyropoulos A, Mahmud U, Keen H. Microalbuminuria as a predictor of clinical nephropathy in insulin-dependent diabetes mellitus. *Lancet* 1982; **1**:1430–2.

43 Mogensen CE. Prevention and treatment of renal disease in insulin-dependent diabetes mellitus. *Semin Nephrol* 1990; **10**:260–73.

44 Joint Working Party on Diabetic Renal Failure of the British Diabetic Association, Renal Association and Research Unit, Royal College of Physicians. Renal failure in diabetics in the United Kingdom. Deficient provision of care in 1985. *Diabetic Med* 1988; **5**:79–84.

45 Mogensen CE. Long-term antihypertensive treatment inhibiting progression of diabetic nephropathy. *Br Med J* 1982; **285**:685–8.

46 Parving HH, Andersen AR, Smidt UM, Svendsen PA. Early aggressive antihypertensive treatment reduces rate of decline in

kidney function in diabetic nephropathy. *Lancet* 1983; **1**:1175–9.

47 Micossi P, Pollavini GG, Raggi U, Librenti MC, Garimberti B, Beggi P. Effects of metoprolol and propanolol on glucose tolerance and insulin secretion in diabetes mellitus. *Horm Metab Res* 1984; **16**:59–63.

48 Olsson G, Wikstrand J, Warnold I et al. Metoprolol-induced reduction in postinfarction mortality: pooled results from five double-blind randomised trials. *Eur Heart J* 1992; **13**:28–32.

49 ISIS-1 (First International Study of Infarct Survival) Collaborative Group. Randomised trial of intravenous atenolol among 16027 cases of suspected acute myocardial infarction. *Lancet* 1986; **ii**:57–66.

50 Parving H-H, Hommel E, Nielsen MD. Effect of captopril on blood pressure and kidney function in normotensive insulin dependent diabetes with nephropathy. *Br Med J* 1989; **299**:533–6.

51 Zucchelli P, Zuccala A, Borghi M et al. Long-term comparison between captopril and nifedipine in the progression of renal insufficiency. *Kidney Int* 1992; **42**:452–8.

52 O'Donnell MJ, Rowe BR, Lawson N, Horton A, Gyde OH, Barnett AH. Comparison of the effects of an angiotensin-converting enzyme inhibitor and a calcium antagonist in hypertensive, macroproteinuric diabetic patients: a randomised double-blind study. *J Hum Hypertens* 1993; **7**:333–9.

53 Kasiske BL, Kalil RSN, Mar JZ, Lee AO, Liao M, Keane WF. Effect of antihypertensive therapy on the kidney in patients with diabetes: a META regression analysis. *Arch Int Med* 1993; **118**: 129–38.

54 Guidi E, Bianchi G, Rivolta E et al. Hypertension in man with a kidney transplant: role of familial versus other factors. *Nephron* 1985; **41**:14–21.

55 Bianchi G, Fox U, Di Francesco GF, Giovanetti AM, Pagetti D. Blood pressure changes produced by kidney cross-transplantation between spontaneously hypertensive rats and normotensive rats. *Clin Sci* 1974; **47**:435–48.

56 Tobian L, Coffee K, McCrea P, Dahl L. A comparison of the antihypertensive potency of kidneys from one strain of rats susceptible to salt hypertension and kidneys from another strain resistant to it. *J Clin Invest* 1966; **45**:1080.

57 Curtis JJ. Hypertension and kidney transplantation. *Am J Kidney Dis* 1986; **7**:181–96.

58 Van Ypersele de Strihou C. Prevalence, aetiology and treatment of late post transplant hypertension. In: Hamburger J, Crosnier J, Grünfeld JP, Maxwell MH, eds. Advances in Nephrology 12. Chicago: Year Book, 1983:41–60.

59 West TH, Turcotte JG, Vander A. Plasma renin activity, sodium balance and hypertension in a group of renal transplant recipients. *J Lab Clin Med* 1969; **73**:564.

60 Popovtzer MM, Pinnggera W, Katz FH et al. Variations in arterial blood pressure after kidney transplantation. *Circulation* 1973; **47**:1297–305.

61 Bachy C, Alexandre GPJ, von Ypersele de Strihou C. Hypertension after renal transplantation. *Br Med J* 1976; **2**:1287.

62 Jacquot C, Idatte MJ, Bedrossian J, Weiss Y, Safar M, Bariety J. Long-term blood pressure changes in renal homotransplantation. *Arch Intern Med* 1978; **138**:223.

63 Bennett WM, McDonald WJ, Lawson RK, Porter GA. Posttransplant hypertension: studies of cortical blood flow and the renal pressor system. *Kidney Int* 1974; **6**:99.

64 Kasiske BL. Possible causes and consequences of hypertension in stable renal transplant recipients. *Transplantation* 1987; **44**:639–43.

65 McHugh MI, Tanboga H, Wilkinson R. Alternate-day steroids and blood pressure control after renal transplantation. *Proc Eur Dial Transpl Assoc* 1980; **17**:496.

66 European Multicentre Trial Group: Cyclosporin A in cadaveric renal transplantation: one year follow-up of a multicentre trial. *Lancet* 1982; **2**:896–989.

67 Myers BD, Sibley R, Newton L et al. The long-term course of cyclosporine associated chronic nephropathy. *Kidney Int* 1988; **33**:590–600.

68 Schacter M. Cyclosprin A and hypertension. *J Hypertens* 1988; **6**:511–16.

69 Muirhead N. Recombinant human erythropoietin in anaemic patients on haemodialysis:

Canada. In: Erslerv AJ, Adamson JW, Winearls GG, eds. *Erythropoietin Molecular, Cellular and Clinical Biology*. Baltimore: John Hopkins University Press: 241–68.

70   Sundal E. Correction of anaemia of chronic renal failure with recombinant human erythopoietin: Safety and efficacy of one year treatment in a European multicenter study in 150 haemodialysis-dependent patients. *Nephrol Dial Transplant* 1989; **4**:979.

71   Schaefer MF, Walter HH, Massry SG. Treatment of renal anaemia with recombinant human erythropoietin. *Am J Nephrol* 1989; **9**: 353–62.

72   Adamson JW, Eschbach JW. Management of the anaemia of chronic renal failure with recombinant erythropoietin. *Q J Med* 1989; **73**:1093–101.

73   Neff MS, Kim KE, Persoff M, Onesti G, Swartz C. Haemodynamics of uraemic anaemia. *Circulation* 1971; **43**:876–83.

74   Coleman TG. Haemodynamics of uraemic anaemia. *Circulation* 1972; **45**:510–11.

75   Lederla RM, Saul F, Klaus D, Achwarze D. Influence of erythropoietin on haemodynamics, left ventricular performance and neurohumoral factors in endstage renal failure. *13th Scientific Meeting of the International Society of Hypertension*, Montreal 1990:224 [abstract].

76   Evans RW, Rader B, Manninnen DL. Cooperative Multicentre Epo Clinical Trial Group. The quality of life of haemodialysis recipients treated with recombinant human erythropoietin. *JAMA* 1990; **263**:825.

77   Fahal IH, Yaqoob M, Ahmad R. Phlebotomy for erythropoietin-induced malignant hypertension. *Nephron* 1992; **61**:214–16.

78   Lifschitz MD, Kirschenbaum MA, Rosenblatt SG, Gibney R. Effect of saralasin in hypertensive patients on chronic dialysis. *Ann Intern Med* 1977; **88**:23–7.

79   Vaughan ED Jr, Carey RM, Ayers CR, Peach MJ. Haemodialysis-resistant hypertension: control with an orally active inhibitor of angiotensin-converting enzyme. *J Clin Endocrinol* 1979; **48**:869–71.

80   Zuchelli P, Santoro A, and Zuccala A. Genesis and control of hypertension in haemodialysis patients. *Semin Nephrol* 1988; **8**:163–8.

81   Kleinknecht C, Laouari D. The influence of dietary components on experimental renal diseases. *Contemp Issues Nephrol* 1986; **14**:17–35.

82   El Nahas AM, Zoob SN, Evans DJ, Rees AJ. Chronic renal failure after nephrotoxic nephritis in rats: contribution to progression. *Kidney Int* 1987; **32**:173–80.

83   SHEP Cooperative Research Group. Prevention of stroke by antihypertensive drug treatment in older persons with isolated systolic hypertension. Results of the Systolic Hypertension in the Elderly Program. *JAMA* 1991; **265**:3255–64.

84   MRC Working Party. Medical research council trial of treatment of hypertension in older adults: principal results. *Br Med J* 1992; **304**:405–12.

85   Ruilope LM, Miranda B, Morales JM, Rodicio JL, Romero CJ, Raij L. Converting enzyme inhibition in chronic renal failure. *Am J Kidney Dis* 1989; **2**:120–6.

86   Raij L, Keane WF. Glomerular mesangium. Its function and relationship to angiotensin II. *Am J Med* 1985; **79**:24–36.

87   Anderson S, Rennke HG, Brenner BM. Therapeutic advantage of converting enzyme inhibitors in arresting progressive renal disease associated with systemic hypertension in the rat. *J Clin Invest* 1986; **77**:1993–2000.

88   Mann JFE, Reisch C, Ritz E. Use of angiotensin-converting enzyme inhibitors for the preservation of kidney function. *Nephron* 1990; **55**(suppl 1):38–42.

89   Rodicio JL, Alcazar JM, Ruilope JL. Influence of converting enzyme inhibition on glomerular filtration and proteinuria. *Kidney Int* 1990; **38**:590–4.

90   ter Wee PM, Epstein M. Angiotensin-converting enzyme inhibitors and progression of nondiabetic chronic renal disease. *Arch Intern Med* 1993; **153**:1749–59.

91   The SOLVD Investigators. Effect of enalapril on mortality and the development of heart failure in asymptomatic patients with reduced left ventricular ejection fractions. *N Engl J Med* 1992; **327**:685–91.

92   Yusuf S, Pepine CJ, Garces C et al. Effect of enalapril on myocardial infarction and unstable angina in patients with low ejection fractions. *Lancet* 1992; **340**:1173–8.

93   ISIS-4 Collaborative Group. Fourth International Study of Infarct Survival: protocol for a large simple study of the effects of oral mononitrate, of oral captopril, and of intravenous magnesium. *Am J Cardiol* 1991; **68**:86D–100D.

94   Pfeffer MA, Braunwald E, Moye LA et al. on behalf of the SAVE investigators. Effect on captopril on mortality and morbidity in patients with left ventricular dysfunction after myocardial infarction. Results of the Survival and Ventricular Enlargement trial. *N Eng J Med* 1992; **327**:669–77.

95   Reams G, Lau A, Knaus V, Bauer JH. The effect of nifedipine GITS on renal function in hypertensive patients with renal insufficiency. *J Clin Pharmacol* 1991; **31**:468–72.

96   Schrier RW, Arnold PE, Van Putten VJ, Burke TJ. Cellular calcium in ischaemic acute renal failure: role of calcium entry blockers. *Kidney Int* 1987; **32**:313–21.

97   Lee SM, Hillman BJ, Clark RL, Michael UF. The effects of diltiazem and captopril on glycerol-induced acute renal failure in the rat: function, pathologic and microangiographic studies. *Invest Radiol* 1985; **20**:961–70.

98   Watson AJ, Gimenez LF, Kassen DK, Stout RL, Whelton A. Calcium channel blockade in experimental aminoglycoside nephrotoxicity. *J Clin Pharmacol* 1987; **27**:625–7.

99   Puschett JB. Calcium antagonists and renal ischaemia. In: Epstein M, Loutzenhiser R, eds. *Calcium Antagonists and the Kidney*. Philadelphia: Hanley and Belfus, 1990:177–85.

100 Russo D, Testa A, Della Volpe L, Sansone G. Randomised prospective study on renal effects of two different contrast media in humans. Protective role of calcium channel blocker. *Nephron* 1990; **55**:254–7.

101 Dawidson I, Rooth P. Effects of calcium antagonists in ameliorating cyclosporine A nephrotoxicity and post-transplant ATN. In: Epstein M, Loutzenhiser R, eds. *Calcium Antagonists and the Kidney*. Philadelphia, P.A. Hanley and Belfus, 1990:233–46.

102 Berg KL, Holdaas H, Endresen L et al. Effects of isradipine on renal function in cyclosporin-treated renal transplanted patients. *Nephrol Dial Transplant* 1991; **6**:725–30.

103 Wagner K, Albrecht S, Neumayer H. Prevention of post-transplant acute tubular necrosis by the calcium antagonist diltiazem. A prospective randomised study. *Am J Nephrol* 1987; **7**:287–91.

104 Neumayer HH, Wagner K. Prevention of delayed graft function in cadaver kidney transplants by diltiazem: Outcome of two prospective, randomized clinical trials. *J. Cardiovasc Pharmacol* 1987; **10**:S170–S177.

105 Yudkin JS, Forrest RD, Jackson CA. Microalbuminuria as a predictor of vascular disease in non-diabetic patients. Islington Diabetes Survey. *Lancet* 1988; **ii**:530–3.

106 Cruickshank JM, Thorp JM, Zacharias FJ. Benefits and potential harm of lowering high blood pressure. *Lancet* 1987; **i**:581–4.

11

Hypertension and cerebrovascular disease

Roger Shinton and Barnabas Panayiotou

This chapter aims to establish the rationale for treating hypertension in stroke patients. It then examines the natural course of blood pressure during and after stroke onset and considers the management of high blood pressure in the acute and chronic phases following a stroke. Lastly, practical problems in dealing with stroke patients are covered. We have sought to offer guidance based on our own clinical practice, backed when appropriate by the scientific evidence gleaned by those working in this challenging field.

Why treat patients with cerebrovascular disease?

The high risk of recurrent stroke

The main benefit from treating high blood pressure is the prevention of disabilities and death caused by stroke. It is widely accepted that patients who have already had a stroke or who have evidence of cerebrovascular disease, such as a transient ischaemic attack, are at a substantially increased risk of a second event. In the large Dutch TIA trial, around 5% of patients who had had a cerebrovascular event went on to develop a stroke every year.[1] Data from the Oxfordshire community stroke project indicated that 30% of stroke patients had suffered a recurrence by 5 years – approximately 10 times the risk of stroke in the general population.[2]

This substantially increased risk is an important consideration in any decision on treatment for hypertension in this group of patients. For both hypertension treatment and other interventions, such as lowering of cholesterol, there is an increasing consensus that any decision to intervene should be related to the baseline risk. Patients at low risk of stroke should probably not have pharmacological interventions, as these carry risks of their own. On the other hand, patients at high risk are more likely to derive benefit from the use of risk-lowering interventions. This balancing of risk and benefit is particularly important in relation to patients with cerebrovascular disease, since these patients tend to be older and to have diseases such as diabetes, ischaemic heart disease, and a history of cigarette smoking, which are all associated with increased risk.

Interpretation of results of existing randomized trials

It is difficult to suggest clear guidelines for blood pressure treatment in patients with cerebrovascular disease because of the lack of substantive trial data in this group, and there is a theoretical problem in generalizing the results from patients predominantly free of overt cerebrovascular disease to those known to have cerebrovascular disease. Some smaller trials in stroke patients have produced conflicting results. In a study of 97 patients, Carter observed a 20% recurrence in patients randomized to treatment compared to 44% in the untreated group,[3] though no significant effect was noted by the Hypertension Stroke Cooperative Study Group in an early randomized trial of 200 patients.[4] With the BEST trial of beta-blockers, treated patients tended to have a worse outcome as measured by discharge alive from hospital.[5] The recent Dutch TIA trial involving around 3000 patients showed no significant improvement in outcome from atenolol.[6]

The data at present, therefore, do not make a strong case for blood pressure treatment but could be consistent with a modest benefit. Lack of data from an adequately sized trial will always mean that decisions on the benefit of treatment are going to be made on inadequate evidence. At present, however, there are few grounds to believe that the occurrence of a minor cerebrovascular event debars a patient from treatment. Indeed, it is inevitable that many patients who have been randomized in the various hypertension trials have had a degree of cerebrovascular disease.

Co-existing clinical problems

The majority of patients who have had a stroke also have a vascular risk factor.[7] These associated clinical conditions (Table 11.1) often determine not only which pharmacological interventions to try but whether or not to treat at all.

Ethics and the decision to treat

The aim of treating high blood pressure is to prevent disabilities and death caused by stroke and, to a lesser extent, cardiac disease. There is an argument, therefore, that once a stroke has occurred it is too late to treat high blood pressure. Major trials of blood pressure treatment have, however, excluded only those

Ischaemic heart disease
Cardiac failure
Atrial fibrillation
Diabetes mellitus
Peripheral vascular disease
Carotid artery disease
Renal disease
Multi-infarct dementia
Epilepsy

Table 11.1
Clinical problems that commonly co-exist with cerebrovascular disease.

patients with a stroke in the preceeding 3 months.[8,9] The decision to treat depends to a substantial extent on where along the spectrum of disability a patient with cerebrovascular disease lies. There seems little logic in denying treatment to a patient who has recovered fully from a cerebral ischaemic event, whether it has lasted for more or less of the 24 hours required by the World Health Organization to classify the event as a definite stroke. The decision whether or not to treat, however, gets more difficult as the level of disability increases. Patients who have had strokes that have put them into the category of persistent vegetative state have been known to have their blood pressure treatment continued via percutaneous gastrostomy. We would consider this inappropriate treatment. For each patient a decision has to be made about the balance of likely useful benefit (Table 11.2). Issues such as the current quality of life and the practicability of administering medication need to be considered. If possible, the views of the patient who has had a stroke on whether or not he or she should continue with medication should be

For	Against
Minor stroke	Major stroke
Good cognition	Poor cognition
Hypertension severe	Hypertension mild
Concurrent angina or cardiac failure	Concurrent peripheral vascular disease (femoral, carotid, renal artery)
Few concerns over compliance	Major concerns over compliance
Treatment well tolerated	Treatment not well tolerated
Few other medications	Complex drug treatment
High patient or carer motivation	Low patient or carer motivation

Table 11.2
Factors for and against the treatment of hypertension in patients with cerebrovascular disease.

sought. This may have to be sensitively probed, and in a significant number of patients it will not be possible. In patients with whom adequate communication is not feasible, the views of relatives and carers should be sought when coming to a conclusion about the merits of antihypertensive drugs.

Blood pressure changes after cerebrovascular events

The phases of blood pressure change

Three phases of blood pressure change following a stroke have been demonstrated.[10] The first 4 days comprise the acute phase. In most patients, blood pressure rises rapidly at the onset of the stroke and usually remains high until the subacute phase. This comprises the period from the 4th to the 10th or 14th day, when in most cases the blood pressure gradually returns

spontaneously to normal levels. In succeeding months or years (the chronic phase) the blood pressure course is more unpredictable, with some patients exhibiting a significant fall and others a significant rise from the blood pressure level at discharge.[11] This pattern of changes in blood pressure have been observed after all types of acute stroke, with the highest levels being noted in patients with haemorrhagic stroke or a previous history of hypertension. Indeed, in the Guy's Hospital score, a very high systolic pressure on admission tends to predict the diagnosis of haemorrhage rather than infarction.[12]

A similar rise and fall in blood pressure is known to occur in transient ischaemic attacks. Recent studies using non-invasive 24-hour ambulatory blood pressure monitoring have also shown that, in both the acute and chronic phases of stroke, the normal circadian rhythm of blood pressure is often disturbed, with a smaller fall or even a rise in nocturnal blood pressure (the 'non-dipping' pattern of blood pressure).[13,14]

Aetiology of initial rise in blood pressure

The initial rise in blood pressure may be explained by a variety of factors,[15] including:

- stimulation of central pressor centres;
- stress due to acute illness;
- hospital admission and 'white coat effect';
- release of cathecholamines and cortico-steroids; and
- a rise in blood pressure secondary to elevated intracranial pressure.

Further explanation for changes in blood pressure after cerebrovascular events has been suggested by reproducible animal experiments, which have demonstrated that a decrease in cerebral perfusion results in a compensatory rise in blood pressure.[10] Given also that cerebrovascular autoregulation is reduced or abolished in acute stroke (especially in patients who are elderly or have pre-existing chronic hypertension),[16] it is now widely believed that the observed acute rise in blood pressure represents, at least in part, a protective response to maintain cerebral blood flow and to minimize brain damage.

Prognosis of hypertension following stroke

Acute phase

In ischaemic stroke most studies have reported that the hypertension observed during the acute illness does not correlate with worse stroke outcome; indeed, recent evidence suggests the opposite may be true.[18]

Data from patients with confirmed subarachnoid haemorrhage suggest that there may be higher rebleeding and mortality rates if the systolic blood pressure is greater than 160 mmHg or the mean blood pressure is greater than 110 mmHg.[17]

In intracerebral haemorrhage with large intracerebral hematomas, there is invariably a rise in intracranial pressure with a secondary rise in systemic blood pressure to maintain cerebral flow. Large or rapid reductions in blood pressure produced by medical intervention are associated with a worse outcome.[17] In many cases of ischaemic stroke, pharmacological reduction of blood pressure has been shown to lead to worsening of the neurological deficit.[15] Furthermore, in animal studies and in some clinical cases, treatments to raise blood pressure have led to improved neurological function. For example, a controlled study of 91 acute stroke patients suggested that raising the blood pressure further using dextrans (up to 210 mmHg systolic) assisted neurological recovery as compared to controls, but no change in mortality was detected.[19]

Chronic phase

In observational studies, patients with cerebrovascular disease and hypertension have sometimes, but not consistently, had a poorer prognosis than those with lower blood pressures. These studies were recently reviewed.[16] Following transient ischaemic attack, the Rochester cohort of 199 patients showed that persistent hypertension was the most significant factor predicting development of stroke. Beevers et al followed 162 stroke patients (mean age 56 years) for a mean of 2 years and found that those with good control of blood pressure (diastolic over 100 mmHg) had a stroke recurrence of 15% as compared to 32% for those with moderately well-controlled blood pressure (diastolic 100–109 mmHg) and 55% for those with poorly controlled blood pressure (diastolic over 110 mmHg). Irie et al in a recent 6-month follow-up of 368 patients (mean age 62 years) reported significantly higher stroke recurrence in those with diastolic pressures > 85 mmHg.[20]

In contrast, neither the patients in the Dutch TIA study[1] nor a study of 1680 stroke patients seen in Minessota between 1950 and 1979[21] showed any benefit from effective treatment of the hypertension.

Asymptomatic cerebrovascular disease

At least 5 recent, detailed studies of elderly hypertensives without a clinical history of stroke revealed a strong correlation between sustained hypertension and a variety of cerebrovascular lesions such as lacunar infarcts, subcortical infarcts, and periventricular infarcts.[22–26] Up to 50% of hypertensive patients were affected, and many had multiple lesions. In those without evidence of left ventricular hypertrophy, vascular cerebral lesions were absent or infrequent.[23] In 1 of these studies, strong correlation was found between high blood pressure and vascular dementia.[26] It is interesting that the presence of cerebrovascular lesions and vascular dementia correlated better with nocturnal than with daytime or 24-hour blood pressure level.[23,25] At present, there is no firm data on whether or not antihypertensive treatment can slow the progression of the vascular dementias. This important question needs to be addressed in a large and carefully planned trial.

Blood pressure management in acute stroke

Indications

It is clear there is no convincing evidence that rapid lowering of elevated blood pressure in acute stroke is beneficial, and more importantly, such intervention can be detrimental. Both the American Heart Association[27] and the Royal College of Physicians of London[28] now recommend that antihypertensive therapy should be instigated rarely and cautiously. It is suggested that markedly elevated pressure after ischaemic stroke (systolic over 200 mmHg or mean blood pressure over 130 mmHg) should be reduced gradually. In intracerebral haemorrhage, treatment for systolic pressures over 200 mmHg or diastolic pressures over 120 mmHg is recommended in order to limit vasogenic oedema.[29] For subarachnoid haemorrhage, systolic blood pressure should be maintained below 160 mmHg, as there is evidence suggesting a greater risk of rebleeding above this level.[17] It is also important to identify those few patients with hypertensive encephalopathy or aortic dissection, whose stroke may be a consequence of these conditions; they need urgent treatment for their high blood pressure.

Blood pressure measurement: which arm to use?

Blood pressure measurement has usually been taken on the arm unaffected by the stroke because of the belief that altered muscle tone influences blood pressure readings. However, a more recent study of multiple simultaneous measurements in acute stroke patients showed no overall difference in blood pressure between the arms of a group of hemiplegic patients.[29] In a minority of patients, an absolute inequality between arms of > 10/8 mmHg was detected, but in some the level was higher in the unaffected arm and in others the level was higher in the hemiplegic arm. These differences were found to be similar to those in elderly patients in general and they are usually due to the presence of occlusive atheromatous vascular disease. It should be remembered the British Hypertension Society recommends measurement of blood pressure in both arms of all patients on at least 1 occasion. If a clinically significant difference is noted, subsequent measurements should be taken using the arm with the higher level.

Which drugs to use?

A number of different compounds can be used effectively if acute severe hypertension does need treatment. Recent reviews of the management of hypertensive emergencies in the USA recommended sodium nitroprusside as the drug of choice in acute ischaemic stroke.[15] This drug is potent and short acting, enabling closely controlled manipulation of blood pressure. In the UK, nifedipine is preferred[30] and can be given sublingually for fast action, or orally or via a nasogastric tube. Intravenous labetalol is an alternative. Drugs that take several days or longer to become effective, e.g. thiazide diuretics, would not be appropriate when a more rapid effect is required. Intravenous hydrallazine, a very effective agent in a variety of other hypertensive emergencies, is contraindicated in acute stroke because it causes cerebral vasodilation and impaired autoregulation.[15]

Patients already on antihypertensive therapy

At least one third of patients admitted with stroke have a history of hypertension and many patients are already on antihypertensive therapy. No studies investigating whether this therapy should be continued have been reported. A reasonable policy is to withdraw antihypertensive drugs after admission and monitor closely the blood pressure level and the patient's condition. If blood pressure remains high after the acute stages of stroke, antihypertensive treatment can be gradually introduced in the same way as in other stroke patients.

Co-existing myocardial infarction

Around 5% of stroke patients are admitted to hospital with concomitant acute myocardial infarction. This is one reason why an electrocardiogram is important in patients with acute stroke. This is particularly important in patients with a history of hypertension. The myocardial infarction may render the blood pressure lower and obviate the need for continued antihypertensive medication. In these patients, it is particularly important to stop current treatment on admission and to monitor the blood pressure in the long term. If drug treatment is then needed, a diuretic or ACE inhibitor should be considered first if there is concern about impaired left ventricular function.

Treatment of chronic hypertension after a stroke
Discussion with patient and carer

For all patients, but particularly those with cerebrovascular disease, it is important to determine the wishes of the patient (or carer) after explanation of the advantages and risks of antihypertensive medication. Early discussion allows the patient or carer to be committed to the planned management. This approach reduces problems with compliance. While discussing the need for treatment the physician should bear in mind that the patient already has a reduced life expectancy. For this reason, the quality of life should remain a high or the highest priority. Overzealous pharmacological management may further reduce the zest for life in patients who are already suffering from the effects of cerebrovascular insults. For these patients, side effects are often less acceptable than they are in fitter patients, who are more easily able to dismiss them as trivial.

Simple regime

For a significant number of stroke patients, remembering to take tablets may be a far more complex problem than in other people. For this reason it is particularly important that any treatment regime is simple. Drugs should be once daily if at all possible. In some cases this may be vital as a drug will need to be given by a carer who may only call once a day. Most classes of antihypertensive medication can now be prescribed as a once-daily dose. At present, it would be sensible to advise that tablets should be taken in the morning. There is no trial data that addresses the question of the time during the day at which medication should be taken. There is, however, concern that medication taken at night could drop the already dipping nocturnal blood pressure to an excessive extent, causing underperfusion of critically ischaemic areas in both the heart and the brain and so lead to further vascular events.

Assess coexisting diseases

A majority of patients with cerebrovascular disease and hypertension are likely to have a concurrent problem such as angina, heart failure or diabetes (see Table 11.1). Assessing these diseases is more difficult in stroke patients and more reliance on investigations such as electrocardiogram and chest x-ray may be required than in fitter people. The baseline investigations required prior to starting treatment for blood pressure are the same as those that should have been already performed to assess someone who is presenting with cerebrovascular disease. Further tests, therefore, are usually not required.

Stroke and concomitant angina

A practical problem with stroke and associated angina is that the assessment of angina is extremely difficult in patients with either cognitive impairment or dysphasia. Close liaison is required with nursing and rehabilitation staff – an electrocardiogram during apparent pain or a trial of treatment may be the only way of determining likely benefit. Patients who suffer from angina but who do not have overt evidence of cardiac impairment may be suitable for calcium channel blocking agents, such as nifedipine, or for a beta-blocker, such as atenolol. Patients with concurrent heart failure potentially benefit from bendrofluazide, from ACE inhibitors, or from ACE inhibitors with bendrofluazide or frusemide.

Stroke and concomitant carotid stenosis

For patients with carotid stenosis it is important to decide on the assessment and possible surgical intervention for this condition.[31] Again, there is little trial data to guide the physician in determining the approach to hypertensive patients with carotid stenosis. Many are cautious about lowering the pressure in cases of severe stenosis as they fear that this may cause critical ischaemia. This concern is based on reports of transient ischaemic attacks related to hypotension.[32] In this situation, however, judicious use of agents would seem justified with systolic pressures over 200 mmHg and diastolic pressures over 115 mmHg. Some recent data from the Systolic Hypertension in Elderly People trial has suggested that treating hypertension can reduce the degree of stenosis.[33]

Stroke and concomitant atrial fibrillation

In patients with atrial fibrillation, early assessment of the possible benefits of wafarin treatment is required. For lone atrial fibrillation, there is accumulating evidence of the useful reduction in stroke with warfarin.[34] The difficulties of monitoring treatment and the not uncommon side effects of gastrointestinal haemorrhage mean the balance of risks has to be weighed carefully for each individual patient. For some patients, aspirin may be the sensible compromise.[35] Atrial fibrillation is not infrequently associated with cardiac failure and this may influence the decision of whether to treat and the choice of therapy. It needs to be remembered that blood pressure is more difficult to measure in patients with atrial fibrillation and this may mean a somewhat high threshold for intervention is used in practice. Again, there are no adequate data addressing the benefits of antihypertensive treatment in patients with atrial fibrillation.

Non-pharmacological approaches

Non-pharmacological approaches both to lowering blood pressure and to reducing the risk of further vascular events are just as important in stroke patients as in others. Stroke patients rarely have the opportunity to discuss the factors that lay behind the occurence of the stroke. In the period following a stroke, any

Intervention	Likely value	Comment
Stop smoking	High	Remains 'unproven' but clearly wise Good compliance Reduces fire hazards
Exercise	High	May be impracticable Encourages well-being Aids rehabilitation
Avoid excessive alcohol	High	Disability and finances dictate compliance Important for carer
Contain weight	Moderate	Important for mobility Compliance poor Immobility a major hindrance Sympathy needed
Reduce salt intake	Moderate	Evidence controversial Can be unpalatable Complex instructions needed
Eat more fruit	Moderate	Easy Many potential benefits
Avoid stress	Low	Importance controversial Practical guidelines hazy
Low-cholesterol diet	Low	Inappropriate for cerebral haemorrhage Association between stroke and cholesterol unclear Reduces risk of coronary heart disease Unpopular dietary change

Table 11.3
Non-pharmacological approaches to lowering blood pressure in stroke patients.

information from the medical team is eagerly picked up by concerned patients and their relatives. For this reason compliance with non-pharmacological approaches can be high. The approaches that may be indicated are illustrated in Table 11.3. Personal experience suggests good compliance with stopping smoking and limiting alcohol intake; patients are often keen to exercise but are now limited by their disability. Some are worried that exercise may be inappropriate and education to correct this myth is important.

Containing or losing weight is particularly difficult for stroke patients. Notable successes, however, can occur in very overweight patients restricted by both their obesity and their stroke. This devastating combination means that strict dietary control can produce substantial weight loss albeit over several months. Weight loss in these instances is more important for rehabilitation than control of blood pressure or diabetes, but the two can be presented as twin benefits.

There is again, no adequate trial evidence that indicates that any of these interventions is 'proven'. Generalization of interventions in other patient groups and a review of data from risk factor studies, however, lead to a conclusion that this area should not be neglected.[36]

Cerebral haemorrhage

It is the experience of neurosurgeons that patients who survive a ruptured cerebral aneurysm rarely return in later years with a repeat event. This reassuring observation should be given to patients who have suffered such an event. It allows physicians to treat such patients on the same basis as other patients with hypertension. (There is a possible exception to this with polycystic kidney disease and associated cerebral aneurysms.)[37] If an aneurysm has been identified but left unclipped

there is a strong case for close supervision of blood pressure.

For primary intracerebral haemorrhage, caused by presumed microaneurysms, there may be a case for more concern over blood pressure control. It would seem sensible in this group to monitor control of blood pressure very carefully. More data is needed on the risks of recurrent intracerebral haemorrhage and its relation to hypertension. Clearly these patients should not have aspirin or anticoagulation. The identification of this subgroup is one of the clear benefits of a policy of performing CT scans on patients who present with stroke.

Commencement and monitoring of therapy

There is no consensus regarding the optimal timing to initiate long-term antihypertensive therapy in patients with persistently raised blood pressure. Provided that the patient is making good recovery and a further ischaemic or haemorrhagic cerebral event has not occurred, therapy could be started from 10 to 14 days after the stroke, although many physicians prefer to wait longer. Patients with blood pressure over 180 mmHg systolic or over 100 mmHg diastolic should have treatment.[16] Those with blood pressure between 160–180 mmHg systolic or 90–100 mmHg diastolic do not always require treatment. Because of altered cerebral autoregulation, the blood pressure should be lowered slowly and reduced to no less than 140 mmHg systolic and 80–90 mmHg diastolic.[16] Overenthusiastic treatment has been shown to lead to higher stroke recurrence in a recent large study.[20]

Whatever the chosen timing, it is important to ensure regular monitoring of the blood pressure level, irrespective of whether the patient is on the acute ward, in a rehabilitation unit, or at home. In more difficult cases (e.g.

borderline hypertension, suspected 'white coat' hypertension, or the presence of orthostatic hypotension), the application of non-invasive 24-hour ambulatory measurement can be useful to reach a decision about treatment and to monitor its effects.

Practical problems with stroke patients

It is always wise to consider problems which may arise in the administration of treatment (Table 11.4).

Impaired motor function

The biggest problem this presents is transport to the blood pressure clinic and pharmacy. The practicability of overcoming these problems should be ensured before treatment is commenced. In some hospitals, stroke patients, particularly if elderly, attend a day hospital for continued rehabilitation and support. This is a highly convenient setting in which to monitor

---

Dysphasia
Cognitive impairment
Motor impairment
Visual impairment
Swallowing problems
Multiple concurrent diseases
Depression and poor motivation
Financial hardship

Table 11.4
Common problems encountered treating stroke patients.

blood pressure. The relaxed state of the patient should reduce the 'white coat' effect seen in the more formal clinic setting.

Dysphagia

In the acute stages of stroke, when dysphagia is most commonly present, treatment for blood pressure can usually be deferred. If the dysphagia persists, medication can be given in several ways. If limited swallowing is possible, the tablet can be crushed and added to thickened fluids. In more severe cases, the crushed tablet may need to be given via nasogastric tube or percutaneous gastrostomy. Care should be taken to avoid formulations unsuitable for crushing, such as those designed for slow release.

Cognitive impairment

If a decision has been made to treat a cognitively impaired patient care is needed to ensure compliance. In hospital 'self-medication' regimes allow the ward team to assess the competence of the patient in this area. If assistance is needed, a designated carer, who is happy with this supervisory role, needs to be appointed. In such patients, the indications for treatment need to be kept under review.

Dysphasia

In patients with dysphasia, it is important to determine to what extent comprehension has been affected (receptive dysphasia). If there are significant difficulties with comprehension, the comments above for cognitive impairment apply.

Visual impairment

Recent onset of visual impairment presents more problems for patients than long-standing blindness, as adaptive stategies will not have been learnt. For these patients, supervision of medication is usually required.

Multiple coexisting problems

Many illnesses often leads to many tablets. To reduce the problems of polypharmacy, careful consideration is required about the relative importance of different treatments. Conditions with lower priority may not justify treatment. These patients usually have a poor quality of life and limited life expectancy. Symptomatic treatment is usually a high priority. In these patients, it is sometimes appropriate to stop antihypertensive medication and to resist the temptation to push non-pharmacological methods too hard.

Financial hardship

Medication may be low in some families' priorities if funds are limited. Entitlement to financial support from the state can be highlighted as appropriate. This is particularly important to people living on their own with no obvious carer.

Conclusion

We believe hypertensive patients with cerebrovascular disease are entitled to careful and sensitive assessment regarding the merits of blood pressure treatment. During the first few days following stroke, treatment should almost invariably not be given. Once into the chronic phase following stroke, the tendency to neglect blood pressure and its treatment needs to be resisted. At present, it seems wise to continue to treat moderate or high pressures with an appropriate agent if there is a consensus for this, including the agreement of the patient or his or her family. The practical problems of ensuring compliance are greater in stroke patients than others and demand extra care.

References

1 The Dutch TIA Trial Study Group. Predictors of major vascular events in patients with a transient ischemic attack or nondisabling stroke. *Stroke* 1993; **24**:527–31.

2 Burn J, Dennis M, Bamford J, Sandercock P, Wade D, Warlow C. Long-term risk of recurrent stroke after a first-ever stroke: the Oxfordshire community stroke project. *Stroke* 1994; **25**:333–7.

3 Carter AB. Hypotensive therapy in stroke survivors. *Lancet* 1970; **i**:485–9.

4 Hypertension Stroke Co-operative Study Group. Effect of anti-hypertensive treatment on stroke recurrence. *JAMA* 1974; **229**:409–17.

5 Barer DH, Cruickshank JM, Ebrahim SB, Mitchell JRA. Low dose beta blockade in acute stroke ('BEST' trial): an evaluation. *Br Med J* 1988; **296**:737–41.

6 The Dutch TIA Trial Study Group. Trial of secondary prevention with atenolol after transient ischaemic attack or nondisabling ischaemic stroke. *Stroke* 1993; **24**:543–8.

7 Sandercock PAG, Warlow CP, Jones LN, Starkey IR. Predisposing factors for cerebral infarction: the Oxfordshire community stroke project. *Br Med J* 1989; **298**:75–80.

8 Medical Research Council Working Party. MRC trial of treatment of mild hypertension: principal results. *Br Med J* 1985; **291**:97–104.

9 Medical Research Council Working Party. Medical Research Council trial of treatment of hypertension in older adults: principal results. *Br Med J* 1992; **304**:405–12.

10 Loyke HF. The three phases of blood pressure in stroke. *South Med J* 1990; **83**:660–3.

11 Harper GD, Castleden CM, Potter JF. When can we diagnose hypertension after stroke? *Age Ageing* 1990; **20**(suppl 1):23–4.

12 Allen CMC. Clinical diagnosis of the acute stroke syndrome. *Q J Med* 1983; **208**:515–23.

13 Fotherby F, Harper G, Panayiotou B, Castleden C, Potter J. 24 hour blood pressure profiles following stroke. *Clin Sci* 1993; **84**(suppl 28):91.

14 O'Brien E, Sheridan J, O'Malley K. Dippers and non-dippers. *Lancet* 1988;**ii**:397.

15 Phillips SJ. Pathophyiology and management of hypertension acute ischemic stroke. *Hypertension* 1994; **23**:131–6.

16 Shuaib A. Alteration of blood pressure regulation and cerebrovascular disorders in the elderly. *Cerebrovasc and Brain Metab Rev* 1992; **4**:329–45.

17 Lavin P. Management of hypertension in patients with acute stroke. *Arch Intern Med* 1986;**146**:66–8.

18 Jorgensen HS, Nakayama H, Raaschou HO, Olsen TS. Effect of blood pressure and diabetes on stroke in progression. *Lancet* 1994; **344**:156–9.

19 Meier F, Wessel G, Thiele R, Gottschild D, Brandstiatt H. Induced hypertension as an approach to treating acute cerebrovascular ischaemia: possibilities and limitations. *Exp Pathol* 1991; **42**:257–63.

20 Irie K, Yamaguchi T, Minematsu K, Omae T. The J-curve phenomenon in stroke recurrence. *Stroke* 1993; **24**:1844–9.

21 Meissner I, Whisnant JP, Garraway WM. Hypertension management and stroke recurrence in a community (Rochester, Minnesota, 1950–1979). *Stroke* 1988; **19**:459–63.

22 Ikeda T, Gomi T, Kobayishi S, Tsuchiya H. Role of hypertension in asymptomatic cerebral lacunae in the elderly. *Hypertension* 1994; **23**(suppl 1):1259–62.

23 Shimada K, Kawamoto A, Matsubayashi K, Mishinaga M, Kimura S, Ozawa T. Diurnal blood pressure variations and silent cerebrovascular damage in elderly patients with hypertension. *J Hypertens* 1992; **10**:875–8.

24 Kawamoto A, Shimada K, Matsubayashi K, Nishinaga M, Kimura S, Ozawa T. Factors associated with silent multiple lacunar lesions on magnetic resonance imaging in asymptomatic elderly hypertensive patients. *Clin Exp Pharmacol Physiol* 1991; **18**:605–10.

25 Shimada K, Kawamoto A, Matsubayashi K, Ozawa T. Silent cerebrovascular disease in the elderly. Correlation with ambulatory pressure. *Hypertension* 1990; **16**:692–9.

26 Tohgi H, Chiba K, Kimura M. Twenty-four-hour variation of blood pressure in vascular dementia of the Binswanger type. *Stroke* 1991; **22**:603–8.

27 American Heart Association Special Resuscitation Situations (part iv): Stroke. (American Heart Foundation). *JAMA* 1992; **268**:2242–4.

28 Royal College of Physicians Working Party. *Stroke – towards better management.* London: Royal College of Physicians, London, 1989.

29 Panayiotou BN, Harper GD, Fotherby MD, Potter JF, Castleden CM. Interarm blood pressure difference in acute hemiplegia. *J Am Geriatr Soc* 1993 **41**:422–3.

30 O'Connell JE, Gray CS. Treating hypertension after stroke. *Br Med J* 1994; **308**:1523–4.

31 European Carotid Surgery Trialist's Collaborative Group. MRC European Carotid Surgery Trial: interim results for symptomatic patients with severe (70–99%) or with mild (0–29%) carotid stenosis. *Lancet* 1991; **337**:1235–43.

32 Ruff R L, Talman W T, Petito F. Transient ischaemic attacks associated with hypotension in hypertensive patients with carotid artery stenosis. *Stroke* 1981; **12**:353–5.

33 Sutton-Tyrrell K, Wolfson SK, Kuller LH. Blood pressure treatment slows the progression of carotid stenosis in patients with isolated systolic hypertension. *Stroke* 1994; **25**:44–50.

34 The Boston area anticoagulation trial for atrial fibrillation investigators. The effect of low dose warfarin on the risk of stroke in patients with nonrheumatic atrial fibrillation. *N Engl J Med* 1990; **323**:1505–11.

35 Stroke Prevention in Atrial Fibrillation Investigators. Warfarin versus aspirin for prevention of thromboembolism in atrial fibrillation: Stroke Prevention in Atrial Fibrillation II Study. *Lancet* 1994; **343**:687–91.

36 Shinton R, Beevers G. Meta-analysis of the relation between cigarette smoking and stroke. *Br Med J* 1989; **298**:789–94.

37 Chauveau D, Sirieix M, Schillinger F, Legendre C, Grunfeld J. Recurrent rupture of intracranial aneurysms in autosomal dominant polycystic kidney disease. *Br Med J* 1990; **301**:966–7.

12

The hypertensive patient and anaesthesia

Scott H Russell and Peter Hutton

Anaesthetists, correctly, still treat hypertensive patients with respect even though their management is much more satisfactory with modern maintenance therapy than it was in the past. The bad reputation that hypertension has in anaesthetic practice dates from 1929, when it was found that 32% of patients with hypertensive cardiac disease died during or shortly after surgery.[1] In 1947, the death rate in hypertensives following sympathectomy was six times that of normotensives.[2] There were similarly worrying reports on the response to spinal blockade.[3,4] In the 1950s and 1960s (the early days of antihypertensive medication), it was found that the combination of rauwolfia or ganglion blockade and general anaesthesia had the capacity to produce profound hypotension refractory to treatment and there was considerable debate as to whether or not to discontinue such medication for some days before surgery.[5-7]

Hypertension is a common condition that reduces life expectancy, increases the risk of morbid events and, if untreated, produces

Timing	Event	Potential problems
Preoperative	Inadequate preoperative assessment	Lack of appreciation of end-organ damage, e.g. left ventricular hypertrophy, renal impairment
	Premedication	If a high dose is prescribed or if a patient is very sensitive to the drugs used, there may be oversedation with hypoxia and hypercarbia, which is especially dangerous in the presence of left ventricular failure and ischaemic heart disease
	Anxiety	Activation of 'fight or flight' response may produce increased blood pressure, tachycardia, increased systemic vascular resistance, and reduced renal blood flow

Table 12.1
Preoperative events to which the hypertensive patient is subject.

Timing	Event	Potential problems
Intraoperative	Administration of intravenous and volatile anaesthetic agents	Almost all these agents affect systemic vascular resistance and myocardial contractility, and compromise autoregulatory mechanisms
	Spinal and epidural blockade	These techniques produce vasodilatation of vascular beds with resultant hypotension. Severe reactions are possible from unintended intravenous administration of drugs
	Drug interactions	These are many but ususally predictable. Treated hypertensive patients may be very sensitive to short-acting alpha- and beta-stimulants given to treat intraoperative hypotension
	Laryngoscopy and intubation	If there is inadequate depth of anaesthesia, the response of increased sympathetic activity can result in hypertension and tachycardia sufficient to have cardiac effects
	Surgical stimulation	If there is inadequate depth of anaesthesia, the response of increased sympathetic activity can result in hypertension and tachycardia sufficient to have cardiac effects
	Intermittent positive pressure ventilation	In the presence of hypovolaemia, this can produce significant falls in mean blood pressure together with pulse pressure variation synchronous with inspiration and expiration
	Blood loss and/or inappropriate fluid replacement	This produces an acute change in circulating fluid volume and haematocrit, with associated changes in oxygen flux, blood pressure, heart rate, and cerebral, coronary, and renal perfusion
	Procedures to reduce blood loss, e.g. use of vasoconstrictors, elective hypotension	May have unpredictable effects with inadequate organ perfusion and ischaemic damage

Table 12.2
Intraoperative events to which the hypertensive patient is subject

end-organ damage. The pathological mechanisms of these processes and the long-term maintenance therapy of hypertension are described elsewhere: only those aspects particularly relevant to the perioperative period will be discussed here. Anaesthesia and surgery impose additional physiological stresses on the hypertensive patient, which, if not anticipated and monitored, increase the likelihood of adverse incidents in the pre-, intra- and

Timing	Event	Potential problems
Postoperative	Inadequate fluid replacement	Renal impairment, hypotension
	Arousal and reawakening	There may be sudden changes in blood pressure and heart rate
	Inadequate pain control	Following upper abdominal incisions, pain can markedly restrict breathing with resultant hypoxia. Severe pain produces sympathetic response with peripheral vasoconstriction, increased blood pressure and tachycardia
	Over-generous analgesia with sedation	This can cause reduced respiratory drive resulting in hypoxia. It is very dependent upon supplementary facemask oxygen when bellows function of lung is poor with low alveolar ventilation
	Sleep on first three nights	Sleeping patterns are disturbed with apnoeas, hypoxia, and induction of myocardial ischaemia
	Gastrointestinal tract temporarily out of action because of surgery or vomiting, etc	This requires parenteral maintenance therapy for the appropriate period, and necessitates change to different drug or change in dosage because of increased bioavailability of parenteral route

Table 12.3
Postoperative events to which the hypertensive patient is subject.

postoperative periods. The causes and effects of these are summarized in broad categories in Tables 12.1, 12.2, and 12.3.

It should be noted by non-anaesthetists in particular that both local and general anaesthetic techniques have complications: the belief that 'local' techniques (spinals and epidurals) are intrinsically safer and less physiologically disturbing is unproven.

Numerically, the two commonest groups of patients are those with essential hypertension and those with systolic hypertension secondary to generalized arteriopathy. Folkow et al,[8,9] working with hypertensive rats, developed the concept that the high vascular resistance in patients with essential hypertension is due to thickening or adaptive hypertrophy of the muscular media of arterioles. This occurs to such an extent that lumen of the arterioles is reduced. Consequently, even at maximal dilatation, the resistance they offer to blood flow is correspondingly greater than in normotensives, and their range of vasodilatation–vasoconstriction activity lies on a different performance curve: for a given change in smooth muscle length, there is a much greater proportional change in vascular resistance in the hypertensive patient. Tables 12.1, 12.2, and 12.3 demonstrate that before, during, and after anaesthesia and surgery there are many events that affect vascular smooth muscle. Thus hypertensive patients are more sensitive than normotensives to anaesthetic agents, vasoactive drugs and perioperative events such as surgical stimulation and laryngoscopy.

In contrast to patients with essential hypertension, patients who have a generalized rigid arteriopathy have normal diastolic pressure, because they do not possess the arteriolar hypertrophy of essential hypertension. Because of the rigidity of their arterial tree, these patients are, however, very sensitive to changes in stroke volume and cardiac output, and it is easy with many of the factors listed in Tables 12.1, 12.2, and 12.3 to produce wild swings in systolic blood pressure.

This potential instability of the cardiovascular system in the perioperative period has to be interpreted in relation to the incidence and risk factors associated with hypertensive disease, which is the single most important accelerator of atherosclerotic processes affecting the brain, heart, and kidney.[10–12] All hypertensive patients presenting for surgery must be assumed to have coronary arterial disease whether or not there is a history of infarct or angina. Hypertension is the commonest cause of left ventricular hypertrophy, and it also contributes significantly to mortality from myocardial infarction, stroke, aortic dissection, ruptured aortic aneurysm, and sudden death.[11,12]

Left ventricular hypertrophy develops as an adaptive response to the increased pressure load, and when left ventricular hypertrophy can be identified on the electrocardiogram, the cardiac output is usually subnormal. In these cases, the risk of congestive failure is tripled and overall mortality increases sixfold.[11] The hypertrophied ventricle is stiff and less distensible and undergoes poor relaxation during diastole, thus requiring higher filling pressures.[13] Blood supply to the myocardium is decreased by high cavity pressures compressing the subendocardial

region, or by low aortic pressures supplying the main coronary arteries (Fig. 12.1). Cardiac output and blood pressure are therefore very sensitive to factors that influence the optimal left ventricular filling pressure (e.g. hypovolaemia, tachycardia, dysrhythmias) and to factors that cause loss of atrial contraction or loss of the ability of the ventricle to pump. In addition, patients with left ventricular failure usually have a chronic dilatation of the coronary vessels, especially in the subendocardial layers.[14,15] The capacity for further coronary vasodilatation is seriously impaired, and this puts the myocardium at considerable risk in the presence of generalized hypoxia.

In normal patients, there is a wide range of pressures over which the cerebral circulation autoregulates the cerebral blood flow. This autoregulation is affected by the vasodilatational effects of anaesthetic agents, which make flow more dependent upon perfusion pressure.[16] In hypertensive patients, the autoregulation curve is shifted to the right,[17] putting them at greater risk of ischaemia at low blood pressures. Even in treated hypertensives, the curve does not return to normal, and ischaemic thresholds are observed at intermediate values (Fig. 12.2).[18] Of particular importance to anaesthesia are the results that were observed when the blood pressure of conscious patients with accelerated hypertension was reduced rapidly.[19] It was demonstrated that the development of neurological complications (which cannot be detected easily in the anaesthetized patient) occurred at pressures well above the 'normal' autoregulation threshold.

Chronic hypertension also causes changes in the kidneys. The renal vascular resistance is elevated out of proportion to the general increase in systemic vascular resistance, and the kidneys sustain a decrease in total blood flow directly related to the duration and severity of the hypertension.[20]

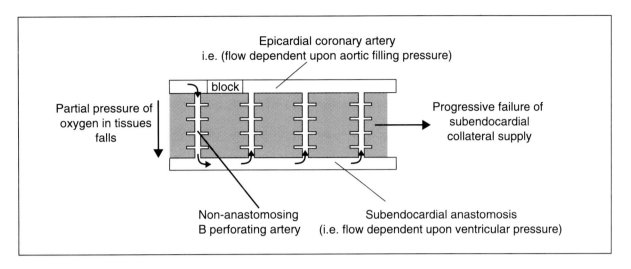

Figure 12.1
Factors affecting perfusion of the left ventricular wall. During diastole (as shown) the subendocardial vessels are patent. During systole they are compressed by ventricular cavity pressure, and collateral perfusion is impossible. The epicardial coronary artery flow is dependent upon aortic filling pressure; flow in the subendocardial region is dependent upon intraventricular cavity pressure. (Adapted from Hutton and Cooper, 1985.[45])

Consequently, the hypertensive patient is at a markedly increased risk from perturbations in the cardiovascular system, and during anaesthesia and surgery, the hypertensive patient is in a situation in which these adverse cardiovascular changes are most likely to occur.

When the hypertensive patient presents for anaesthesia

General principles

From the early 1970s onwards, the management of hypertensive disease during anaesthesia and surgery has received considerable attention. There have been a number of groups who have published in this area.[21-24] Some of their findings have been contradictory, and this has led to the publication of editorials and critical reviews.[25-27] However, there does appear to be increasing evidence that intraoperative cardiovascular instability (to which hypertensive patients are very susceptible) is related to overall outcome. At particular risk are the heart, brain, and kidneys. For example, both hypotension and hypertension adversely affect renal function,[28,29] and patients with a preoperative mean blood pressure of 110 mmHg or over have been reported to be at increased risk of intraoperative falls in blood pressure that cause postoperative complications.[28] Hypertensive patients with cardiomegaly,[30] previous myocardial infarction, valvular disease, or episodes of cardiac failure,[31] are at greater risk of postoperative

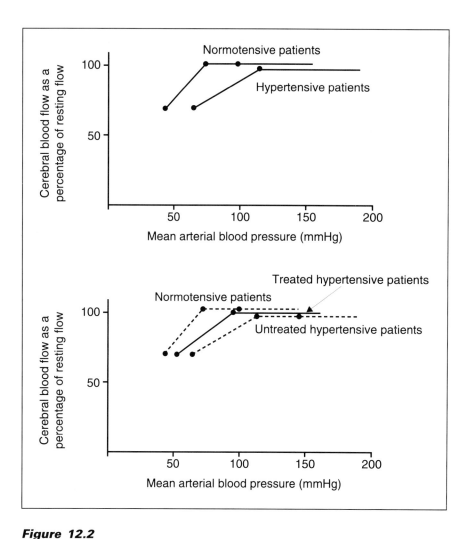

Figure 12.2

Cerebral autoregulation in normotensives, hypertensives and treated hypertensives. The top graph shows the average curves of cerebral blood flow in normotensive and severely hypertensive patients. Each curve is defined by the mean values of resting blood pressure, the lower limit of cerebral blood flow autoregulation, and the lowest tolerated blood pressure. There is a clear shift of the hypertensive patients' curve to the right. The lower graph superimposes onto the upper graph the average curve of cerebral blood flow autoregulation in patients with previously severe hypertension which at the time of the study was controlled effectively by antihypertensive treatment. It can be seen that the curve for the treated patients falls between those of the normotensives and hypertensives. (From Strandgaard, 1976.[18])

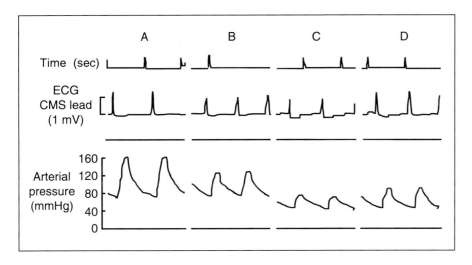

Figure 12.3
Onset of myocardial ischaemia caused by hypotension in a treated hypertensive patient. Progressive deterioration of ST segment depression in relation to decreasing arterial pressure in a treated hypertensive patient with pre-existing coronary arterial disease. The arterial hypotension occurred during elective hypotension for parotid surgery. Note particularly the increased PR interval in panel C associated with the ischaemic response, and the resolution of both the PR interval and the ST segment with the increase in arterial pressure (panel D). (From Prys-Roberts, 1982.[36])

complications if they had mean intraoperative blood pressure changes of 20–40 mmHg for sustained periods.[30,31] Although there has been one report of deliberate hypotension being used safely in well-controlled hypertensives,[32] it is the authors' opinion that deliberate hypotension should not be offered as a routine technique for hypertensive patients. The aim should be to maintain cardiovascular stability.

There are, however, some general principles and guidelines for the management of hypertensive patients who require general or regional anaesthesia:

1. No particular anaesthetic techniques or specific drug combinations have been shown to be better than others for the hypertensive patient.
2. Antihypertensive drug therapy should be continued throughout the perioperative period and given on the day of surgery.
3. Hypertensive patients, whether on treatment or not, are more likely to have fluctuations in blood pressure during anaesthesia, and the extremes of blood pressure can be associated with electrocardiographic evidence of myocardial ischaemia (Fig. 12.3). These changes can result from a variety of causes as listed in Tables 12.1, 12.2, and 12.3).
4. Adequate monitoring is essential for all patients, since malignant physiological

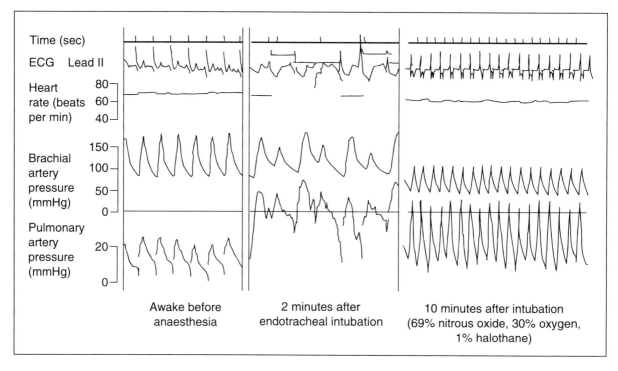

Figure 12.4
Onset of cardiovascular instability during induction and endotracheal intubation in a treated hypertensive patient. Bidirectional junctional tachycardia and hypertension following laryngoscopy and intubation in a treated hypertensive patient. Myocardial ischaemia, indicated by ST segment depression and T wave inversion (right hand panel), persisted during the subsequent maintenance anaesthesia despite the cessation of dysrhythmia. (From Prys-Roberts et al, 1971.[52])

changes can occur rapidly (Fig. 12.4), and monitoring is required not only for the detection of these changes but also to monitor the effects of therapy. The threshold for instituting invasive monitoring should be very low.

Elective surgery and the hypertensive

The well-controlled patient
A well-controlled, fit hypertensive patient with no other risk factors usually behaves predictably during anaesthesia and surgery and, when appropriate, can be operated on as a day case. The commonest problem presented by well-controlled patients is when the surgery prevents oral medication being taken in the postoperative period. This is considered later.

A normotensive or well-controlled hypertensive patient taking a monoamine oxidase inhibitor has traditionally been thought to be at risk of developing a hypertensive crisis in the perioperative period. Accepted practice used to be to withdraw the monoamine oxidase inhibitor 2 weeks before surgery. However, recent findings indicate that the dangers may well have been overstated, and the current recommendation is that the monoamine oxidase inhibitors should be continued up to surgery as with other drugs.[33] If a patient is on a monoamine oxidase inhibitor, pethidine may precipitate a hypertensive crisis and should be avoided. Morphine is the analgesic of choice.[33]

The untreated or poorly controlled patient

There are no universally accepted guidelines to indicate what level of hypertension should warrant elective surgery being delayed. Raised blood pressure on admission is often found to be spurious and to settle over a few hours, so repeated measurements should be made. If it does not settle and if there are no contraindications, even a short period of antihypertensive medication on a beta-blocker may be beneficial in preventing excessive sympathetic responses. Otherwise, the risks of immediate surgery must be weighed against the risks of postponement.

A reasonable view, distilled from the available literature[25,26,34–36] and our own clinical experience, is that patients with diastolic pressures up to 110 mmHg are probably acceptable for anaesthesia, provided that there is nothing abnormal in the history (especially no history of episodic states suggestive of phaechromocytoma) and provided that careful clinical examination reveals no evidence of end-organ damage (especially no signs of left ventricular failure) or of pregnancy. In addition, the following should be normal:

ECG, Echocardiogram, and chest x-ray	(no evidence of severe LVH, conduction abnormalities or dysrhythmias)
Full blood count	(no evidence of polycythaemia)
Urea and electrolytes	(no evidence of renal or endocrine involvement)
Serum glucose	(not diabetic)

If there are any positive findings, the patient should be referred for investigation and treatment. It is also necessary, of course, to consider other factors such as the patient's age, the magnitude and the site of the proposed surgery, and the presence of pulmonary disease and obesity. Ultimately, in difficult cases it must be the experienced clinician who balances the pros and cons of proceeding with surgery or delaying it.

When untreated or poorly controlled hypertensive patients come to anaesthesia, they must have their blood pressures carefully controlled and be well monitored throughout the perioperative period, as described below.

Patients with diastolic pressures above 110 mmHg should be referred for further investigation and treatment.

Patients with the generalized rigid arteriopathy referred to earlier usually present with a high systolic pressure but with a normal or low diastolic pressure. They also need careful preoperative assessment. However, since the disturbed pathology cannot be materially altered by a short course of antihypertensive therapy, no advantage is to be gained by delaying surgery.

Urgent surgery and the hypertensive

If surgery cannot be postponed, an anaesthetic will be needed even if the blood pressure is very high. Meticulous preoperative assessment and preparation are of course mandatory, but the only indications for a rapid reduction in blood pressure are encephalopathy, acute left ventricular failure, and very severe pre-eclampsia or eclampsia.

Otherwise, the risks of rapid reduction (retinopathy and cerebral episodes),[19] are greater than any potential benefits. The key to success with these patients is careful, well-monitored anaesthesia by an experienced clinician and an awareness that the dangers continue well into the postoperative period (see below).

The choice and management of anaesthesia

The management of anaesthesia and the choice of anaesthetic agent in hypertensive patients have been considered in detailed reviews[25,26,34–36] and only general principles will be discussed here.

General anaesthesia

Points for consideration are:

- premedication
- monitoring
- induction
- laryngoscopy and endotracheal intubation
- maintenance anaesthesia
- extubation and immediate recovery

Premedication

Because the hypertensive patient demonstrates exaggerated arterial pressure responses to those events that would cause an increase of pressure in a normal patient, an anxiolytic premedication is often useful. If for any reason an antisialogogue is required, it is better to use intramuscular glycopyrollate or hyoscine rather than atropine, which has a propensity to cause tachycardia.

Monitoring

In order to meet the approved minimal standards, all patients require monitoring and non-invasive blood pressure measurement, pulse oximeter, and electrocardiogram should be established before the induction of anaesthesia and subsequently carried on throughout anaesthesia. For major surgery and for poorly controlled hypertensives, the advantages of invasive pressure monitoring outweigh any disadvantages, and information on the cardiovascular system is gained on a beat-by-beat basis. The establishment of pulmonary artery pressure monitoring and cardiac output will always be a personal decision of the anaesthetist, but the decision needs to be guided by the degree of end-organ damage in the patient – it is especially useful in left ventricular hypertrophy, left ventricular failure, and ischaemic heart disease – and the degree and duration of the physiological insult proposed by the surgery.

Induction

The induction agent chosen is not critical, but it should be given slowly to minimize changes in blood pressure and it should be titrated against individual response.

Laryngoscopy and endotracheal intubation

During light general anaesthesia and under the action of muscle relaxants, laryngoscopy and endotracheal intubation provoke activity of the sympathetic nervous system, which causes the characteristic haemodynamic pressor responses and increased plasma catecholamine concentrations. These unwanted effects can be minimized by skilful adjustment of the depth of anaesthesia and by pretreatment with beta-blockers, potent opioids such as fentanyl or anfentanil, and topical local anaesthesia of the pharynx and larynx.

Maintenance anaesthesia

The choice of drugs for maintenance anaesthesia is not critical, but their appropriate use and a knowledge of drug interactions is.[53] The response to intermittent positive pressure ventilation needs to be observed closely because it can produce unexpectedly large falls and swings in blood pressure. As described above, hypertensive patients show marked responses to changes in circulating fluid volume. There is, therefore, an erosion of the safety margin that is present in a normal patient. Particular attention needs to be given to replacement of blood and evaporative loss and to the maintenance of renal perfusion.

As events occur (e.g. myocardial ischaemia, dysrythmias, hypotension, fall in urine output), the cause should be diagnosed and treated accordingly (see Table 12.2). If drug interventions are necessary, the drugs used should be short acting and given well diluted and by infusion, e.g. glyceryl trinitrate, sodium nitroprusside, metaraminol, phentolamine, phenylephrine, dopamine.

It is vital that cardiovascular abnormalities caused by anaesthetic errors (e.g. hypoxia from disconnected ventilator, hypertension from inadequate depth of anaesthesia, dysrhythmias from hypercarbia) should be recognized early and corrected appropriately.

Extubation and immediate recovery

The immediate postoperative period can be one of considerable haemodynamic instability, often associated with residual effects of anaesthetic agents. The combination of hypoxia and hypercarbia with tachycardia and hypertension or hypotension is no less dangerous in the postoperative period than is is intraoperatively. Additional oxygen should be administered and frequent monitoring continued until the patient is well recovered and stable.

If the tracheal tube is removed while the patient is still deeply anaesthetized the process does not cause significant pressor responses. However, if the patient is extubated when awake or if the patient awakes suddenly and is frightened, systolic and diastolic pressures and heart rate can rise dramatically. Once extubation has been completed, most exaggerated responses result from inadequately supressed

pain (which can also affect the ability to breathe properly) or bladder distention.

Unstable patients or those with untreated hypertension should be nursed in a high-dependency ward, or (depending upon the type of surgery) in an intensive care unit.

The use of intermittent positive pressure ventilation occasionally masks the presence of pulmonary oedema, and heart failure that develops intraoperatively may only become manifest in the recovery room. Emergency reintubation may be necessary, and the anaesthetist should be immediately available until this possibility has been excluded.

Renal failure caused by intraoperative insults may only become obvious postoperatively. Urine output must be monitored carefully, with early intervention if the flow rate is inadequate. It is vital to keep these patients well hydrated: renal perfusion *must* be maintained at high levels.

Regional anaesthesia

The principles of preoperative assessment, monitoring and intraoperative and postoperative care described above for general anaesthesia are of course essential for the management of regional blockade as well, particularly if the two are combined as part of a balanced technique. There is relatively little data on the response of well controlled hypertensives to spinal or epidural blockade, although is has been reported several times that untreated hypertensives showed a more unpredictable and profound fall in blood pressure than their normotensive counterparts.[26]

Following studies on patients maintained on beta-blockers, the combination of extradural block with light general anaesthesia was recommended for intra-abdominal surgery, hip surgery and lower limb vascular surgery, given the proviso that careful monitoring was used.[26,34]

The postoperative period

The postoperative period is a time of some concern, because once the immediate operative period is over is is easy to forget that dangers subsequent to anaesthesia and surgery persist for several days.

Attention must be given to analgesia, fluid balance (by measurement of urine output), and oxygenation. Efforts should be made to prevent or reduce vomiting, using antiemetics if necessary. Postoperative blood pressure control is not a problem in the majority of instances, even if the the patient cannot take oral medication because of the combined effects of bed rest, sedation, and analgesics.

However, if the gastrointestinal tract is to be out of action more than a few days, or if the patient's hypertension is particularly brittle, parenteral antihypertensive therapy will need to be prescribed. There are a variety of preparations that can be chosen for this purpose. More important than the drug chosen is the fact that it should be given sensibly, with the patient well monitored (preferably in a high-dependency area).

The greatest dangers are unexpected side effects because of a change of drug (e.g. asthma from intravenous labetalol), or the whole of a day's dosage being delivered intravenously over a very short time period. It is recommended that patients requiring this type of therapy should receive it via a dedicated line (preferably centrally placed) from a positive displacement syringe driver or a volumetric pump.

Hypoxaemia in the postoperative period is always a concern because of its potential contribution to postoperative morbidity and mortality[37] but this is especially so in the hypertensive patient who may have borderline myocardial ischaemia, compromised renal function, and widespread atheroma. Postoperative hypoxaemia can be broadly categorized into early (first 12 hours) and late (up to 4 days).

The early phase of hypoxaemia is dominated by the residual effects of drugs (general anaesthetics, opioids, neuromuscular blockers) and intraoperative atelectasis that developed during surgery.

Late-phase hypoxaemia has only been recognized relatively recently. It may be prolonged and profound, with oxygen saturations as low as 60%.[37] It is dominated by the combined effects of atelectasis and opioid induced abnormalities of respiratory control, the latter being exacerbated by sleep. When the effects of different postoperative analgesic regimens and sleep were studied, it was found that all the hypoxaemic episodes (peripheral oxygen saturation under 80%) occurred during sleep, all were associated with obstructive apnoea, and all occurred in every patient receiving morphine.[38] This is almost certainly due to the loss of tonic muscular activity in the upper airway.[37] In fully awake, normal humans a large negative pressure (as much as 8 kPa) is needed to close the upper airway completely wheras during sleep or sedation a pressure of less than 1 kPa is sufficient.

Various patterns of hypoxia have been described,[39] some of which show gross disorganization of breathing action with profound desaturations lasting for considerable periods. Events similar to these have been shown to be associated with ischaemic changes in the electrocardiograph, and these are reversed by the administration of oxygen.[41,42] They can continue until the third postoperative night.[42] Myocardial ischaemia also occurred in some patients at night even when the saturation of oxygen was in the normal range. Other studies have demonstrated either a temporal relationship between hypoxaemia and the development of ischaemia[43] or have suggested that myocardial ischaemia is more likely to occur if an episode of hypoxaemia is prolonged (over 5 minutes) and severe (85% oxygen saturation or less).[44] Although direct evidence is still lacking that outcome is improved by reducing the frequency and severity of postoperative ischaemia, an understanding of the pathophysiology and clinical implications of hypertension suggest that hypertensive patients are a high risk population who need careful postoperative care.

Special situations

Endocrine problems

Hypertension associated with endocrine problems is considered in detail in chapters 9 and 13. Outside specialist units, anaesthetists meet these patients only rarely. Detailed management of endocrine problems and anaesthesia can be found in standard textbooks.[45,46] The importance of hypertension associated with endocrine dysfunction is that there are often additional anaesthetic problems which have to be overcome.

Acromegaly

Acromegalics have a high incidence of hypertension. It is an important disease for the anaesthetist because of difficult airway management. These patients have large lips, jaw, tongue, and epiglottis. Facemask ventilation may be impossible. Hypertrophy of pharyngeal and laryngeal structures may make the anatomy difficult to interpret, the vocal cords may not be seen, and the larynx may be resistant to external manipulation. All these factors result in a difficult intubation with its potential for a hypertensive and tachycardic response.

Cushing's syndrome

Hypertension is common in this disorder. There may be cardiac enlargement and hypokalaemia.

Postoperatively, patients need specific steroid replacement therapy.

Conn's syndrome

In addition to the problems associated with all hypertensive patients, hypokalaemia should be checked for and corrected.

Phaeochromocytoma

These cases present major anaesthetic problems with difficult pre-, intra-, and postoperative problems.[47] There is still a range of opinions as to how they should best be managed. There are always severe cardiovascular disturbances during dissection and removal of the tumour, and skilful management is needed with rapidly acting drugs that have a short duration of effect.

Acute aneurysms

Patients presenting with acute aortic dissection or imminent rupture of an aortic aneurysm can have blood pressures ranging from severe hypotension to marked hypertension depending upon pain, circulating fluid volume and underlying pathology. Following immediate supportive measures (intravenous access, facemask oxygen, pain control, etc), hypertension should be controlled by a rapid-onset, short-acting drug (e.g. glyceryl trinitrate, sodium nitroprusside) titrated against blood pressure recordings from an arterial line. A urine catheter is mandatory to ensure adequate renal function, and a proper neurological assessment must be undertaken before therapy is instituted to establish baseline spinal cord damage. The optimal management of these cases is not easy and perioperative anaesthetic strategies are complex.[48]

Endoscopy

Gastrointestinal endoscopy is a common procedure and it is generally regarded as safe. There is, however, an incidence of serious complications of about 1 in 1000 associated with diagnostic upper gastrointestinal endoscopy,[49] and the mortality rate exceeds that of general anaesthesia. Recently, guidelines have been published for the management of endoscopic procedures[49,50] and blood pressure is recommended as being part of the risk assessment for all patients.[50] To the present authors' knowledge, there is no literature on hypertensive patients undergoing endoscopy. Since over 50% of serious reactions during endoscopy are cardiopulmonary, since falls in oxygen saturation frequently occur, and since it is thought that most cardiac dysrhythmias are related to hypoxia,[49] it seems reasonable to assume that a hypertensive patient is at increased risk.

Pregnancy

Hypertensive disease of pregnancy can range from a mild elevation of blood pressure through to full-blown eclampsia or the HELLP syndrome (haemolysis, elevated liver enzyme activity and low platelet count).[51] Many of these patients have Caesarean deliveries and some require anaesthesia for intercurrent conditions. It is important, when hypertension is detected unexpectedly preoperatively in a young woman, to exclude pregnancy as a cause because its presence implies other risk factors related to anaesthesia, which also need to be assessed (e.g. deep vein thrombosis, coagulopathy, aspiration pneumonia, supine hypotension).

Conclusion

The hypertensive patient about to undergo general or regional anaesthesia and surgery is at increased risk compared with the normotensive patient. The appropriate management does not depend upon using particular agents and avoiding others but rather on following certain principles. These are:

1. Whenever possible, hypertensive patients should be recognized early and ideally their blood pressure should be controlled and stable before surgery is undertaken.
2. Careful preoperative assessment is essential and should include a full evaluation of cardiac and renal function.
3. Before, during, and after surgery, the aim should be to avoid marked swings in blood pressure.
4. During anaesthesia and postoperatively, careful monitoring is mandatory and every effort should be made to ensure that adequate oxygenation and perfusion of vital organs is maintained.
5. Although there are no universally accepted guidelines, untreated or poorly controlled patients with diastolic blood pressures up to 110 mmHg can probably be accepted for anaesthesia and surgery provided that (as described in the text) there is nothing abnormal in the history and careful clinical examination and basic investigations reveal no evidence of end-organ damage or pregnancy.

References

1 Sprague HB. The heart in surgery. An analysis of results of surgery on cardiac patients during the past ten years at the Massachusetts General Hospital. *Surg Gynecol Obstet* 1929; **49**:54.

2 Smithwick RH, Thompson JE. Splanchnicectomy for essential hypertension. *JAMA* 1953; **152**:501.

3 Kety SS, King BD, Horvath SM et al. The effects of an acute reduction in blood pressure by means of differential spinal sympathetic block on the cerebral circulation of hypertensive patients. *J Clin Invest* 1950; **29**:402–7.

4 Pugh LGC, Wyndham CL. The circulatory effects of high spinal anaesthesia in hypertensive and control subjects. *Clin Sci* 1950; **9**:189–203.

5 Coakley CA, Alpert S, Boling JS. Circulatory responses during anesthesia of patients on rauwolfia therapy. *JAMA* 1956; **161**:1143–4.

6 Crandell DL. The anesthetic hazards in patients on antihypertensive therapy. *JAMA* 1962; **179**:495–500.

7 Katz RL, Weintraub HD, Papper EM. Anesthesia, surgery and rauwolfia. *Anesthesiology* 1964 **25**:142–7.

8 Folkow B. The haemodynamic consequences of adaptive structural change of the resistance vessels in hypertension. *Clin Sci* 1971; **41**:1–12.

9 Folkow B. Cardiovascular structural adaptation: its role in the initiation and maintenance of primary hypertension. *Clin Sci Mol Med* 1978; **55**:3s–22s.

10 Kaplan NM. Systemic hypertension: mechanisms and diagnosis. In: Braunwold E, ed. *Heart Disease: A Textbook of Cardiovascular Medicine*, 3rd edition. Philadelphia: WB Saunders, 1988:849–901.

11 Kreger BE, Kannel WB. Influence of hypertension on mortality. In: Amery A, ed. *Hypertensive Cardiovascular Disease: Pathophysiology and Treatment*. Boston: Martinus Nijhoff, 1982:451–63.

12 Roberts SC. The hypertensive disease: Evidence that systemic hypertension is a greater risk factor to development of other cardiovascular diseases than previously suspected. *Am J Med* 1975; **59**:523

13 Fouad FM, Tarazi RC, Gallagher JH et al. Abnormal left ventricular relaxation in hypertensive patients. *Clin Sci* 1980; **59**:411s.

14 Wicker P, Tarazi RC. Coronary blood flow in left ventricular hypertrophy; a review of experimental data. *Eur Heart J* 1982; **3**:111.

15 Strauer BE. Ventricular function and coronary haemodynamics in hypertensive heart disease. *Am J Cardiol* 1979; **44**:999.

16 Campkin TV, Turner JM. Intracranial effects of anaesthetic agents. In: Campkin TV, Turner JM, eds. *Neurosurgical Anaesthesia and Intensive Care*, 2nd edition. London: Butterworths, 1986:48–72.

17 Campkin TV, Turner JM. The cerebral circulation. In: Campkin TV, Turner JM, eds. *Neurosurgical Anaesthesia and Intensive Care*, 2nd edition, London: Butterworths, 1986:3–20.

18 Strandgaard S. Autoregulation of cerebral blood flow in hypertensive patients. *Circulation* 1976; **53**:720–7.

19 Ledingham JG, Rajagopolan B. Cerebral complications in the treatment of accelerated hypertension, *Q J Med* 1979; **48**:25.

20 Pedersen F, Kornerup HJ. Renal haemodynamics and plasma renin in patients with essential hypertension. *Clin Sci Mol Med* 1976; **50**:409.

21 Prys-Roberts C, Meloche R, Foex P. Studies in relation to hypertension. 1: Cardiovascular responses of treated and untreated patients. *Brit J Anaesth* 1971; **43**:122–37.

22 Goldman L, Caldera DL. Risks of general anesthesia and elective operation in the hypertensive patient. *Anesthesiology* 1979; **50**:285.

23 Bedford RF, Feinstein B. Hospital admission blood pressure: A predictor for hypertension following endotracheal intubation. *Anesth Analg* 1980; **59**:367.

24 Asiddao CB, Donegan JH, Whitesell RC et al. Factors associated with perioperative complications during carotid endarterectomy. *Anesth Analg* 1982; **61**:631.

25 Roizen MF. Anesthetic implications of concurrent diseases: Diseases involving the cardiovascular system. In: Miller RD, ed. *Anesthesia* 3rd edition. New York: Churchill Livingstone, 1990:820–4.

26 Prys-Roberts C. Anaesthesia and hypertension. *Brit J Anaesth* 1984; **56**:711.

27 Mangano DT. Perioperative Cardiac Morbidity. *Anesthesiology* 1990; **72**:153–84.

28 Charlson ME, MacKenzie R, Gold PG, Ales KL, Topkins M, Shires GT. Preoperative characteristics predicting intraoperative hypotension and hypertension among hypertensives and diabetics undergoing non-cardiac surgery. *Ann Surg* 1990; **212**:66–81.

29 Charlson ME, MacKenzie R, Gold PG, Ales KL, Shires GT. Postoperative renal dysfunction can be predicted. *Surg Gynecol Obstet* 1989; **169**:303–9.

30 Charlson ME, MacKenzie R, Gold PG et al. The preoperative and intraoperative haemodynamic predictors of postoperative myocardial infarction or ischaemia in patients undergoing noncardiac surgery. *Ann Surg* 1989; **210**:637–48.

31 Charlson ME, MacKenzie R, Gold PG, Ales KL, Topkins M, Shires GT. Risk for postoperative congestive heart failure. *Surg Gynecol Obstet* 1991; **172**:95–104.

32 Sharrock NE, Mineo R, Urquhart B. Haemodynamic effects and outcome analysis of hypotensive extradural anaesthesia in controlled hypertensive patients undergoing total hip arthroplasty. *Brit J Anaesth* 1991; **67**:17–25.

33 Stack CG, Rogers P, Linter SPK. Monoamine oxidase inhibitors and anaesthesia. A review. *Brit J Anaesth*. 1988; **60**:222–7.

34 Dagnino J, Prys-Roberts C. Strategy for patients with hypertensive heart disease. In: Foex P, ed. *Anaesthesia for the Compromised Heart. Ballieres Clinical Anaesthesiology* June 1989:261–89.

35 Savege T. The patient with cardiovascular disease. In: Stevens J, ed. *Preparation for Anaesthesia. Clinics in Anaesthesiology* July 1986:705–34.

36 Prys-Roberts C. Hypertension and Systemic Arterial Diseases. In: Vickers MD, ed. *Medicine for Anaesthetists* 2nd edition. Blackwell, 1982:74–100.

37 Mangat PS, Jones JG. In: Kaufman L, ed. *Perioperative Hypoxaemia in Anaesthesia Review 10.* Churchill Livingstone,1993:83–106.

38 Catley DM, Thornton C, Jordon C, Lehane JR, Royston D, Jones JG. Pronounced episodic oxygen desaturation in the postoperative period; its association with ventilatory pattern and analgesic regimen. *Anesthesiology* 1985:**63**:20–8.

39 Entwistle MD, Roe PG, Sapsford DJ, Berrisford RG, Jones JG. Patterns of oxygenation after thoracotomy. *Brit J Anaesth* 1991; **67**:704–11.

40 Reeder MK, Muir AD, Foex P, Goldman MD, Loh L, Smart D. Postoperative hypoxia: temporal associations with myocardial ischaemia. *Brit J Anaesth* 1991; **67**:626–31.

41 Reeder MK, Goldman MD, Loh L, Muir AD, Casey KR, Lehane JR. Late postoperative nocturnal dips in oxygen saturation in patients undergoing major abdominal vascular surgery. *Anaesthesia* 1992: **47**:110–15.

42 Muir AD, Reeder MK. Postoperative oxygen desaturation and myocardial ischaemia in patients presenting for vascular surgery. *Brit J Anaesth* 1991; **66**:369P.

43 Rosenberg J, Rasmussen V, van Jensen F, Ullstad T, Kehlet H. Late postoperative episodic and constant hypoxaemia and associated ECG abnormalities. *Brit J Anaesth* 1990; **65**:684–91.

44 Gill NP, Wright B, Reilly CS. Relationship between hypoxaemic and cardiac ischaemic events in the perioperative period. *Brit J Anaesth* 1992; **68**:471–3.

45 Hutton P, Cooper GM. *Guidelines in Clinical Anaesthesia.* Oxford: Blackwell Scientific, 1985:209–47.

46 Stoelting, RK, Dierdorf SF, McCammon RL. *Endocrine Disease in Anesthesia and Co-existing Disease*, 2nd edition. Churchill Livingstone, 1988:473–515.

47 Hull CJ. Phaeochrocytoma. Diagnosis, preoperative preparation and anaesthetic management. *Br J Anaesth*, 1986; **58**:1453–68.

48 McLeod T, Hutton P. Anaesthetic management of thoracic aorta disease. *Curr Anaesth Crit Care*, in press.

49 Bell GD, McCloy RF, Charlton JE et al. Recommendations for standards of sedation and patient monitoring during gastrointestinal endoscopy. *Gut* 1991; **32**:823–7.

50 Royal College of Surgeons of England. *Guidelines for Sedation by Non-Anaesthetists*. London: Royal College of Surgeons of England, 1993.

51 Gutsche BB, Cheek TG. Anesthetic considerations in pre-eclampsia and eclampsia. In: Scnider SM, Levinson G, eds. *Anesthesia for Obstetrics*, 3rd edition. Baltimore: Williams and Wilkins, 1993:305–36.

52 Prys-Roberts C, Greene LT, Meloche R, Foex P. Studies of anaesthesia in relation to hypertension II: haemodynamic consequences of induction and endotracheal intubation. *Br J Anaesth* 1971; **43**:531–47.

53 Ty Smith N, Corbascio AN. *Drug Interactions in Anesthesia*, 2nd edition. Philadelphia: Lea and Febiger, 1986.

13

The management of hypertension in patients with concomitant disorders

Martin J Kendall and Iris Rajman

Hypertension is predominantly a disorder of middle-aged and older people, many of whom suffer from other disease. Some of these are particularly relevant to the management of the patients high blood pressure (Table 13.1).

First, they may suggest that the patient already has diffuse vascular disease and therefore, particularly if the patient is relatively young and otherwise well, indicate that considerable efforts should be made to correct all risk factors including hypertension.

Table 13.1

Disorders and conditions that merit specific attention when they occur in patients with hypertension.

```
Disorders that suggest the presence of advanced atheromatous
disease
      Ischaemic heart disease
            Angina
            Previous myocardial infarct*
            Congestive cardiac failure
      Cerebrovascular disease
            History of transient ischaemic attacks*
            Previous stroke*
      Vascular disease
            Aortic aneurysms
            Peripheral vascular disease
Disease that increases the risk of developing ischaemic heart
disease
      Diabetes mellitus*
      Hyperlipidaemia
Disorders that influence the choice of antihypertensive therapy
      Cardiovascular disorders (see above)
      Respiratory disease
            Asthma
            Obstructive airways disease
      Metabolic disorders
            Diabetes mellitus*
            Hyperlipidaemia
            Gout
Renal disease*
Pregnancy* (not a disorder but a special circumstance)

*These disorders and pregnancy have their own specific chapters
which address the problems raised.
```

Second, in the patients who are at increased risk of developing coronary artery disease because they smoke or have a positive family history, hypercholesterolaemia, or diabetes mellitus, all the reversible risk factors should be addressed and the blood pressure should be reduced to well into the normal range. Failure to take appropriate action over risk factors such as smoking or a raised plasma cholesterol, or failure to consider hormone replacement therapy where appropriate, would be to fail to manage the patient properly.

Third, the disease states already discussed and a number of others will influence the choice of antihypertensive therapy. In some, there is a positive need to choose a particular form of drug therapy; in others, certain treatments need to be avoided because they may cause unwanted effects.

There are a number of instances in which a relatively common disorder coexisting with hypertension has a major impact on the way the hypertension is managed. These are considered in specific chapters elsewhere in this book. In this chapter, an attempt is made to give an overview of the problem of coexisting disorders and to present some guidance on the management of those disorders not considered elsewhere. These will be considered under three headings: respiratory, cardiovascular and metabolic disorders.

Respiratory disorders

The potentially severe bronchospasm that may occur if a beta-blocker is given to an asthmatic patient[1] is probably the best known and most serious consequence of not taking seriously the presence of a coexisting disease when treating a hypertensive patient. Problems arise because doctors are in a hurry or fail to ask about respiratory symptoms in a way that is readily understood by the patient. Occasionally, drugs are prescribed using trade names and, particularly if a combination preparation is used, the

doctor forgets or does not appreciate that the active ingredient is a beta-blocker. Finally, there may be confusion over the spectrum of disease states – from mild bronchitis to very reactive asthma – and the spectrum of drug actions – from those caused by large doses of non-selective-beta-blockers to those caused by low doses of controlled-release preparations of beta$_1$-selective beta-blockers.

If patients have had asthma or have suffered from spontaneous wheezing at any time in their life, they should not be given a beta-blocker. Patients with chronic obstructive airways disease are much less sensitive than true asthmatics. Patients who usually smoke or have smoked and have started to suffer from early morning cough and who get exacerbations of cough with sputum accompanied by increasing dyspnoea in the winter months may benefit from a bronchodilator and may deteriorate on a beta-blocker. Such patients should not be given a non-selective beta-blocker, though often they can tolerate low doses of a beta$_1$-selective beta-blocker,[2] particularly if plasma concentrations are kept low by using a controlled release preparation.[3] Alternatively, a beta$_1$-blocker with beta$_2$-agonist properties, such as celiprolol[4] may be prescribed.

Cardiovascular disease
Ischaemic heart disease – angina and postmyocardial infarction

Hypertensive patients who also have angina or who have recovered from a myocardial infarct have established coronary artery disease and a persisting risk factor. Every effort should therefore be made to treat the hypertension very effectively and to address other correctable risk factors.

In those with angina, it is logical to choose an antihypertensive agent such as a beta blocker or a calcium antagonist, which effectively helps to reduce the frequency and severity of anginal attacks. There are no agreed guidelines for the management of angina. However, it would seem logical to suggest beta-blockers for those patients who are particularly anxious about their angina and those who tolerated the vasodilatory effects of nitrates poorly. Calcium antagonists would obviously be chosen for patients for whom beta-blockers are contraindicated or who have been adversely affected by beta-blockers in the past. However, in patients with angina or a history of myocardial infarction, one of the key aims of treatment is to improve the patient's prognosis.

Both hypertension[5] and established coronary artery disease[6] predispose to sudden death, myocardial infarction, or reinfarction. There is therefore a strong argument for choosing an antihypertensive agent that has the potential to reduce the risk of sudden death and infarction. Beta-blockers, perhaps particularly lipophilic beta-blockers, are the antihypertensive drugs for which there is evidence that they have this cardioprotective potential.[7] This is particularly true for the post infarct patient.[8-12] ACE inhibitors also reduce reinfarction rates, episodes of heart failure, and hospital admissions, but probably do not reduce the rate of sudden death.[13]

The evidence that beta-blockers have a cardioprotective effect is not universally accepted. The data have accumulated over a number of years, and some of the relevant clinical trials were performed over 10 years ago. The recent literature has concentrated on newer agents, which have proved less effective. The evidence that beta-blockers are cardioprotective is summarized in Table 13.2. The consistency of the beneficial

Table 13.2
Evidence for a cardioprotective role of beta-blockers.

Impact on the pathological processes that lead to death from coronary artery disease
Beta-blockers
- reduce haemodynamically induced endothelial damage[14,15]
- impede atheroma formation[16,17]
- have a beneficial impact on some clotting processes[18,19]
- reduce the risk of ventricular fibrillation in animal models with myocardial ischaemia[20-22]

Beta-blockers in clinical trials
  Primary prevention
    Non-randomized trials
      - DHSS Hypertension Care Computing Project[23]
      - Puget Sound Case Control Study[24]
    Randomized trials with positive results in males
      - MRC Trial (propranolol)[25,26]
      - IPPPSH Collaborative Group[27]
      - MAPHY Study[28]
  Acute postinfarction studies
      - Atenolol – ISIS 1[8]
      - Metoprolol – MIAMI Trial[29]
  Longer term post infarction studies
      - Timolol – Norwegian Multicentre Study[9]
      - Metoprolol – Gothenberg Study[12]
      - Propranolol – BHAT Study[10]

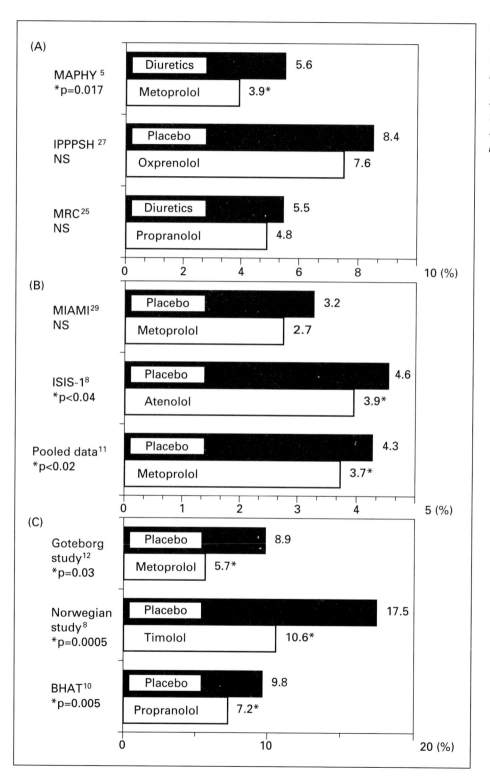

Figure 13.1
(A) Coronary events rate (%) in primary prevention trials; (B) 7 days' mortality in acute postinfarction trials; (C) Cumulative mortality in chronic post infarction trials.

impact can be seen by presenting the primary prevention trial results and the acute and chronic postinfarct results together (Fig. 13.1).

Congestive cardiac failure

Though hypertension is an important cause of heart failure, patients who develop this complication rarely retain the potential to produce a markedly raised blood pressure, though in the past prolonged untreated or inadequately treated severe hypertension caused heart failure. Today this is rare.

If hypertension and heart failure should coexist, it is logical to avoid negatively inotropic drugs; these include particularly beta-blockers but also verapamil and diltiazem. Diuretic therapy or ACE inhibitors can both be recommended, as they effectively lower the blood pressure and improve the symptoms of heart failure.

Cerebrovascular disease

The problem of controlling hypertension in patients with cerebrovascular disease is reviewed in detail in chapter 11.

Hypertension is the major risk factor for stroke, and the control of hypertension has been shown many times to reduce the risk of having a stroke.[30–32] Adequate blood pressure control is the most effective means of preventing strokes and should be a particularly important part of the strategy for managing those at increased risk of having a stroke. Those who have had one or more transient ischaemic attacks and those who have had a stroke from which they have recovered or are recovering are high-risk patients in this context.

The standard advice is to withold treatment at the time of a cerebral infarction but thereafter to lower the pressure effectively, taking care to avoid acute falls in pressure and postural hypotension. This might suggest trying to avoid the use of alpha-blockers and ACE inhibitors.

Vascular disease

The management of aortic dissections

In 1958, Hirst et al[33] reviewed 505 patients with aortic dissections that were untreated or offered supportive medical treatment. The mortality rate was 21% within 24 hours, 49% at 4 days, 74% at 2 weeks, and 93% at 1 year. Subsequently, more effective surgical treatments were introduced by DeBakey et al,[34,35] and more rational medical management was described by Wheat et al.[36]

Treatment strategies are now determined by the availability of skilled surgeons and intensive care facilities and also by the type of dissection to be treated. Proximal dissections, involving the ascending aorta (Stanford type A) have a bad prognosis and are usually treated surgically, whereas distal dissections (type B) involving the descending aorta may be treated either medically or surgically.[37,38] In some type B dissections, the patient is not well enough to undergo surgery and these have a significant mortality.[39,40] However, surgery may be required if there are acute complications, such as rupture with bleeding into the pericardium or peritoneum, or if the blood supply to the lower limbs or any of the major abdominal viscera becomes impaired. Since the more seriously ill patients tend to require surgery their inhospital mortality is high – 25–75% – whereas those well enough to be treated medically have an inhospital mortality of 10–20%.[41] It follows that 80–90% of those who have relatively uncomplicated type B dissections and are given effective medical therapy may survive long enough to leave hospital.

The decision to operate electively at a later date to prevent late rupture is influenced by a number of the factors already discussed, but in addition the size of the aorta is important. Patients whose aorta is more than 5 cm maximum diameter or whose chronic dissected aorta starts to enlarge should be offered surgery.[38,41]

If medical treatment is chosen, the aim should be to provide close monitoring and effective antihypertensive therapy in an intensive care unit. The systolic blood pressure should be reduced to between 115 and 135 mmHg: the exact figure will be determined by the need to reduce the pressure in the aorta to the lowest possible level whilst maintaining reasonable cerebral, coronary and renal perfusion. This may require intravenous infusions of sodium nitroprusside (starting with 0.3 μg/kg/min) if the situation is serious and the patient is deteriorating rapidly. If less drastic measures are needed, then the use of beta-blockers intravenously or orally is usually advocated[41] as they reduce the force of ventricular contraction. However, they may not reduce the blood pressure enough and the addition of a calcium channel blocking drug, perhaps sublingual nifedipine initially, may assist in reducing the blood pressure further and in helping to maintain tissue perfusion.

The choice of a beta-blocker in this situation can be supported by reference to the literature. For example, Halpern et al[42] in 1971 suggested that beta-blockers should be used in Marfan's syndrome. They noted that in malignant hypertension, reducing the blood pressure without reducing the rate of change of intra-arterial pressure (dP.dt) did not prevent aortic dissection; in fact, it apparently increased the risk.[36] By comparison, beta-blockers have been shown to be effective in the management of aortic dissections in early studies[36] and in more recent studies.[43] In further studies in turkeys prone to die from aortic rupture, propranolol was found to be protective.[44,45] Though the haemodynamic effects are believed to be the most important factor, it may be relevant that propranolol increases collagen-cross linking in animals bred to suffer from aortic rupture,[46,47] reduces collagen breakdown in patients with hyperthyroidism,[48] and increases collagen deposition in the lung.[49]

A recent comparison of propranolol and no treatment in young patients with Marfan's syndrome showed convincingly that the growth in the ascending aortic diameter was reduced by beta-blockade.[50] Oral beta-blockade has also been shown to reduce the rate of growth of aortic aneurysms.[51] Thus, although the literature is not extensive, there are reasonable theoretical reasons for choosing a beta-blocker in patients with aneurysms, and some clinical trial data confirm the efficacy of this approach.

Peripheral vascular disease

All types of atherosclerotic vascular disease are associated with hypertension. This relationship is most pronounced with cerebrovascular disease, less pronounced with coronary artery disease, and least with peripheral vascular disease.[52] Those with peripheral vascular disease and hypertension often have a history of heavy cigarette smoking, many have hyperlipidaemia and some have diabetes mellitus. The management therefore consists of:

- a careful evaluation of the vascular risk factors;
- the choice of an antihypertensive regimen that does not adversely affect blood flow to the feet.

There is little or no evidence to suggest that good control of the patient's blood pressure will improve the peripheral vascular disease. However, it may be expected to reduce the patient's risk of having a stroke and it might have some favourable impact on the progress of the patient's coronary artery disease.

The standard undergraduate-level advice on the management of patients with hypertension and peripheral vascular disease is to avoid beta-blockers and choose a vasodilator antihypertensive agent. There are two reasons put forward to support his advice.

First, beta-blockers are said to reduce cardiac output and probably limb perfusion, and they have a reputation for causing cold extremities. It seems likely that limb perfusion is influenced by the pressure in more proximal vessels and therefore that perfusion will be reduced by any agent that effectively reduces arterial blood pressure, irrespective of the mean by which this is achieved.

The second concern, namely that beta-blockers exacerbate symptoms from peripheral vascular disease, has now been well investigated and there is clinical data to suggest that beta-blockers do not cause such problems.[53] The arguments in favour of vasodilators suggest that if perfusion is reduced because of arterial narrowing, vasodilation should help. However, the vasodilator may prove more effective in dilating relatively normal vessels rather than diseased vessels. This may have an adverse effect and cause the so-called steel phenomenon. However, if the vasodilator helps to open up collateral vessels this would be an advantage.

Clinical experience and clinical trial data, however, do suggest that beta-blockers tend to reduce the walking distance of patients with intermittent claudication,[52] whereas captopril[54] and nifedipine[55] have no adverse effects, and doxazosin may increase walking distance.[56]

Interestingly, there is some evidence that celiprolol (a beta$_1$-blocking drug with beta$_2$-agonist properties) also tends to increase pain-free walking distances.[57]

The advice must be that blood pressure should be reduced cautiously in hypertensives with peripheral vascular disease. A vasodilator drug should probably be used, and an alpha-blocker may be the best option.

Metabolic disorders

Diabetes mellitus

Hypertension in a diabetic patient merits particular attention and is considered in detail in chapter 9. It may be helpful to consider that the problem has 3 quite separate facets.

Hypertension is approximately twice as common in diabetic as in non-diabetic patients.[58] Diabetes mellitus and hypertension are both major risk factors for coronary artery disease; furthermore, patients with both these risk factors who have a myocardial infarct have a poor prognosis. Careful control of the diabetes may reduce the risk of having a coronary event,[59] but modest improvements in overall control have little impact. Good control of the hypertension is more important, and it would seem logical to choose an antihypertensive agent with some potential to reduce coronary risk. This might suggest the use of a beta$_1$-selective beta-blocker[60] (as discussed above), though many prefer not to use beta-blockers in diabetics because of concern about the metabolic effects of beta-blockers, including the risk of masking hypoglycaemic symptoms.

The second problem relates to the desirability of choosing an antihypertensive drug that does not adversely affect plasma glucose control, insulin resistance, and plasma lipids.

This suggests a metabolically neutral drug, such as a calcium antagonist; a drug believed to reduce insulin resistance, such as an ACE inhibitor;[61] or a drug that tends to improve the plasma lipid profile, such as an alpha blocker.

The third aim of treatment is to avoid making the important complications of diabetes worse. These are predominantly caused by macrovascular disease and microvascular disease. A vasodilator seems a sensible choice, and it may be that a drug like captopril (or other ACE inhibitors) with a specific advantage because of a useful intrarenal effect, should receive serious consideration. It is the drug for which the evidence that it delays renal deterioration is most persuasive at the time of writing.[62,63]

Diuretics, which have adverse metabolic effects and also cause impotence, are usually considered unsuitable and non-selective beta-blockers are likely to do more harm than good.

It is clear that there are a number of options available. The choice of therapy will be determined in part by the perceived needs of the particular patient and in part by the importance attached to each of the above problem areas (see Chapter 9).

Hyperlipidaemia

The management of hypertension in patients with hyperlipidaemia has been a source of considerable controversy. This can in part be attributed to the comments and criticisms directed at certain antihypertensive drugs by the manufacturers of competitor products who perceive that they have a marketing advantage which needs to be exploited.

The facts are that both hypertension and hyperlipidaemia are important risk factors for coronary artery disease, and when both coexist the treatment of each should be more rigorous than if either occurred alone. Although some antihypertensive drugs do produce changes in the plasma lipids that are generally considered to adversely affect the patient's risk, the changes are usually modest and there is no evidence that drug induced changes in plasma lipids are necessarily associated with an adverse effect on prognosis.

There is no universally agreed strategy for treating hypertension in patients with hyperlipidaemia. Most prescribers would agree that since thiazide diuretics and non-selective beta-blockers tend to make the plasma lipid profile worse, they should probably be avoided.[64,65] By contrast, alpha-adrenergic blocking drugs (alpha-blockers) tend to improve the plasma lipids and could be recommended. They generally decrease the levels of triglycerides, total cholesterol, VLDL cholesterol, and LDL cholesterol and increase HDL cholesterol levels (Fig. 13.2).[66-71] Long term comparative studies have confirmed the antihypertensive efficacy of prazosin and the newer selective alpha-blockers, such as doxazosin and terazosin, which have comparable antihypertensive effects to beta-blockers and diuretics.[71,72] In practice, if the prescriber does not normally use alpha-blockers in his or her antihypertensive armamentarium, there is a tendency not to use them in this situation.

As an alternative, calcium channel blockers and ACE inhibitors are usually recommended, as they have little or no effect on cholesterol and triglyceride levels and are 'biochemically neutral'. Furthermore, combination therapy consisting of a calcium antagonist and an ACE inhibitor has been reported to be effective in severe hypertension. It is of interest that the combination of an ACE inhibitor with a low dose of thiazide diuretics provides very effective blood pressure control, and the ACE inhibitor reduces some of the adverse effects of diuretics, including hypercholesterolaemia.[61]

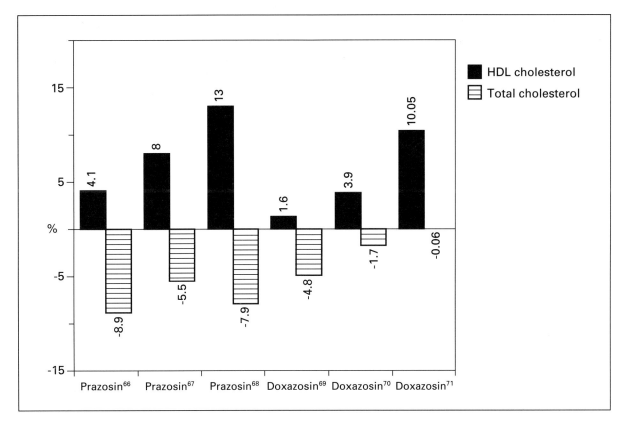

Figure 13.2
Percentage of change from the baseline for the total and HDL cholesterol with prazosin and doxazosin.

Many who treat hypertension would argue that to give a drug that may cause any adverse effects on plasma lipids is illogical, and therefore the lipid-neutral drugs or alpha-blockers are considered preferable. Another viewpoint leading to a quite different therapeutic strategy would argue that patients at high risk of developing and suffering from coronary artery disease should be given treatment that has been shown to reduce coronary risk, i.e. beta-blockers. The aim should be to find beta-blockers with little or no adverse effect on plasma lipids.

The evidence that beta-blockers are cardioprotective is not universally accepted, but it is persuasive (see above). The clinical data of primary prevention is controversial but the MAPHY trial, the IPPSH trial and the MRC trial all showed a reduction in coronary events in men. Immediately postinfarction, both atenolol and metoprolol have been shown to improve mortality rates and in the long-term, postinfarction patients on timolol, propranolol, or metoprolol have a better prognosis.[7-11] There is therefore a strong argument for carefully assessing the magnitude of the adverse effects of atenolol or metoprolol on plasma lipids. Furthermore, in this context a drug with beta$_1$-blocking and beta$_2$-agonist properties, such as celiprolol, looks attractive.[73] The drug for which there is most clinical evidence on cardioprotective effects is metoprolol, and the drug with the most acceptable effects on lipids is celiprolol (Fig. 13.3).

The normal guidelines suggest that hypertensive hyperlipidaemic patients should be treated with drugs that will not make the hyperlipidaemia worse (Table 13.3). We would suggest that a selective beta blocker is more likely to address the problem facing the patient, i.e. the risk of early and severe coronary artery disease. Alpha-blockers affect plasma lipids most favourably, but their possible benefit in preventing coronary artery disease will only be established when appropriate long-term clinical trials have shown that they reduce coronary events. We would further suggest that careful assessment of other risk factors is needed, and that other treatments like aspirin or hormone replacement therapy should be considered, as should life-style changes – particularly those that lead to less smoking, lower body weight, and more exercise.[74]

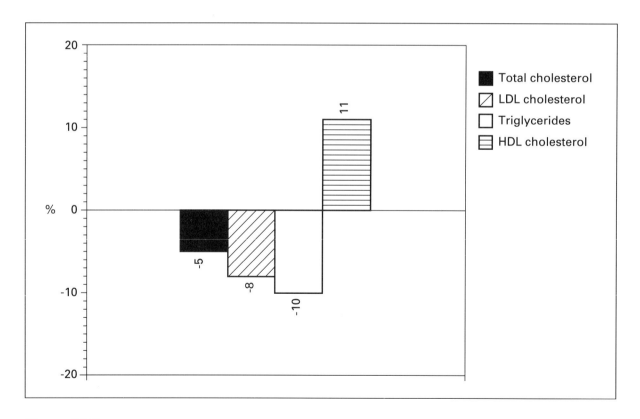

Figure 13.3
Pooled data on the effects of celiprolol on plasma lipids demonstrate reduction in triglyceride, total, and LDL cholesterol levels and increase in HDL cholesterol level.[73]

Thiazide diuretics	triglycerides ↑, LDL cholesterol ↑
Non-selective beta-blockers	triglycerides ↑, HDL cholesterol ↓↓
Beta₁-selective beta-blockers and beta-blockers with intrinsic sympathomimetic activity	smaller changes than non-selective beta-blockers
Celiprolol (third generation beta-blocker)	triglycerides ↓, total cholesterol↓ LDL cholesterol ↓, HDL cholesterol ↑
ACE inhibitors	no important effects on lipid profile
Calcium antagonists	no important effects on lipid profile
Alpha-blockers	triglycerides ↓, total cholesterol ↓, HDL cholesterol ↑

Table 13.3
The effects of different antihypertensive drugs on lipid profile

Gout

Hypertensive patients with gout should not be treated with thiazide diuretics.

Conclusion

Patients with hypertension have a risk factor for coronary artery disease and this should be managed in the light of the presence of other coronary risk factors. In addition, they should be carefully evaluated to determine what other concomitant diseases they have and what other treatments they may be taking. These other treatments will markedly influence the management strategy. As indicated in this chapter, if the patient has signs of developing coronary artery disease or has already developed it, then the hypertension should be treated with particular care, and every effort should be made to ensure that the blood pressure is well controlled. The presence of other diseases will influence the choice of drugs that may be used. Failure to take note of these other disorders will lead to inappropriate management, which may have serious consequences.

References

1 McNeil RS, Ingram CG. Effect of propranolol on ventilatory function. *Am J Cardiol* 1966; **18**:473–5.

2 Thiringer G, Svedmyr N. Interaction of orally administered metoprolol, practolol and propranolol with isoprenaline in asthmatics. *Eur J Clin Pharmacol* 1976; **10**:163–70.

3 Lofdahl CG, Dahlof C, Westergren G, Olofsson B, Svedmyr N. Controlled release metoprolol compared with atenolol in asthmatic patients: Interaction with Terbutaline. *Eur J Clin Pharmacol* 1988; **33** (suppl):S25–S32.

4 Kendall MJ, Rajman I. A risk benefit assessment of celiprolol in the treatment of cardio-vascular disease. *Drug Safety* 1994; **10**(3):220–32.

5 Olsson G, Tudmilehto J, Berglund G et al. Primary prevention of sudden cardiovascular death in hypertensive patients: mortality results from the MAPHY Study. *Am J Hypertens* 1991; **4**:151–8.

6 O'Rourke RA. Role of myocardial infarction in sudden cardiac death. *Circulation* 1992; **85** (suppl 1):I112–I117.

7 Rajman I, Kendall MJ. Sudden cardiac death and the potential role of beta adrenoceptor blocking drugs. *Postgrad Med J* 1993; **69**:903–11.

8 ISIS-1 Collaborative Group. Randomised trial of intravenous atenolol among 16027 cases of suspected acute myocardial infarctions: ISIS-1. *Lancet* 1986; **ii**:57–66.

9 The Norwegian Multicentre Study Group. Timolol-induced reduction in mortality and reinfarction in patients surviving acute myocardial infarction. *N Engl J Med* 1981; **304**:801–7.

10 Beta Blocker Heart Attack Trial Research Group. A randomized trial of propranolol in patients with acute myocardial infarction. *JAMA* 1982; **247**:1707–14.

11 Olsson G, Wikstrand J, Warnold I et al. Metoprolol induced reduction in postinfarction mortality: pooled results from five double blind randomised trials. *Eur Heart J* 1992; **13**:28–32.

12 Hjalmarson A, Elmfledt D, Herlitz J et al. Effect on mortality of metoprolol in acute myocardial infarction. *Lancet* 1981; **ii**:273–7.

13 The Acute Infarction Ramipril Efficacy (AIRE) Study Investigators. Effect of ramipril on mortality and morbidity of survivors of acute myocardial infarction with clinical evidence of heart failure. *Lancet* 1993; **342**:821–8.

14 Kaplan JR, Manuck SB, Adams MR et al. Propranolol inhibits coronary atherosclerosis in behaviorally predisposed monkeys fed an atherogenic diet. *Circulation* 1987; **76**:1364–72.

15 Strawn W, Bondjers G, Kaplan JR et al. Endothelial dysfunction in response to psychosocial stress in monkeys. *Circ Res* 1991; **68**:1270–9.

16 Oslund Lindqvist AM, Lindquist P, Brautigam J, Olsson G, Bondjers G, Nordborg C. The effect of metoprolol on diet induced atherosclerosis in rabbits. *Arteriosclerosis* 1988; **8**:40–4.

17 Spence JD, Perkins DG, Klein RL, Adams MR, Haust MD. Hemodynamic modifications of aortic atherosclerosis: Effects of propranolol versus hydralazine in hypertensive hyperlipidemic rabbits. *Atherosclerosis* 1984; **50**:325–33.

18 Larsson PT, Wiman B, Olsson G, Angelin B, Hjemdahl P. Influence of metoprolol treatment on sympatho-adrenal activation of fibrinolysis. *Thromb Haemost* 1990; **63**:482–7.

19 Frishman WH, Christodoulou J, Weksler B, Smithen C, Killip T, Scheidt S. Abrupt propranolol withdrawal in angina pectoris: Effects on platelet aggregation and exercise tolerance. *Am Heart J* 1978; **95**:169–79.

20 Parker GW, Michael LH, Hartley CJ, Skinner JE, Entman ML. Central β-adrenergic mechanisms may modulate ischaemic ventricular fibrillation in pigs. *Circulation Research* 1990; **66**:259–70.

21 Ablad B, Bjuro T, Bjorkman JA, Edstrom T, Olsson G. Role of central nervous beta-adrenoceptors in the prevention of ventricular fibrillation through augmentation of cardiac vagal tone. *J Am Coll Cardiol* 1991; **17**:165A.

22 Dellsperger KC, Martins JB, Clothier JL, Marcus ML. Incidence of sudden cardiac death associated with coronary artery occlusion in dogs with hypertension and left ventricular hypertrophy is reduced by chronic β-adrenergic blockade. *Circulation* 1990; **82**:941–50.

23 Fletcher A, Beevers DG, Bulpitt C et al. Beta adrenoceptor blockade is associated with increased survival in male but not female hypertensive patients: A report from the DHSS Hypertensive Care Computing Project (DHCCP). *J Human Hypertens* 1988; **2**:219–27.

24 Psaty BM, Koepsell TD, LoGergo JP, Wanger EH, Inui TS. Beta-blockers and primary prevention of coronary heart disease in patients with high blood pressure. *JAMA* 1989; **261**:2087–94.

25 Medical Research Council Working Party: MRC trial of treatment of mild hypertension: Principal results. *Br Med J* 1985; **291**:97–104.

26 Green KG. British MRC Trial of Treatment for Mild Hypertension – a more favourable interpretation. *Am J Hypertens* 1991; **4**:723–4.

28 The IPPPSH Collaborative Group. Cardiovascular risk and risk factors in a randomized trial of treatment based on the beta blocker oxprenolol: The International Prospective Primary Prevention Study in Hypertension (IPPPSH). *J Hypertens* 1985; **3**:379–92.

29 Wikstrand J, Warnold I, Olsson G, Tuomilehto J, Elmfeldt D, Berglund G. Primary prevention with metoprolol in patients with hypertension. Mortality results from the MAPHY study. *JAMA* 1988; **259**:1976–82.

29 The MIAMI Trial Research Group: Metoprolol in acute myocardial infarction (MIAMI). A randomized placebo controlled international trial. *Eur Heart J* 1985; **6**:199–226.

30 MacMahon SW, Cutter JA, Neaton JD et al. Relationship of blood pressure to coronary and stroke morbidity and mortality in clinical trials and epidemiological studies. *J Hypertens* 1986; **4** (suppl 6); 14–17.

31 SHEP Cooperative Research Group. Prevention of stroke by antihypertensive drug treatment in older persons with isolated systolic hypertension: final results of the Systolic Hypertension in the Elderly Program (SHEP). *JAMA* 1991; **265**:3255–64.

32 MRC Working Party: Medical Research Council trial of hypertension in older adults: principal results. *Br Med J* 1992; **304**:405–16.

33 Hirst AE, Johns VJ, Kime SW. Dissecting aneurysms of the aorta: review of 505 cases. *Medicine* 1958; **37**:217–79.

34 DeBakey ME, Cooley DA, Creech O. Surgical considerations of dissecting aneurysms of the aorta. *Ann Surg* 1955; **142**:586–612.

35 DeBakey ME, Henly WS, Cooley DA, Morris GC, Crawford ES, Beall AC. Surgical management of dissecting aneurysms of the aorta. *J Thorac Cardiovasc Surg* 1965; **49**:130–49.

36 Wheat MW, Parlmer RF, Bartley TD, Seelman RC. Treatment of dissecting aneurysms of the aorta without surgery. *J Thorac Cardiovasc Surg* 1965; **50**:364–73.

37 Glower DG, James I, Speier RH et al. Comparison of medical and surgical therapy for uncomplicated descending aortic dissection. *Circulation* 1990; **82**(suppl IV):IV39–IV46.

38 Masuda Y, Yamada Z, Morooka N, Watanabe S, Inagaki Y. Prognosis of patients with medically treated aortic dissections. *Circulation* 1991; **84**(suppl III):III-7–III-13.

39 Wholfe WG, Oldham HN, Rankin JS, Moran JF. Surgical treatment of acute ascending aortic dissection. *Ann Surg* 1983; **197**:738–42.

40 Miller DC, Mitchell RS, Oyer PE, Stinson EB, Jamieson SW, Shumway NE. Independent determinants of operative mortality for patients with aortic dissections. *Circulation* 1984; **70**(suppl I):I-153–I-164.

41 Hara K, Yamaguchi Y, Kurokawa K. The role of medical treatment of distal type aortic dissection. *Int J Cardiol* 1991; **32**:231–40.

42 Halpern BL, Char F, Murdoch JL, Horton WB, McKuisick VA. A prospectus on the prevention of aortic rupture in the Marfan syndrome with data on survivorship without treatment. *Johns Hopkins Med J* 1971; **129**:123–9.

43 DeSanctis RW, Doroghazi RM, Austen WG, Buckley MJ. Aortic dissection. *N Engl J Med* 1987; **317**:1060–7.

44 Simpson CF, Kling JM, Palmer RF. β-Aminopropionitrile induced dissecting aneurysms of turkeys: treatment with propranolol. *Toxicol Appl Pharmacol* 1970; **16**:143–53.

45 Simpson CF, Boucek RJ, Noble NL. Influence of d-, l- and dl-propranolol and practolol on β-aminopropionitrile-induced aortic ruptures of turkeys. *Toxicol Appl Pharmacol* 1976; **38**:169–75.

46 Brophy CM, Rilson JE, Tilson MD. Propranolol stimulates the cross linking of matrix components in skin from the aneurysms-prone blotchy mouse. *J Surg Res* 1989; **46**:330–2.

47 Boucek RJ, Gunja Smith Z, Noble NL, Simpson CF. Modulation by propranolol of the lysyl cross links in aortic elastin and collagen of the aneurysm-prone turkey. *Biochem Pharmacol* 1983; **32**:275–80.

48 Beylot M, Borson F, David L, Sautot G, Riou JP, Mornex R. Reduction by propranolol of urinary hydroxyproline excretion in human hyperthyroidism: a beta-receptor blockade effect or a membrane stabilizing mechanism? *Metabolism* 1984; **33**:124–8.

49 Lindenschmidt RC, Witschi HP. Propranolol-induced elevation of pulmonary collagen. *J Pharmacol Exp Ther* 1985; **232**:346–50.

50 Shores J, Berger KR, Murphy EA, Pyeritz RE. Progression of aortic dilatation and the benefit of long-term beta-adrenergic blockade in Marfan's syndrome. *N Engl J Med* 1994; **330**:1335–41.

51 Leach SD, Toole AL, Stern H, DeNatale RW, Tilson MD. Effect of β-adrenergic blockade on the growth rate of abdominal aortic aneurysms. *Arch Surg* 1988; **123**:606–9.

52 Dawber TR. *The Framingham Study: the Epidemiology of Atherosclerotic Disease.* Cambridge: Harvard University Press, 1980:91.

53 Solomon SA, Ramsay LE, Yeo WW, Parnell L, Morris-Jone W. Beta-blockade and intermittent claudication: placebo controlled trial of atenolol and nifedipine and their combination. *Br Med J* 1991; **303**:1100–4.

54 Roberts DH, Tsao Y, Breckenridge A. Placebo controlled comparison of captopril, atenolol, labetolol and pindolol in hypertension complicated by intermittent claudication. *Lancet* 1987; **2**:650–4.

55 Breckenridge A, Roberts DH. Antihypertensive treatment in concomitant peripheral vascular disease: current experience and the potential of carvedilol. *J Cardiovasc Pharmac* 1991; **18** (suppl 4):578–81.

56 Catalo M, Libretti A. A multicentre study of doxasozin in the treatment of patients with mild or moderate essential hypertension and concomitant intermittent claudication. *Am Heart J* 1991; **121**:367–71.

57 Weber MA. Hypertension with concomitant conditions: the changing role of beta adrenoceptor blockade. *Am Heart J* 1991; **121**:716–23.

58 The Working Groups on Hypertension in Diabetes. Statement on hypertension in Diabetes Mellitus. Final Report. *Arch Intern Med* 1987; **147**:830–42.

59 Hypertension in Diabetes Study (HDS) II. Increased risk of cardiovascular complications in hypertensive type 2 diabetic patients. *J Hypertens* 1993; **11**:319–25.

60 Fogari R, Lazzari P, Zoppi A et al. The effects of celiprolol in the short term treatment of hypertensive patients with type 2 diabetes. *Curr Ther Res* 1990; **47**:879–88.

61 Frishman WH. Comparative pharmacokinetic and clinical profiles of ACE inhibitors and calcium antagonists in systemic hypertension. *Am J Cardiol* 1992; **69**:17c–25c.

62 Ventura HO, Frolich ED, Messerli FH, Kobrin I, Kardon MB. Cardiovascular effects and regional blood flow distribution associated with ACE inhibition (captopril) in essential hypertension. *Am J Cardiol* 1985; **55**:1023–6.

63 Sakemi T, Baba S, Yoshikava S. Angiotensin-converting enzyme inhibition attenuates hypercholesterolemia and glomerular injury in hyperlipidemic rats. *Nephron* 1992; **62**:315–21.

64 Weinberger MH. Antihypertensive therapy and lipids. Evidence, mechanism and implications. *Arch Intern Med* 1985; **145**:1102–5.

65 Weidman P, Vehlinger DE, Gerber A. Antihypertensive treatment and serum lipoproteins. *J Hypertens* 1985; **3**:297–2.

66 Leren P, Foss PO, Helgeland A et al. Effects of propranolol and prazosin on blood lipids. *Lancet* 1980; **ii**:4–6.

67   Lowenstein J, Neusy AJ. Effects of prazosin and propranolol on serum lipids in patients with essential hypertension. *Am J Med* 1984; **76:** (suppl 2A):79–84.

68   Rouffy J, Jaillard J. Effects of two antihypertensive agents on lipids, lipoproteins A and B. *Am J Med* 1986; **80** (suppl 2A):100–3.

69   Lehtonen A and Finnish Multicentre Study Group. Lowered levels of serum insulin, glucose and cholesterol in hypertensive patients during treatment with doxazosin. *Curr Ther Res* 1990; **121:**251–60.

70   Frick MH, Halttunen P, Himanen P et al. A long term double blind comparison of doxazosin and atenolol in patients with mild to moderate essential hypertension. *Br J Clin Pharmacol* 1986; **21:**55S–62S.

71   Castrignano R, D'Angelo A, Pati T et al. A single blind study of doxazosin in the treatment of mild to moderate essential hypertensive patients with concomitant non-insulin-dependent diabetes mellitus. *Am Heart J* 1988; **116:**1778–84.

72   Stamler R, Stamler J, Gosch GC, Berkson DM, Dyer A, Hershinon P. Initial antihypertensive drug therapy: Alpha blocker or diuretic. Interim report of a randomized, controlled trial. *Am J Med* 1986; **80** (suppl 2A):90–3.

73   Hunninghake DB. Effects of celiprolol and other antihypertensive agents on serum lipids and lipoproteins. *Am Heart J* 1991; **121:**696–701.

74   Lakka TA, Venalainen JM, Rauramaa R et al. Relation of leisure time physical activity and cardiorespiratory fitness to their risk of acute myocardial infarction in men. *N Engl J Med* 1994; **330:**1549–54.

SECTION IV

THE DECISION MAKING

14

The development of a new antihypertensive agent

Ali Raza, Donald Stribling and Anthony F Nash

Introduction

The specific focus of this book is the 'difficult' hypertensive patient. The development of new antihypertensive agents is not specifically focused upon such patients: to target such patients as a primary aim of development would be not only impractical but also not commercially viable. However, it is the great variety of antihypertensive agents already available today and the future introduction of new members of this therapeutic class that increasingly allows the physician to select an appropriate therapy, or combination of therapies, in order to treat these patients adequately.

The development of any new medicine to the point where it can be routinely prescribed by the practising physician is a long and complex process about which most of the general public has a low level of awareness. Indeed, many practising physicians have only a limited appreciation of the processes that govern the evolution of a molecule from discovery, through animal testing, human volunteer studies, and finally to the large patient studies that are necessary to characterize a compound before it can be used as a medicine.

The last 30 years or so have seen many significant changes that have had a dramatic effect upon the way new medicines are developed. Most of the antihypertensive agents available today have been developed during this period of change.

Up to the early 1960s, the development of a medicine was governed by relatively few rules or guidelines. The thalidomide phocomelia cases caused a public outcry for governments to take measures that would help to safeguard against similar tragedies in the future. Changes were enacted in the UK by the 1968 Medicines Act, although most reputable companies had already incorporated the various animal tests and extended trial programmes necessary to deliver safer medicines. Since those early days, it is fair to say that western governments and the ethical pharmaceutical industry have continued to work together to achieve the goal of delivering safe, effective medicines of a guaranteed quality.

Bringing a new antihypertensive agent, and indeed any new chemical entity (NCE), to the market is a long and complex process involving many stages. Although very few NCEs have been launched within 7–8 years of discovery of the parent molecule, the average length of time for this process is 10–12 years, and some NCEs take up to 14 years or more.

Given the formal patent life of 20 years, this can leave a very short time in which to recoup the investment made in research and development. However, it is reassuring to note that governments in many of the developed countries, and most notably within the European Union, have taken this issue seriously. In an attempt to prevent effective patent-life erosion and the knock-on effect of

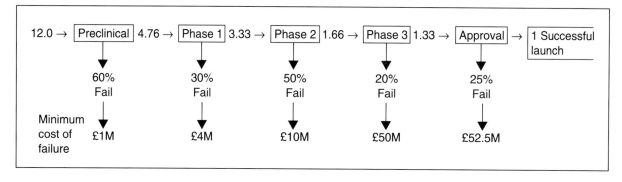

Figure 14.1
Compound attrition rates (for each product achieving launch). For every 12 candidate products entered into the preclinical phase of research, only 1 product reaches the launch stage.

reduced investment in research and development, governments have introduced measures that extend the period, to differing degrees, for which medicines can retain their patent. The average cost of bringing an NCE to launch is variously estimated as ranging from about £50 million to over £200 million. These figures depend on the milestones used for the calculations and whether the cost of all the failures on the way are taken into account when estimating the cost of bringing an NCE to a successful launch. Whatever the method of calculation, the costs of research and development are high and inexorably increasing. The cost of failure at various stages is summarized in Fig. 14.1.

The focus of research companies in the recent past has been to reduce the time taken on research and development. The target is to deliver a quality medicine, rigorously tested for safety and efficacy, in the shortest feasible time. Within most pharmaceutical companies, the development of a medicine follows a generalized template such as the one represented in schematic form in Fig. 14.2. It is important to note that each company has its own schema and these inevitably differ in some aspects. Furthermore, each medicine will have a development schedule tailored to the needs of that particular programme. This chapter will touch upon the main steps involved in this process, from discovery of the chemical entity through to successfully establishing the medicine, including the introduction of line extensions, into the practising physician's armamentarium.

Choosing the right candidate

Given the great number of compounds or products already within this area of medicine, choosing a new research candidate is a decision that requires careful matching of the technical attributes of the target product with the commercial environment into which it will be delivered several years down the line.

Too often in the past many pharmaceutical companies have spent significant amounts of technical time and resources on a research programme before actually involving appropriate commercial colleagues. Predictably, this has

	Research (4–10 years)			Exploratory development (3+ years)		Regulatory development (3+ years)			Commercialization (3+ years)	
Phase		Biological evaluation / Integrated research	Process development	Phase 1 clinical	Phase 2 clinical	Phase 3 clinical	Manufacturing	Registration	Launch and sales	
Stage	Research target									
Activities	• Medical need • Market research • Technical feasibility (commercial viability)	• Therapeutic areas • Research projects • Synthesis • Biochemical/pharmacological screening	• Candidate drug identified • Initial pharmacology • Formulation • Patents	• Safety testing – short term • Pharmacology • Pharmaceutical development	• Safety • Clinical pharmacology • Reproduction safety • Drug kinetics • Bulk drug scale up	• Efficacy • Dosage • Formulation development • Special toxicology	• International clinical trials • Safety testing – long term	• Establish manufacturing processes • Build manufacturing plant • Develop commercialization platform	• Submission to Health Authorities • Sales force training • Evaluation of health economics	• Health Authority approvals • First international launches	• Post-marketing monitoring – safety and efficiency • Further launches worldwide • Further clinical studies worldwide

Figure 14.2
The research and development process.

resulted in the curtailment of many research programmes that should perhaps not have been allowed to start in the first place. The most successful companies, and indeed the most successful products, have been built upon the basis of strong links between the commercial and technical sides of the business. It is now a prerequisite for any organization that has a serious approach to drug discovery and development to involve early input from commercial colleagues in order to underpin the future success of the antihypertensive agent.

One of the first steps is to agree on the target profile of what will be the desired antihypertensive agent in the medical community several years from now. Although built to a great degree of market research and experience, there is inevitably a significant degree of speculation in the assessment of the target profile. Major questions are raised at this stage:

- Will the agent have to be once daily or could it be dosed more often and still be an attractive option?
- What additional properties, other than a simple antihypertensive action, would increase the attractiveness of this medicine to the future prescriber?
- Are there other possible indications within the cardiovascular field, or indeed in other therapeutic areas, where the agent may be of use?

Even more fundamental questions are asked by the most senior decision makers within the company. Some companies have questioned whether they should continue to develop further agents in a field that is already fairly crowded, bearing in mind the potentially crippling costs of bringing an NCE to the market place only to discover in due course that it has failed to secure a sufficient segment of the market to have justified its development costs. This type of thinking has resulted in the exodus of a number of significant players from the field of hypertension research. At the same time, others have gone through a similar reasoning process and come to the very different conclusion that the hypertension area still offers a favourable risk–benefit ratio for future development programmes.

Current areas of research

The search for new antihypertensive agents remains remarkably active. Indeed, a recent review of the available literature revealed about 250 different candidates that are under active investigation. The great majority of these are at the preclinical stage, with about 60 in Phase I research or beyond. This vast array of 'hopefuls' can be broken down into a number of different classes of agents (Table 14.1).

It is noteworthy that a number of companies are continuing to invest resources in the development of yet more beta-blockers, calcium channel blockers, diuretics, alpha-adrenoceptor antagonists, and ACE inhibitors, despite the fact that these classes already dominate the antihypertensive market. There is likely to be a very limited space for new agents in these categories, unless they offer some significant additional advantage. Therefore, recent interest in antihypertensive agents has focused on 2 main approaches:

- exploiting an existing mechanism with added effect on an associated risk factor (e.g. calcium channel blockers with lipid lowering activity); or
- pursuing a novel pathway offering a potential improvement in profile or outcome over established therapy (e.g. endothelin receptor antagonists or possibly angiotensin II antagonists).

Established classes
• Diuretics
• Beta-blockers
• Calcium channel blockers
• Alpha-adrenoceptor antagonists
• ACE inhibitors
Major new classes
• Angiotensin II antagonists
• Renin inhibitors
• Potassium channel activators
• Endothelin receptor antagonists
• Endothelin converting enzyme inhibitors
• ANF antagonists
• Insulin resistance mediators
Other potential approaches
• Vasopressin antagonists
• Adenosine A$_2$ receptor antagonists
• 5HT2A receptors agaonists and antagonists
• Sodium–lithium exchange inhibitors
• Sodium–potassium ATPase inhibitors
• Atrial peptide clearance inhibitors
• cGMP phosphodiesterase inhibitors

Table 14.1
Current areas of antihypertensive research for new NCEs.

The greatest area of activity is still focused upon the renin–angiotensin–aldosterone system. The advent of the ACE inhibitors is generally regarded as having made one of the most significant impacts on cardiovascular medicine in the last decade. These agents were first introduced for the treatment of hypertension and symptomatic heart failure. Their use has now extended to the treatment of left ventricular dysfunction, diabetic nephropathy, and myocardial infarction; further indications are being explored. Given this spectacular success, pharmaceutical research has continued to focus upon the renin–angiotensin–aldosterone system as a central pathway in the regulation of the cardiovascular system.

This investment of effort continues to yield results, as evidenced by the approaching introduction of a number of angiotensin II antagonists. There are currently more angiotensin II antagonists in phase I to III research than any other category of agents. The thinking that has driven this research is not only the commercial success of the ACE inhibitors, but also the potential for achieving additional clinical benefit through a more complete inhibition of the angiotensin II effects. It is already being claimed that these agents produce a lower incidence of cough because, unlike ACE inhibitors, they do not potentiate the action of bradykinin which has been implicated as the mediator of ACE-inhibitor-associated cough. However, it is this same potentiation of the bradykinin pathway that may be responsible for some of the beneficial actions of ACE inhibitors, including regression of left ventricular hypertrophy and improvement of congestive heart failure. It therefore remains difficult to predict what degree of success these new agents will enjoy.

Another possible approach, and indeed an area of active research, has been to interrupt the action of renin at the beginning of the renin–angiotensin–aldosterone pathway. Although this has an attractive scientific rationale, difficulties have been experienced in producing an agent that can be absorbed from the gastrointestinal system to give satisfactory bioavailability. Due to the peptidic nature of these agents and the multistep synthesis process, some companies have moved away from this area of research. However, a number of candidates have apparently overcome these hurdles and are being tested in early human studies. It is difficult, at this stage, to predict with certainty any significant benefits that these agents may have over ACE inhibitors or AII antagonists.

There are a number of potassium channel activators in the research and development pipeline. Their relative popularity is based upon the number of indications, in addition to hypertension, in which these agents may have efficacy. These indications include peripheral vascular disease, congestive heart failure, ischaemic heart disease and dysrhythmias, asthma and urinary incontinence. Again, it is difficult to highlight any significant new advantage that these agents would bring to the treatment of hypertension *per se*.

Although there are intriguing data that insulin resistance or hyperinsulinaemia may play a pathogenetic role in hypertension, it remains to be demonstrated that amelioration of these effects with any mediators will translate into a suitable antihypertensive effect on a broad-based population basis. There may be advantages in certain population subsets of the hypertensive population, and on this basis patents have been filed by a number of companies pursuing this approach.

A number of other approaches, too numerous to discuss individually in this chapter, are currently under exploration. It is clear that the pharmaceutical research community is continuing to invest a great deal of resource into the discovery and development of new antihypertensive agents.

The research phase

Having selected the research target, the challenge is to identify a lead compound. Although computer-assisted molecular modelling has perhaps accelerated the optimization of existing leads, it has not found general application in predicting or selecting compounds likely to have activity where there is no precedent.

In the field of hypertension, biotechnology has allowed screening against the human enzyme or receptor, which removes one possible variable in moving from animal models to man. However, there is currently little scope for a genetically engineered peptide product in a field dominated by orally active once-daily products. As with many fields, there has been a recent return to high throughput screening of collections of synthetic chemicals and natural products to find elusive leads that can then be optimized.

A range of animal models of hypertension (e.g. the spontaneously hypertensive rat) can be used to characterize the profile of lead compounds. Sometimes these models are 'tuned' to detect the particular mechanism (renal artery clip). Most initial testing is completed in rodents but effects are compared in other animals (often dogs, sometimes marmosets) to ensure that the activity crosses species. These models also confirm that the selected mechanism and lead compound achieves the expected effect on blood pressure *in vivo*, correlate time course of effect with plasma drug levels, and optimize the half-life–therapeutic ratio before committing to a specific development candidate.

The cascade of tests to optimize the primary pharmacology is supplemented by tests of systematic general pharmacology to optimize or confirm selectivity. If a specific aspect of toxicology has been identified as an issue, this can be addressed as part of the test cascade, thereby reducing the risk of early failure in development. A typical test cascade using the AII antagonists as an example is shown in Fig. 14.3.

Where compounds with dual actions are being sought, or fixed combinations of 2 antihypertensive molecules are being developed, the testing cascade is inevitably complicated by

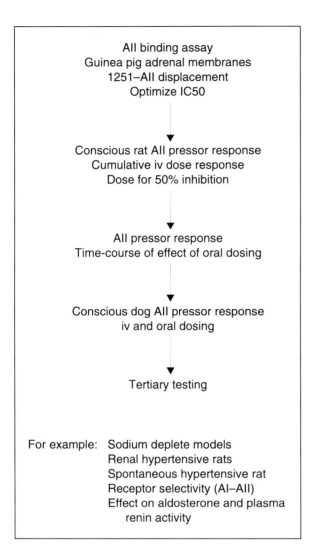

AII binding assay
Guinea pig adrenal membranes
125I–AII displacement
Optimize IC50

Conscious rat AII pressor response
Cumulative iv dose response
Dose for 50% inhibition

AII pressor response
Time-course of effect of oral dosing

Conscious dog AII pressor response
iv and oral dosing

Tertiary testing

For example: Sodium deplete models
Renal hypertensive rats
Spontaneous hypertensive rat
Receptor selectivity (AI–AII)
Effect on aldosterone and plasma
renin activity

Figure 14.3
Test cascade for angiotensin II antagonists

Preclinical and exploratory development

Once the development candidate has been chosen, a package of systematic pharmacology has to be completed to determine effects on the function of the cardiovascular, renal, central nervous, respiratory, and immune systems, etc. These studies have to be completed with compound of equivalent purity to the final sales material. Since they complement the toxicology package they have to be conducted to Good Laboratory Practice standard with the source data available for inspection if required.

Regulatory agencies require that as a chronic therapy, antihypertensive agents are tested in a full programme of toxicology tests including 6–12 month studies in 2 species (rodent and non-rodent), and lifetime oncogenicity studies in 2 species. For oncogenicity studies, the top dose group has to show signs of general toxicity – and for the USA, the Food and Drugs Administration (FDA) expects to agree the doses before the study starts.

The compound must also be assessed for effects on male and female reproductive performance and teratogenic effects when dosed during gestation. This reproductive toxicology needs to take into account that mammalian reproduction is a very complex process involving a number of stages. Data therefore need to be gathered on the process, from gametogenesis and fertilization, through implantation, embryogenesis and fetal growth, to parturition and postnatal development.

The schedule of tests *in vivo* is supplemented by *in vitro* studies, such as the Ames test, looking for evidence of interference with DNA replication, and a test on human lymphocytes, looking for evidence of clastogenicity at concentrations above those predicted to be required for antihypertensive activity in man.

the need to characterize the 2 activities and their interaction across the dose range. Compounds with dual action carry the additional risk that the ratio of effects may not carry across species.

Accompanying this toxicology work, the absorption, distribution, metabolism and excretion of the drug and its metabolites have to be characterized in the primary toxicology species. In part, this provides a warning of potential issues with absorption, distribution, metabolism, and excretion in humans. It also serves to validate the toxicology by showing the level of exposure to the drug and metabolites. Where early studies in volunteers fail to show a similar pattern of exposure and metabolism, the choice of toxicology species has to be revisited and additional species may have to be included to provide toxicological information on the particular compounds found to be circulating in man. For Japan, it is customary to have to characterize the major metabolite and evaluate the toxicology and pharmacology. This is not a general requirement in the West except where the compound is a prodrug (which is metabolized to an active moiety *in vivo*), in which case additional toxicology, ADME, and pharmacology are required to characterize both chemical entities.

With novel antihypertensive agents, it is important to distinguish between toxicology and excess pharmacology during the preclinical evaluation. In the case of ACE inhibitors and angiotensin II antagonists, rabbits showed a particular sensitivity to these classes of compounds with a combination of reflex responses in aldosterone secretion, changes in plasma potassium, a reduction in water intake, and consequent renal failure. These effects were enhanced in pregnant females and this limited the dose that could be evaluated in the teratology studies looking for an effect on fetal development. The adverse effects on the kidney were shown to be attenuated by dosing saline and this allowed higher doses to be evaluated. Where there are species-specific effects, additional studies are required to explore the mechanism and indicate early markers that

would predict problems in humans. As a result, the usual programme of studies will have to be completed in a third species on many occasions.

The pharmaceutical formulation is developed progressively – initial studies use a simple formulation (e.g. a solution or a lactose mixture in a capsule), and the eventual sale formulation is introduced only when the effective dose range has been clarified. Each formulation requires data to confirm its stability and dissolution characteristics. In order to link the clinical efficacy and safety data generated with an early formulation to a new presentation, a definitive bioequivalence study is required to demonstrate that the maximum plasma drug levels, the area under the plasma concentration–time curve, and the elimination half-life are unchanged.

The package of preclinical work has evolved over the years with additional tests being added to detect new mechanisms of toxicity. For example, the rabbit teratology study is included because, after the event, it was shown to detect the activity of thalidomide. The tests required differ between countries – often for historical reasons. However, the ICH (International Congress on Harmonization) is seeking to agree common protocols and standards to avoid needless duplication.

The preclinical safety programme is generally expanded progressively through development in such a way that initial human studies may be supported by 2-week or 1-month studies in 2 species and are restricted to male volunteers. Six-month toxicology studies that have shown a clear safety margin over human exposure are generally sufficient to support chronic dosing during clinical trials, but the oncogenicity studies have to be complete by the time the regulatory package is ready for filing with the agency. Once the reproduction and teratology package is available, studies can expand into females, although there are generally clauses in protocols to exclude the chance of dosing during pregnancy until the safety of the drug is clearly established.

Development strategies

There are many different strategies that can be applied, depending on the resources of the company, their national location, the timing objectives, and the accepted degree of risk. Some sponsors choose to complete short (14-day) toxicology studies with an intravenous formulation to allow single-dose studies in normal male volunteers. This allows an early, low-cost decision on kinetics and pharmacodynamics without possible confusion from a variable rate and extent of absorption. During this work, a further batch of bulk drug, formulation development, and longer term toxicology by the oral route need to be scheduled to avoid delay if the compound proves to be of interest. Alternatively, some sponsors take a higher degree of risk and assume that the compound will pass the early hurdles and proceed directly with oral studies. In both cases, the objective is to start the human studies as soon as possible and to keep the preclinical work off the critical path. Shortening the time to market by one year provides a faster payback but can also have a dramatic effect on competitive position in a new therapeutic class, influencing the speed of regulatory review as well as market share. The earlier that critical 'go' or 'no-go' decisions can be made, the better.

The preclinical pharmacology and the expanding programme of toxicology studies has to be documented and submitted to regulatory agencies, ethical committees and trialists, together with an expert comment on the implications for human safety in order to allow the initiation and expansion of volunteer and clinical studies.

Phase I evaluation

Once the initial preclinical package of work has been satisfactorily completed, the sponsor company will decide whether it is safe to proceed with human studies and if so to what dose. The maximum dose given to humans is calculated based on the animal toxicology data. Generally, the upper limit of the dose will be one fifth of the 'no-effect dose' or one tenth of the lowest toxic dose in the more sensitive of the 2 species tested in the toxicology studies. Alternatively, the calculation can be based on plasma concentration rather than dose.

Following the decision to proceed to human studies, a programme of volunteer studies is initiated. These studies constitute the so-called 'Phase I' studies. There is no regulatory requirement to carry out studies in volunteers at all, and indeed some companies proceed directly into patient studies without any volunteer work.

The exact programme of studies carried out during the course of the phase I evaluation of the compound varies from company to company. However, there are a number of fundamental objectives that underpin this phase of evaluation:

- to establish the safety of the agent on single and multiple dosing (symptoms and laboratory parameters);
- to characterize the kinetic profile of the agent on single and multiple dosing;
- to characterize the pharmacodynamic profile of the agent using blood pressure and/or a surrogate endpoint on single and multiple dosing; and
- to characterize the dose–response curve of the agent on these parameters.

A scheme that could form the basis of a phase I programme of studies for a new antihypertensive agent is shown in Fig. 14.4.

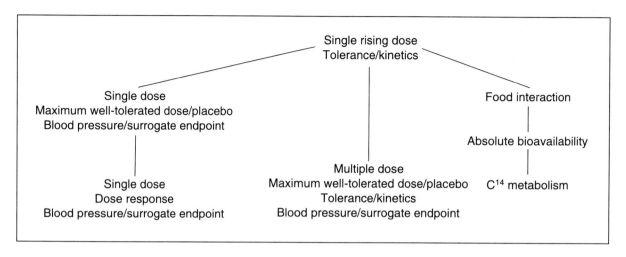

Figure 14.4
Phase I studies for an antihypertensive agent.

All of these studies use an oral formulation with the exception of the absolute bioavailability study, which requires both oral and intravenous formulations. Alternatively, an intravenous formulation may be used for early studies in order to characterize the properties of the drug, thus avoiding any potential problems in drug absorption related to the oral formulation rather than to the drug itself.

The first study in humans takes the form of a rising dose design whereby groups of volunteers are given single oral doses of the compound. Generally, very low doses of the compound are given initially. Dose escalation proceeds until either the drug is no longer tolerated or the threshold dose or plasma concentration calculated from the animal toxicology studies has been reached.

At this stage the maximum well-tolerated dose is given to a further group of volunteers in a crossover design with placebo to further substantiate the safety profile of the agent, and also to provide kinetic data on the maximum plasma concentration, half-life, and area under the curve after a single dose of the agent.

Having established the maximum well-tolerated dose and assuming that the kinetic profile of the compound is adequate, the agent will undergo a pharmacodynamic evaluation, the nature of which will be dependent upon the class of compound being investigated, e.g. blood pressure response to intravenous angiotensin II in the case of angiotensin II antagonists, intravenous angiotensin I challenge in the case of ACE inhibitors, and so on.

This evaluation is initially carried out using the maximum well tolerated dose from the initial rising-dose tolerance studies. Prior knowledge of the significance of such surrogate endpoints, in terms of correlation with blood pressure response in patients, enables such a study to provide a 'go' or 'no-go' decision on the further clinical development of the compound. For example, if the maximum well tolerated dose of an angiotensin II antagonist produced minimal or no inhibition of the blood pressure response to intravenous angiotensin II, a decision would be taken to terminate further development of the drug. Dynamic challenges can therefore be carried out at specific timepoints, especially 24 hours postdose, to provide information on whether a once daily profile is likely.

Assuming significant activity is seen with the maximum well-tolerated dose, the next step is to perform a similar study with lower doses in order to characterize the dose response of effect on these surrogate endpoints. Having completed these single oral dose studies, a multiple dose study is conducted to establish the tolerability and kinetic profile on multiple dosing, using the appropriate surrogate pharmacodynamic endpoint to demonstrate that the pharmacodynamic effects are sustained upon multiple dosing, i.e. that there is no evidence of tachyphylaxis.

Additional studies carried out during the Phase I evaluation of the agent would include the following:

1. Food interaction study – the presence of a significant food interaction would influence the timing of dosing with respect to ingestion of food in future studies.
2. An absolute bioavailability study, which compares the kinetics of an oral and an intravenous formulation of the agent.
3. A radiolabelled C^{14} metabolism study providing detailed information on the absorption, distribution, metabolism, and excretion of the agent.

This Phase I programme of studies should generally be completed in 6–9 months. If the drug under investigation is to enter Phase II in patients, it needs to have been shown to have a pharmacokinetic and pharmacodynamic profile consistent with the target product profile previously identified, prior to embarking upon studies in patients.

Phase II evaluation

The principal objective of this phase of evaluation is to establish the therapeutic dose range necessary for the treatment of patients with hypertension. In the past, the dose ranging work with many antihypertensives has clearly been inadequate. This is evidenced by the change in dosing regimen following widespread use of the agent by practising physicians once the agent has been registered.

The dose selected from the Phase II work is taken forward into the Phase III programme of clinical studies, at which stage proving efficacy studies and long-term efficacy and safety studies are conducted. Again, the nature of a Phase II programme for investigation of antihypertensives tends to vary markedly from company to company. A simple programme is as follows.

Ten-day dose response study
The objectives of this study are to provide preliminary evidence of efficacy in the target population – i.e. mild to moderate hypertension (supine diastolic 95–115 mmHg) – and preliminary dose response information in the target population, and to define the time course of effect. This study would typically involve 40 to 50 hospitalized patients with mild to moderate hypertension (95–115 mmHg diastolic). In the UK, it would customarily be supported by 1-month toxicology studies in a rodent and non-rodent species, and would be conducted under a Clinical Trial Certificate Exemption (CTX) scheme (UK regulatory authority clinical trial approval system).

Three or 4 dose levels plus placebo are studied, with careful measurement of blood pressure, serum electrolytes, and other relevant variables such as angiotensin, renin, and aldosterone, throughout the 10-day period of hospitalization.

The results of this study, in conjunction with the Phase I clinical pharmacology data, forms the basis of a key 'go/no-go' decision point on the future development of the drug. The lack of blood pressure response (as defined by a placebo-subtracted reduction in blood pressure of ≥ 5 mmHg diastolic at the end of the dosing interval) precludes the further evaluation of the compound.

Six-week dose response study

This study is designed to provide definitive dose–response information on blood pressure in the target population. It may also serve as one of the 2 pivotal efficacy studies required by regulatory authorities such as the FDA for registration of a new agent.

The study is of 6 weeks' duration, preceded by a 2- to 4-week placebo run-in. It involves 3 or 4 dose levels, plus placebo and a positive control, with each group containing approximately 60 patients. The doses are selected from the clinical pharmacology study data and the 10-day dose ranging dose response study. The inclusion of a positive control helps to put into context the magnitude of blood pressure reduction seen with the agent of interest. It is typically either a licensed agent in the same class or, if this is not available, a popular agent from an alternative class of treatment.

Both systolic and diastolic blood pressure are measured at the end of placebo run-in at peak and trough plasma concentrations (trough being 12 hours postdose for a twice-daily compound and 24 hours post-dose for a once-daily compound). Blood pressure is measured at intervals throughout the study and at peak and trough at the end of the study. The peak–trough ratio of blood pressure effect is important, and indeed the FDA stipulates that the blood pressure effect at trough should be no less than two thirds of that at peak. This is to ensure that drugs are given in an appropriate dosing regimen and to avoid the problem of 'front loading', in which a drug is given in an inappropriately large dose in order to ensure an effect at the end of the dosing interval, but effectively overdosing at peak.

Ideally, the study will show a clear dose–response on blood pressure reduction with comparable or superior efficacy to the positive control. The results from the study form the basis of another key 'go/no-go' decision point on the further development of the drug. If the study results are positive, a suitable titratable dose regimen will be chosen for the phase III programme, which forms the most costly single element of the Regulatory Development phase of the programme.

Regulatory development
Phase III studies

The principal objectives of the phase III programme of studies includes, but is not limited to, the following (Fig. 14.5):

- to confirm efficacy at the chosen dose in the target population and also in particular subgroups (e.g. the elderly, renally impaired, black population);
- to demonstrate evidence of safety and efficacy over longer term exposure in the target population;
- to demonstrate comparative efficacy and safety with agents in the same class or other classes of antihypertensives;
- to investigate the effect of concomitant drugs and diseases on the pharmacokinetic/pharmacodynamic profile of the agent.

The key efficacy study in this part of the programme is the second pivotal study against

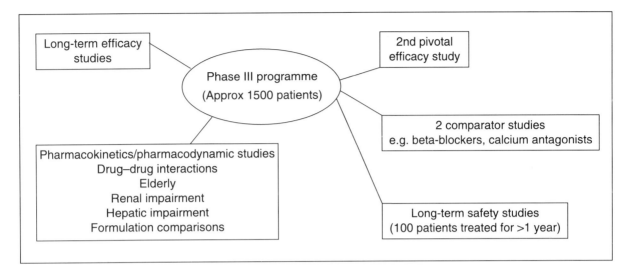

Figure 14.5
Outline of a typical phase III programme for development of an antihypertensive.

placebo. However, comparative efficacy studies are also required for the registration of an antihypertensive in the European Union; these typically involve the most popular product in at least 1 other class of antihypertensive agents. The data from these studies are also of vital importance for marketing purposes once the drug has been registered. These studies are typically of a parallel group design with a dose–titration phase; the study duration would usually be approximately 3 months. The efficacy studies should generally be designed so that they include particular subgroups of patients (e.g. blacks, elderly patients, renally impaired patients) in order that definitive statements on efficacy (and safety) are applicable to these groups. Specific studies in these subgroups can also be carried out especially if the intention is to profile the drug for a specific population with difficult-to-treat hypertension.

There is a European Union regulatory requirement that at least 100 patients should be exposed for 1 year or longer to the agent. Specific studies can be set up to provide these data, or open label extensions to the efficacy studies can be added. The idea here is to demonstrate that the agent is acceptably safe when used as long-term therapy and that efficacy is maintained over this period of time.

There is at present no requirement to provide information to regulatory authorities on the effect of a new agent on the 24-hour blood pressure profile as detected by ambulatory blood pressure monitoring and it is likely that until more information becomes available on the correlation between blood pressure reduction as detected by ambulatory blood pressure monitoring and morbidity and mortality, this situation will not alter. Nevertheless, most companies now conduct studies using ambulatory blood pressure monitoring as supportive evidence for the chosen dosing regimen and efficacy. Moreover, these type of data are again useful for marketing purposes.

Pharmacodynamic studies are conducted, the specifics of the studies depending on the nature of the agent. For example, agents with effects on the conducting system of the heart would usually undergo a detailed electrophysiology study. Invasive left and right heart monitoring studies are also frequently done in order to characterize the effect of the agent on specific haemodynamic parameters. A typical phase III programme as outlined above will generally take approximately 2–3 years to conduct, and at the end of this period there should be sufficient information to register the drug as an antihypertensive agent.

Regulatory submission

It is now a prerequisite for any clinical trial work performed by a pharmaceutical company that this work be performed according to the principles of 'Good Clinical (Research) Practice', i.e. GC(R)P. These principles apply equally to the investigator performing the work and to the sponsor company. The ethical, technical, and scientific quality of a trial is underpinned by adherence to GCP. This covers all stages of the process, including protocol generation, recruitment and consent of patients, conduct of the trial, data collection and documentation, and subsequent source verification, culminating in the production of a written report, which may then be used as part of a submission for registration with the regulatory authorities.

Adherence to GCP helps to ensure the credibility of the data. Indeed, regulatory agencies may refuse to accept data unless they are satisfied that the work was done to GCP.

The exact structure and details of a regulatory submission can clearly vary from one package to another. However, the general content of each package has a number of common features. (Fig. 14.6).

This 'pyramid' of documentation is common to most regulatory authorities around the

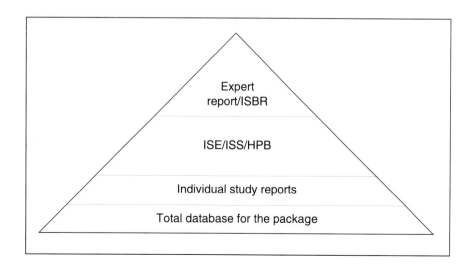

Figure 14.6
General structure of the clinical part of an international regulatory submission.

ISBR=Integrated summary of benefits and risks
ISE=Integrated summary of efficacy
ISS=Integrated summary of safety
HPB=Human pharmacokinetics and bioavailability

world. The clinical expert report is written by a nominated physician who can be an external expert or a company medical adviser. The expert is expected to provide a critical appraisal of the clinical data in the package and give a reasoned opinion on the adequacy of the data to support the proposed indication(s) for the product. The expert report is replaced by the Integrated Summary of Benefits and Risks (ISBR) in regulatory submissions to the FDA in the USA.

Commercialization phase

The registration of a new chemical entity for its indication in hypertension is usually only the first step in the so-called 'commercialization' of the product. It is increasingly apparent that receiving approval from the regulatory authorities is not in itself a guarantee of future success for the product. Additional data needs to be generated from further clinical trials in order to give the product the necessary competitive advantage in the hypertension market.

More and more, this commercialization of the product is planned at the very early stages of development of a compound. At the same time as the phase III studies are being conducted with the aim of securing a hypertension indication, plans will be laid for the phase IIIb studies, which will supplement the IIIa data available to the physician in the postlaunch period. These studies concentrate on increasing the knowledge of the product's relative performance against competitor products or its performance in patient subgroups of particular interest.

Once the product has been launched, the product is further supported by a programme of phase IV market support studies. The purpose of these studies should be to supplement the growing database of knowledge and experience about the products efficacy and safety profile in its registered indication. For instance, there is an increasing awareness of the need to demonstrate mortality benefits for the newer agents. The lack of mortality data for the calcium channel blockers and ACE inhibitors has proven to be something of an Achilles' heel for these classes of therapy in the field of hypertension. Large-scale trials are currently underway to address this, but the pharmaceutical companies have generally accepted the need for trials that demonstrate mortality benefits for the new antihypertensive agents. Clearly, these data are unlikely to be available for the initial registration package. Nevertheless, the registration dossier for the future antihypertensive may well have to contain data supporting claims for beneficial effects on the other cardiovascular risk factors.

With the rapidly evolving healthcare scene, there is also an increasing focus on the economic aspects of treatments. Although the impact of health economics has been more acute in other therapeutic areas, the general principles are also applicable to the hypertension field. All health care systems have an ultimate 'payer'. This may be the patient themselves, the government supporting the national health system (as with the NHS in the UK) or Health Management Organizations, which are increasingly influencing the managed care sector of the US system. The concept of 'value for money' is clearly important to any 'payer'. The 'payer' now increasingly requires clear demonstration that the therapy prescribed is not only the most efficacious and safe but also the most cost effective. This may take the form of demonstrating that patients given a particular therapy have fewer hospitalizations or doctor visits, or fewer subsequent complications of disease, all of which will generate additional costs down the line to the 'payer'. The generation of relevant health-economics data is now becoming a priority for many classes of therapy, including antihypertensive agents.

Line extensions
The pharmacology of the molecule may well lend itself to potential use in other cardiovascular indications such as congestive heart failure, angina, myocardial infarction, and so on. Indeed, the product can occasionally be registered for the treatment of non-cardiovascular conditions, in the way that propanolol is registered for the treatment of anxiety. This expansion of indications and the possible introduction of improved formulations, including the introduction of different delivery systems that deliver a better pharmacokinetic profile linked to clinical benefits, is all part of the broader commercialization of a product.

For a hypertensive agent, an integral part of the development and commercialization of the product is often to combine it with another established antihypertensive agent with a different pharmacology of action.

Combination products

Response to antihypertensive monotherapy varies from as low as 30% up to about 60% of patients. Patients who do not respond to monotherapy may exhibit an improved response to combination of 2 different classes of agent. This practice has led to the development of a number of different types of fixed combinations. The relative success of these products is based upon both the improved efficacy and response rate together with the improved compliance that results from the use of a final combination in a single pill. The pharmacological rationale for fixed combination therapy is based upon the following factors:

- the mechanism of the antihypertensive effects are complementary;
- the kinetic profiles of the 2 agents are compatible;
- the reduction in arterial pressure is greater than with either agent alone, thereby controlling the blood pressure for more of the treated population;
- the incidence or severity of the adverse events are reduced or not significantly increased compared to monotherapies; and
- the dosing regimen can be simplified, facilitating use of the lowest effective doses of the two agents.

A number of different combinations are available. The most popular currently are ACE inhibitors combined with diuretics and calcium channel blockers combined with beta-blockers. A number of new combinations will also be available in due course, such as calcium channel blockers with ACE inhibitors and angiotensin II antagonists with diuretics. Fixed combinations are generally used as second-line agents for those patients who have been established on the respective doses of the monocomponents. Clearly, the clinician does face some restriction in choice of dosage when prescribing fixed combinations compared to the free combinations. However, some fixed combinations offer a choice of dosage ratios, especially with ACE inhibitor–diuretic combinations.

Development of fixed combinations
The key step in the development of a fixed combination is choosing the right dosage ratio. This is most expediently done using a dose matrix design study, which assesses the efficacy and safety of a number of different doses of the 2 monotherapies (Table 14.2). The optimal dosage combination can then be studied in a further trial, and it can be compared against placebo or a competitor product, or against both.

	Antihypertensive A (e.g. diuretic)			
Antihypertensive B (e.g. ACE inhibitor)	6.25 mg	12.5 mg	25 mg	Placebo
10 mg	10/6.25	10/12.5	10/25	10/0
20 mg	20/6.25	20/12.5	20/25	20/0
Placebo	0/6.25	0/12.5	0/25	Placebo

Table 14.2
Example of a dose matrix design study for assessing combination therapy of two antihypertensives (antihypertensive A – e.g. a diuretic – and antihypertensive B – e.g. an ACE inhibitor). This study design would allow an initial assessment of the most appropriate combinations of the two monocomponents.

As most fixed combination products are based on monocomponents which have an established role in the treatment of hypertension, there is no further need for oncogenicity studies, although a limited toxicology programme is required to underpin the safety of the dosage combination used. The clinical part of the regulatory dossier for such a product will be a slimline package centred around the kinetic profile of the monocomponents, the dose matrix efficacy studies and the long-term ('100 patient years') efficacy and safety follow-up study.

In the past, the patent expiry strategy for NCEs generally centred upon the introduction of line extensions, as discussed above. However, the growing challenge of generic substitution, fuelled by the ever-sharpening focus on increasing health care costs, has resulted in a significant change of strategy by the pharmaceutical industry in recent years. It is now accepted by most of the research-and-development-based companies that the most effective response to the introduction of generic substitution following a product's patent expiry is indeed to generate further new products from the research and development pipeline to replace those being lost to generic competition. This increasing investment in innovation is resulting in rapidly escalating costs of research and development. These rising costs will inevitably lead to a continued shake-out in the pharmaceutical industry, the ultimate outcome of which is difficult to predict, other than to expect a more slimline industry with a smaller number of large companies and a larger number of 'niche' players.

Concluding remarks

To be successful in the future, new antihypertensive medicines will also have proven significant additional benefits such as lipid-lowering ability, antiatherogenic properties, beneficial effects on microalbuminuria, insulin resistance, or other recognized risk factors.

The continued development of new antihypertensive agents is a process which has come under close scrutiny in many of the cardiovascular companies. In a market-place that already has over 10 representatives of the ACE inhibitor class alone, and well over 100 different brands of different antihypertensive products, the practising physician is in danger of being overwhelmed for choice. However, it is this very choice of different agents already available and to be further augmented over the coming years that helps the physician to treat the 'difficult' hypertensive patient more efficiently.

15

Determining the impact of antihypertensive drugs on quality of life

Astrid Fletcher and Christopher Bulpitt

The benefits of treating hypertension have been established from several large randomized controlled trials that show that active treatment produces a 40% reduction in strokes and a 14% reduction in coronary heart disease compared with placebo.[1] The few trials that compare different antihypertensive treatments have not found a clear advantage or disadvantage from beta-blockers or diuretics on mortality or major cardiovascular events,[2-4] although the results of one trial suggested that diuretics were more effective than beta-blockers in the elderly.[5] The comparative benefits of more recently developed drugs on cardiovascular events is currently unknown, although large-scale trials are planned.

In the absence of data on reduction in cardiovascular events, other factors – such as costs and adverse effects – influence the choice of treatment. Adverse effects include morbidity, e.g. gout from an elevated uric acid, or diabetes from glucose intolerance, as well as the more diffuse side effects that impair well-being and cause some patients to discontinue treatment.

Psychological well-being may be affected by drug treatment, and in this chapter, results from antihypertensive trials that have used a formal measurement of quality of life will be discussed.

Quality of Life measures in comparative trials of ACE inhibitors

In 1986, Croog et al published the results of the first major trial using Quality of Life (QOL) methods in hypertension, which was conducted in the USA.[6] This was a randomized double blind trial of 6 months' duration in 626 men with mild to moderate hypertension who had been randomized to receive captopril, methyldopa, or propranolol. Hydrochlorothiazide was added if needed to control the blood pressure. The trial employed interviewers and used a large number of measures of QOL. After 6 months' treatment, a significant benefit for captopril compared to methyldopa was shown in a measure of overall well-being, physical symptoms, and self-rated work performance, in a measure of cognitive function, and in an overall measure of life satisfaction. There were fewer differences between captopril and propranolol, though there were significant differences in favour of captopril in general well-being, sexual dysfunction, and physical symptoms. Patients on propranolol did better than those on methyldopa in work performance.

Certain reservations were expressed about the trial, primarily in the choice of comparator

Study	N	Length (months)	Trial drugs
Croog et al[6]	540	6	Captopril, propranolol, methyldopa
Herrick et al[7]	147	3	Enalapril, atenolol
Fletcher et al[8]	125	2	Captopril, atenolol
Steiner et al[9]	360	2	Captopril, enalapril, atenolol, propranolol
Croog et al[10]	306	2	Captopril, atenolol, verapamil
Palmer et al[11]	296	1.5	Captopril, atenolol (cross-over)
Fletcher et al[12]	540	6	Cilazapril, atenolol, nifedipine
Moeller et al[13]	360	2	Lisinopril, metoprolol
TOMHS[14]	900	12	Enalapril, acebutolol, amlodipine, doxazosin, chlorthalidone, placebo
Os et al[15]	828	6	Lisinopril, nifedipine

Table 15.1
Randomized trials using QOL measurements to evaluate ACE inhibitors

drugs and the exclusion of women. Since this trial, several other trials have examined whether these benefits for ACE inhibitors are also found when compared to newer drugs (Table 15.1).[7-15] In many of the studies, atenolol was one of the comparator drugs and in 4 trials a calcium channel blocker was one of the comparator drugs. In the Treatment of Mild Hypertension Study (TOMHS)[14] over 2000 patients aged 45–69 years were randomized to one of 5 active treatments (acebutolol, amlodipine, doxazosin, chlorthalidone, enalapril) or to placebo.

Similar dimensions of QOL were assessed in all trials; these dimensions included those aspects which might potentially be affected by antihypertensive treatment: psychological well-being, work performance, sexual and sleep dysfunction, and symptomatic complaints. Objective tests of cognitive function were included in some trials.

Global measures

The trials found no differences between the ACE inhibitors and atenolol in global measures of psychological and general well-being and life satisfaction. The adverse effect of propranolol suggested in the 1986 Study by Croog et al[6] was confirmed in the trial by Steiner et al.[9] Both atenolol and enalapril were associated with positive changes on the life-satisfaction scale whereas propranolol was associated with negative changes. In the TOMHS study,[14] patients on acebutolol appeared to fare better than those on placebo.

The Psychological General Well-Being Index (PGWB) was used in four of the trials (Table 15.2). In the original Croog study[6] significant differences of 3.8 units were observed between captopril and methyldopa, and of 2.5 units between captopril and propranolol. In general, the differences observed between ACE

Study	Drug comparison	Change (95% confidence if available)	Effect size if available
Croog et al[6]	Captopril–Methyldopa	3.8	0.3
	Captopril–Propranolol	2.5	0.2
Steiner et al[9]	Captopril–Propranolol	1.7	
	Captopril–Atenolol	0.3	
	Enalapril–Atenolol	0.7	
Croog et al[10]	Captopril–Atenolol	1.0 (men)	
		−0.8 (women)	
	Captopril–Verapamil	3.4 (men)	
		1.0 (women)	
	Atenolol–Verapamil	2.4 (men)	
		1.8 (women)	
Fletcher et al[12]	Cilazapril–Atenolol	0.7 (−1.9, 3.4)	0.04
	Atenolol–Nifedipine	−0.3 (−2.9, 2.4)	−0.01
	Cilazapril–Nifedipine	0.5 (−2.2, 3.1)	0.03

Table 15.2
Changes in the Psychological General Well-Being Index measured at the end of trials that compared antihypertensive treatments for their effects on QOL.

inhibitors and atenolol were of a smaller order than those seen between ACE inhibitors and either propranolol or methyldopa.

In the trial comparing cilazapril with atenolol and nifedipine[12] (the largest of the recent trials and of the same duration as the 1986 Croog study), the average result showed only a very small difference between the ACE inhibitor and atenolol (0.7 units), and nifedipine (0.5 units). The 95% confidence intervals excluded an effect between cilazapril and atenolol and between cilazapril and nifedipine of the size seen for captopril and for methyldopa (i.e. 3.8 units), but they did not exclude the difference of 2.5 between captopril and propranolol.

In the trial in black hypertensives,[10] men on captopril or atenolol showed greater improvements in the PGWB index (3.4 and 2.4 units

respectively) compared to men on verapamil. The differences were of less magnitude in women but in the same direction (see Table 2). These differences were not significant at the 5% level, reflecting the smaller size of this trial compared with the original Croog study;[6] moreover in this later trial,[10] the results are given for men and women separately.

Mood

Measures of overall well-being may conceal specific effects on mood. Steiner et al[9] found that both captopril and enalapril were significantly different from atenolol and propranolol in the depressed mood subscale although the effect for atenolol was less than for propranolol. None of the other trials reviewed found significant differences in overall measures of depression. An analysis of the individual 30 items of the General Health Questionnaire (a screening questionnaire for psychiatric disorders) found a difference in favour of lisinopril compared with metoprolol in four items, though the overall measure was not significant.[13]

Differences between ACE inhibitors and beta blockers may also reflect improvements in mood as a result of ACE inhibition. In the early days of ACE therapy there were suggestions of an anti-depressant[16] or indeed potentially euphoric effect of ACE inhibitors. Steiner et al[9] found similar improvements in vitality and positive well-being with ACE inhibitors and atenolol but not propranolol. Little change in measures of vigour was observed with ACE inhibitors compared to either atenolol or nifedipine. Overall, these results do not support an association of ACE inhibitors with mood elevation but the instruments used may not have been sensitive to subtle effects.

A key issue in looking at the results from QOL trials is interpretation of the importance and meaning of changes resulting from treatment, especially as most clinicians are unfamiliar with the scales used. Effect size is a parameter that provides a measure of the relative importance of changes observed in a QOL dimension as a result of treatment. In general, effect sizes are calculated as the difference between pretreatment and post-treatment means divided by the standard deviation between patients of the pretreatment means. Within a study, effect size can be used as an indicator of effects likely to be noticed by patients. It is likely that effect sizes greater than 0.3 would be detected by patients. Effect sizes can act as reference values or as benchmarks against which newer drugs can be assessed.

Table 2 shows effect sizes for between drug differences in a measure of psychological well-being in 2 studies of antihypertensive drugs.

Small to moderate effect sizes were observed for the differences between captopril and methyldopa (0.3) and between captopril and propranolol (0.2)[6] whereas studies comparing more recent classes of drugs with angiotensin converting enzyme (ACE) inhibitors found negligible differences, with effect sizes ranging from −0.01 to 0.04.[6] The effect sizes accorded with clinical experience of these drugs.

Cognitive function

Psychomotor speed and concentration

Trail Making B is a test of the time taken to join letters and numbers in sequence, and was used in several of the trials (Table 15.3).[6] Significant differences were found between captopril and methyldopa (8 seconds in favour of captopril) but not between propranolol and captopril (2 seconds). Again the differences expressed as effect sizes show a small adverse effect of both methyldopa and (to a lesser extent) propranolol on psychomotor speed; this effect is likely to be detected by patients.

In the larger trial of Fletcher et al[12] very small differences were observed between cilazapril, atenolol and nifedipine, with patients treated with atenolol and nifedipine being 2–3 seconds faster than patients on cilazapril. The 95% confidence intervals for the differences ranged from −6 to +7 excluding the size of difference between captopril and methyldopa observed in the trial by Croog et al. This suggests that the differences previously observed reflected adverse effects of methyldopa rather than improvements with captopril.

Other workers have found differences between ACE inhibitors and beta blockers in other measures of psychomotor speed and alertness. For example, Herrick et al[7] reported that, in the Digit Symbol Substitution Test and Paced Auditory Serial Addition Task, hypertensive patients treated with enalapril showed

Study	Drug comparison	Change in seconds (95% CI if available)	Effect size if available
Croog et al[6]	Captopril–Methyldopa	8	0.3
	Captopril–Propranolol	2	0.2
Croog et al[10]	Captopril–Atenolol	–12 (men)	
		4 (women)	
	Captopril–Verapamil	–14 (men)	
		10 (women)	
	Atenolol–Verapamil	–2 (men)	
		6 (women)	
Fletcher et al[12]	Cilazapril–Atenolol	–2 (–6, 3)	0.04
	Atenolol–Nifedipine	0 (–4, 5)	0
	Cilazapril–Nifedipine	–3 (–2, 7)	0.03

Table 15.3
Changes in Trail Making B measured at the end of trials comparing antihypertensive treatments.

significantly greater improvement compared to baseline than patients treated with atenolol.

Verbal and visual memory
In 3 trials[6,7,10] verbal memory was assessed using Digit Span Tests (repetition of digits both forwards and backwards). No differences were found between ACE inhibitors, propranolol, atenolol or verapamil. Steiner et al[9] also showed no comparative effects on a range of other tests of verbal memory, and both Croog et al[6] and Herrick et al[7] reported no differences between ACE inhibitors, beta-blockers and methyldopa in tests of visual memory.

How important for patients are the changes noted with cognitive testing? No differences in a scale of self-reports of problems with memory or concentration were found between ACE inhibitors and atenolol in two large trials,[11,12] while a benefit for both captopril and propranolol in comparison with methyldopa[6] in self-reported work performance was found, which confirms that an effect size of 0.3 is compatible with a small adverse effect likely to be noticed by patients. Lisinopril significantly improved self-reports of work activity compared with metoprolol.[13]

There have been two trials that have compared two different ACE inhibitors with each other – the trial by Steiner et al,[9] and a recent publication by Testa and colleagues.[17] Steiner et al[9] found a significant advantage in favour of enalapril compared with captopril in one of the subscales of the PGWB, with no indication of an adverse effect on any other subscale or measure. In contrast, the study by Testa et al[17] conducted in nearly 400 men, found significant advantages for captopril compared with enalapril in a range of QOL subscales, including overall quality of life, perceived general health, vitality, health status, and sleep. Calculation of effect sizes suggested that these differences were very small for overall well-being (0.15), but compatible with the differential effects of methyldopa and captopril for the vitality subscale (0.35). These surprising results do not seem to accord with clinical experience of the drug and the conclusion has to be that any relative benefits of captopril compared with enalapril are still unknown.

It is also worth remembering that for many years ACE inhibitors were considered to be effectively free of side effects. It is now accepted that cough, typically an irritating, persistent, dry cough, is the most common side effect of ACE treatment.[18] There is considerable variation in estimates of the occurrence of cough; this variation reflects study design, methods of ascertaining cough, methods of measuring occurrence, and size of study. Growing awareness of the cough caused by ACE inhibitors has also influenced the level of reporting. Cough was either not mentioned in early review articles of ACE inhibitors or the evidence was considered inadequate to associate the cough with the drug. Estimates from early postmarketing survey studies gave low figures for the prevalence of cough (0.2%, 0.8% and 1.1%), based on spontaneous reports of suspected adverse reactions with captopril and enalapril. The incidence of cough in hospital clinic series has been higher, ranging from 6% to 16%. Double blind randomized trials, using a standard, patient-assessed questionnaire on side effects, provide more reliable results; bias is reduced and the net increase from baseline is measured for both ACE inhibitors and a comparator drug. In such trials, the increase in cough over baseline was between 13% and 25% – much higher than the 2% or less reported for the comparator drug. Cough caused by ACE inhibitors appears to be more common in women and disappears on average 3–6 days after drug withdrawal. One measure of the disturbance to the patients is the number of patients who are withdrawn from treatment because of cough. In one hospital-based study, 6% of patients stopped the drug over a 4-year period because of cough; this is about 40% of those who developed a cough. Little is known about the reduction in quality of life caused by this side effect. In one study, a high proportion of patients reported the cough as moderate to severe (71%), present both during the day and at night (81%), and disturbing sleep (71%). In 21% the cough caused vomiting. Sore throat (10% excess) and voice changes (14% excess) were also reported more frequently in patients on enalapril. Another study found that cough due to ACE inhibitors was associated with some deterioration in well-being: depression and sore throat are significantly associated with the cough, as is a tendency to increased fatigue.

Quality of Life measures in comparative trials of calcium channel blockers

Four of the trials discussed in the previous section included a calcium channel blocker in the comparison with an ACE inhibitor.[10,12,14,15] The results of the study by Croog et al in black hypertensives[10] suggested greater benefits in psychological well-being in patients treated with atenolol or captopril compared with verapamil. However, the results were presented separately for men and women and the sample sizes were rather small, so no firm conclusion can be drawn. The results of the trial comparing nifedipine with atenolol and cilazapril showed mixed effects.[12] Symptomatic complaints (especially flushing and oedema) were more frequent throughout the trial in the patients on nifedipine, and they also accounted for a significantly higher discontinuation rate on this treatment (17% on nifedipine discontinued compared to 8% on atenolol and 5% on cilazapril). On the other hand, patients on nifedipine reported significantly fewer problems in the fatigue score than patients on either cilazapril or atenolol. There were small differences in the PGWB between nifedipine and atenolol, and between nifedipine and cilazapril (see Table 15.2). In the trail making tests, patients on nifedipine had a similar performance to those on atenolol and were marginally faster than those on cilazapril (see Table 15.3).

Testa et al[19] reported the results of a 24-week comparison of atenolol with nifedipine gastrointestinal therapeutic system (GITS). Only men were included and nifedipine was used in a novel preparation. Their results, showing significant benefits for nifedipine compared to atenolol across a range of QOL dimensions, were based only on the patients who completed the trial, even though a large proportion of patients on nifedipine (40%) and atenolol (32%) withdrew. Analysis of all randomized subjects indicated very little difference in QOL between the two drugs. Withdrawal due to adverse effects was commoner on nifedipine (16%) than on atenolol (4%); $p < 0.001$. A similar finding of a high withdrawal rate and an increase in side effects for nifedipine when compared with lisinopril has been reported.[13]

There have been a few other trials in which calcium channel blockers have been evaluated against other therapies. One trial randomized patients to double blind treatment with verapamil (n=47) or propranolol (n=47) for 4 months.[20] The QOL questionnaire for this trial has been described by Bulpitt et al.[21] In brief, symptomatic side effects of treatment were evaluated from a checklist. An activity and

well-being index (Health Status Index) was derived from responses to questions on work, absence from work due to sickness, and interference with lifestyle caused by treatment. The Symptom Rating Test assessed psychiatric morbidity, both overall and for five subscales: anxiety, depression, somatic, cognitive performance, and hostility. The QOL results showed an overall trend of improvement with verapamil and deterioration with propranolol. Little change was observed in the patients on verapamil in the reporting of symptoms and side effects, compared to an increase in the patients on propranolol ($p < 0.05$). The Health Status Index increased on verapamil and fell on propranolol ($p < 0.05$) – a rise indicates an improvement. Psychiatric morbidity tended to improve in patients on verapamil, while patients taking propranolol showed deteriorations in all the psychological scores except hostility. However, only the somatic scale was significantly different between the drugs.

QOL was evaluated in a 6-month double blind trial in 6 European countries.[22] Patients who were already on a diuretic were randomized to receive additional pinacidil (n=110) or nifedipine slow-release (n=107). The measurements of QOL were essentially the same as in the trial by Fletcher et al[20] described above, but there were additional questions on expected side effects, such as hirsutism and heartburn. Eighteen patients on pinacidil and 12 on nifedipine withdrew because of side effects such as oedema (both drugs) and flushing (nifedipine). The average number of symptomatic complaints fell on both drugs, with significant decreases in the reporting of headaches, sleepiness, and blurred vision on nifedipine. Complaints of heartburn increased significantly on nifedipine as did complaints of body hair on pinacidil. The drugs differed in their effect on psychiatric morbidity as measured by the Symptom Rating Test. At the end of the trial patients on pinacidil showed a significant improvement in the total and cognitive scores compared to nifedipine ($p < 0.05$). The Health Status Index improved on both drugs.

The trials described above have shown different results on the effects of calcium channel blockers on QOL. A part of this difference may be attributed to the different pharmacological properties of the drugs used. Nifedipine and nitrendipine (both calcium channel blockers of the dihydropyridine class) are potent vasodilators, whereas verapamil has greater chronotropic and inotropic depressant action. The results of a randomized controlled trial that directly compared verapamil slow release with nifedipine retard have been published.[23] The increase in symptoms on nifedipine was due mainly to swollen ankles and flushing. Measures of psychiatric morbidity tended to improve on verapamil and to deteriorate on nifedipine. Only the change in cognitive function was significant between the drugs, being worse on nifedipine ($p=0.05$).

Quality of Life on diuretics

QOL was not formally measured in two large placebo-controlled trials in the elderly that employed a diuretic.[24,25] Checklists of side effects were used in both trials. In the trial of the European Working Party on High Blood Pressure in the Elderly (EWPHE),[24] triamterene was used as the first-line drug and methyldopa was required additionally in one third of patients. Certain symptoms were significantly commoner on active treatment than placebo: dry mouth, and the complaint that this symptom interfered with eating, nasal stuffiness, and diarrhoea. Symptoms significantly associated with active treatment were further investigated by comparing patients on active

diuretic with those on active diuretic plus methyldopa at 1, 2, and 3 years. Dry mouth was significantly related to treatment with methyldopa plus diuretic (57% at 1 year and 60% at 3 years; $p < 0.001$) compared to diuretic only (27% at 1 year and 40% at 3 years; $p < 0.05$). Dry mouth interfering with eating was reported consistently more by patients on methyldopa plus diuretic (23%, 20% and 19% at 1, 2 and 3 years) than by patients to diuretic alone (6%, 11% and 8%) ($p < 0.05$). Diarrhoea was also associated more with methyldopa plus diuretic (36%, 30% and 34% at 1, 2 and 3 years) compared to diuretic only (25%, 21% and 16%) ($p < 0.05$ at 3 years).

In the Systolic Hypertension in Older Adults Program (SHEP),[25] which used chlorthalidone as first-line treatment and atenolol as second-line treatment, symptoms were characterized as either troublesome or intolerable. No symptoms were significantly associated with placebo. Falls and faints increased from around 10% on placebo to nearly 13% on active treatment. Problems with memory and concentration were reported by 26% of patients on active treatment and 20% on placebo.

In the pilot study for the trial,[26] cognitive status, depression, and disability were measured. Four hundred and forty-three subjects who received active treatment (usually chlorthalidone alone) and 108 subjects who received placebo were eligible for assessment after one year, and 87% were actually assessed. No effect of treatment on depression was found in a multivariate analysis. An independent effect of treatment on a measure of psychomotor speed and alertness was found, but this disappeared in the multivariate analysis.

The Trial of Antihypertensive Interventions and Management (TAIM)[27] randomized 697 patients aged 21–65 years to chlorthalidone, atenolol, or placebo. Patients were additionally randomized to 1 of 3 diets (normal diet, a low-sodium–high-potassium diet, or a weight-loss diet). No differences between the drugs were found in measures of mood, fatigue, or overall life satisfaction. This suggests that both the diuretic and ACE inhibitor are similar to placebo. In contrast, in the TOMHS study,[14] patients on chlorthalidone appeared to fare better than those on placebo.

Little is known about the effects of diuretics on cognitive function. One trial found that diuretics interfered with cognitive function in the elderly,[28] but no differences in a range of standard cognitive tests were observed between atenolol, hydrochlorothiazide, and placebo in the first 9 months of treatment in the MRC trial of hypertension in older people.[29]

Sexual function and antihypertensive treatment

Reports of problems with various aspects of sexual response and function are not uncommon in patients on antihypertensive drug treatment. The difficulty lies in ascertaining the extent (if any) to which these may be attributed to the actual drugs being used, since sexual problems are also commonly reported in the general population and in untreated hypertensives. Moreover, until relatively recently, there was a dearth of good-quality research in this area. For many antihypertensive drugs, there is little information other than anecdotal reports. Questions on sexual dysfunction have been included in a few double blind randomized trials of antihypertensive agents, mainly the more recently developed drugs such as ACE inhibitors. Even these studies provide only limited information.

Most attention has focused on male compared to female sexual dysfunction, probably because problems such as impotence, or failure of ejaculation can be elicited by direct questions. Also, there has tended to be a reluctance to ask women (especially older ones) about the quality of their sexual experiences. A problem of interpretation is that sexual dysfunction may not be directly due to the drug itself but to some other side effect of the drug, e.g. tiredness or depression. The evidence that different antihypertensive agents may adversely affect sexual function is reviewed below.

Diuretics

In the large Medical Research Council Trial[30] on the treatment of mild to moderate hypertension, using questionnaires completed by patients, impotence was reported twice as commonly on bendrofluazide as on placebo (16% at 12 weeks and 23% at 2 years on bendrofluazide, compared to around 10% on both occasions on placebo). Impotence caused the withdrawal of 2% of the patients on bendrofluazide, but only a negligible number of patients on placebo. Other diuretics also appear to cause problems with impotence. In the Hypertension Detection Follow Up Program,[31] 5% of males treated with the first-line drug chlorthalidone withdrew from treatment because of sexual problems, mostly impotence (4.4%), and 1.6% of males on spironolactone were withdrawn because of sexual dysfunction. It must be remembered that both in this study and the MRC trial, the investigators knew each patient's treatment, and therefore bias cannot be discounted. Even so, these effects have been confirmed in several double blind trials. In the TOMHS study,[14] 17% of men on chlorthalidone reported problems with obtaining an erection and a similar number reported problems in maintaining an erection. The comparable figures for placebo were 7% for both problems. The

TAIM study[27] included 3 questions on sexual dysfunction: inability to have an orgasm, loss of sexual interest, and inability to have an erection. More men reported problems with erection on chlorthalidone than on placebo and atenolol. Several interesting findings emerged in the diet groups and in the interactions with diet and antihypertensive treatment groups. Substantial reductions in the reporting of the 3 sexual problems were found in the weight-loss group (both for men and women). In this group, men on chlorthalidone were similar to those on placebo and atenolol in the reporting of problems with impotence. In women, the reporting of sexual problems was the same on chlorthalidone from placebo when averaged over all the diet groups. Among women receiving chlorthalidone, those on their usual diet reported a worsening of sexual problems compared with those on a weight-loss diet. Although one needs to be cautious about the data, they do suggest that the adverse effects of chlorthalidone may be countered by weight loss, although the mechanisms for this are unclear. The trial also included a questionnaire on sexual satisfaction over the previous 6 months in terms of quality of sex life, frequency of sex, strength of sex drive, and arousal. This scale did not reveal any differences between any of the diet or drug groups for men or women. However, given the results reported above it is possible that this scale was insensitive to changes.

In a randomized double blind trial comparing 3 antihypertensive agents (propranolol, methyldopa, and captopril) in 626 hypertensive men, sexual symptoms worsened in patients on propranolol and methyldopa who required additional diuretic (hydrochlorothiazide) to control the blood pressure.[33] This effect was not observed in patients on captopril. The interpretation of this is not clear, but an adverse effect of taking 2 drugs with sexual side effects (methyldopa and diuretic or propranolol and diuretic) may be more troublesome than diuretic alone or diuretic and captopril.

In the SHEP study[25] a significantly greater number of patients on active treatment (4.8%) reported problems in sexual function as troublesome or intolerable compared to those on placebo (3.2%). Further details on the nature of these sexual problems have not yet been published.

Beta blockers

An association between propranolol and erectile problems has been frequently reported. It is less clear how common the problem is and whether other aspects of sexual function are also affected. In the MRC trial,[30] the prevalence of impotence in patients taking propranolol, based on questionnaires completed by patients, was not significantly different from placebo at both 12 weeks and 2 years (13% compared to 10%). Significantly more patients on propranolol were withdrawn from the trial because of impotence compared to placebo (0.6% compared to 0.01%). This figure was much lower than that observed for bendrofluazide (2%).

In another trial,[33] the Sexual Symptom Distress Index was used. This index is derived from patient assessment of 4 symptoms on a 5-point scale of distress: reduction in sexual desire, problems in obtaining an erection, problems in maintaining an erection, and problems in ejaculation. Using this index, hypertensive men treated with propranolol showed a significant deterioration compared with men treated with captopril after 6 months. At this stage, 22% of the propranolol group and 33% of the captopril group were also taking hydrochlorothiazide. The comparison of the 12-week data when all patients were still on monotherapy showed no statistically significant differences between the treatment groups, although there was a tendency for a deterioration on propranolol and methyldopa and little change on captopril. As discussed above, the addition of the diuretic further increased the reporting of sexual problems by those on methyldopa and propranolol but not by those on captopril. The biggest differences were in the group on propranolol.

The association of propranolol with impotence was not confirmed in another smaller trial[9] of 360 male hypertensives randomized to 1 of 4 groups: propranolol, atenolol, captopril, or enalapril. Eight aspects of sexual function were measured: interest, arousal, enjoyment, obtaining an erection, maintaining an erection, morning erection, intercourse, and orgasm. There was no evidence of any differences between the groups after 8 weeks treatment, except that patients on propranolol reported erections on awakening more frequently than the other treatment groups. This may be associated with vivid dreams, a well-known side effect of propranolol, or it may be due to some other underlying mechanism. It is possible that this trial missed differences because it was small but the changes in the four groups were very similar. Moreover, this trial did detect some adverse effects of propranolol, including adverse effects on general well-being.

The effects of beta-blockers other than propranolol have also been investigated. In the TAIM study,[27] no significant effect of atenolol on aspects of sexual function was observed either in men or women or in different diet groups. In the TOMHS study,[14] a similar percentage of men reported problems with erection on acebutolol (7%) as on placebo.

Other antihypertensives

From the results of the comparative trials of antihypertensive agents discussed above, it seems that ACE inhibitors do not adversely affect sexual function. In most trials, ACE inhibitors have been the same as the comparator drug with the exception of an advantage for ACE inhibitors in comparison with propranolol. In the TOMHS study,[14] enalapril was similar to placebo in reports of problems with erection.

Calcium channel blockers have been less frequently investigated with respect to sexual dysfunction. None of the comparative trials described above found any adverse effects, but it is possible that a small effect may have been missed. In the TOMHS study,[14] men treated with amlodipine had similar reporting rates of impotence as men on placebo.

In general, alpha-blockers such as prazosin are considered to have a low reporting rate of impotence. In an open study,[34] 80% of men with impotence from previous treatment with methyldopa or clonidine reported improvement when treated with prazosin.

The results of the TOMHS study[14] have suggested that alpha-blockers may in fact be better than placebo. Patients treated with doxazosin had slightly lower reporting rates for difficulties in obtaining an erection (4.2%) compared to placebo (6.8%) and there were significantly fewer reports of problems with maintaining an erection on doxazosin (2.8%) compared to placebo (6.8%). There is some support for the notion that doxazosin might act therapeutically in men with erectile problems. Alpha$_2$-adrenergic antagonists have been used with some success in the treatment of non-psychogenic erectile dysfunction. However, the Veterans Administration Cooperative Study Group on Antihypertensive Agents,[35] in a trial of 232 men, found that the reporting of impotence in patients already receiving thiazides and additionally randomized to prazosin or hydralazine was 28% on prazosin compared to 18% on hydralazine.

Conclusions

In this chapter, some results from comparative trials that used QOL assessments in hypertensive patients have been described. It is important to be aware that it is impossible to make a direct interpretation of the absolute effects of the antihypertensive agents on quality of life without a comparison with a placebo group. In most of the studies described, the interpretation is based on the relative effects of drugs in the trial. Thus, apparent benefits for captopril on quality of life in an early trial were mainly due to the poor performance of methyldopa, and to a lesser extent propranolol. When ACE inhibitors and atenolol were compared, neither drug appeared to offer any important benefits over the other. Although lack of power may have been a factor in some of the trials, the suggestion that atenolol, at least in low doses, has minimal adverse effects on QOL is supported by the results from the TAIM study comparing atenolol with placebo. The question of whether atenolol produces more subtle effects (both beneficial and disadvantageous) on mood and cognition still remains. Likewise, the possibility of similarly subtle effect with ACE inhibitors cannot be completely discounted.

Whether the results for atenolol can be extrapolated to other beta-blockers (apart from propranolol) remains uncertain. Most randomized trials using QOL measurements have used atenolol as the beta-blocker comparator, and there is far less information on the effects of drugs such as metoprolol or acebutolol.

The results from comparative trials with nifedipine are consistent in showing a high withdrawal rate and a high level of reporting of side effects. Those patients who can tolerate nifedipine do not appear to suffer any impairment in their quality of life, and may even do better than they would on the comparator drug (atenolol or cilazapril). Benefits for verapamil were suggested in comparisons with propranolol and nifedipine; however, Croog's trial in black hypertensives[10] leaves some uncertainty about the effects of this drug on QOL.

Although diuretics have been the mainstay of antihypertensive therapy for many years, few studies have undertaken a formal evaluation of their effect on QOL. Two large trials[14,27] that have employed a diuretic in comparison with a placebo have shown that the diuretic used (chlorthalidone in both trials) was the same or better than placebo for measures of general well-being. Other diuretics such as bendrofluazide or hydrochlorothiazide may not give a similar result. Studies of the effects of diuretics on QOL are required, especially in view of the high proportion of the elderly receiving this type of medication.

The data suggesting no impairment of well-being with chlorthalidone may seem to be inconsistent with the evidence that this and other diuretics, such as the thiazides, increase the incidence of impotence, with reporting rates of around 17% compared to a background placebo rate of between 3% and 10% in patients under 65. The effect of these drugs on female sexual function is uncertain, with only the TAIM study[27] so far suggesting any possible adverse effect. It is possible either that the interference with sexual function by the diuretics is not reflected in impaired well-being or that the scales used are insensitive. The average changes across patient groups may include small subsets (< 20%) with poor well-being due to sexual problems.

Although propranolol appears similarly to interfere with erectile function, the proportion of patients affected are somewhat lower (13%) than the thiazides. The effect of propranolol in women is not known. Newer beta-blockers such as atenolol have minimal adverse effects (if any). The effect of ACE inhibitors has been investigated in several large trials with no evidence for an association with dysfunction. Similar results may be true for the calcium channel blockers but the number of trials examining sexual effects with this drug group is smaller. The TOMHS study suggests that alpha-blockers may be usefully employed in men at risk of developing impotence either through increased age, or because of a previous history of impotence on antihypertensive medication. This finding however should be confirmed in other trials.

References

1 Collins R, Peto R, MacMahon S et al. Blood pressure, stroke and coronary heart disease. Part 2, short term reductions in blood pressure: overview of randomised drug trials in their epidemiological context. *Lancet* 1990; **335**:827–38.

2 IPPPSH Collaborative Group. Cardiovascular risk and risk factors in a randomised trial of treatment based on the beta blocker oxprenolol: the International Prospective Primary Prevention Study in Hypertension (IPPPSH). *J Hypertens* 1985; **3**:379–92.

3 Wilhelmsen L, Berglund G, Elmfedt D et al. Beta blockers versus diuretics in hypertensive men: main results from the HAPPHY trial. *J Hypertens* 1987; **5**:561–72.

4 Wilkstrand J, Warnold I, Olsson G, Tuomilheto J, Elmfedt D, Berglund G. Primary prevention with metoprolol in patients with hypertension. Mortality results from the MAPHY Study. *JAMA* 1988; **259**:1976–82.

5 Medical Research Council trial of treatment of hypertension in older adults: principal results. *Br Med J* 1992; **304**:405–12.

6 Croog SH, Levine S, Testa MA et al. The effects of antihypertensive therapy on the quality of life. *N Engl J Med* 1986; **314**:1657–64.

7 Herrick AL, Waller PC, Bern KE et al. Comparison of enalapril and atenolol in mild to moderate hypertension. *Am J Med* 1989; **86**:421–6.

8 Fletcher AE, Bulpitt CJ, Hawkins CM et al. Quality of life on antihypertensive therapy: a randomised double blind controlled trial of captopril and atenolol. *J Hypertens* 1990; **8**:463–6.

9 Steiner SS, Friedhoff AJ, Wilson BL, Wecker JR, Santo JP. Antihypertensive therapy and quality of life: a comparison of atenolol, captopril, enalapril and propranolol. *J Hum Hypertens* 1990; **4**:217–25.

10 Croog SH, Kong W, Levine S, Weir MR, Baume RM, Saunders E. Hypertensive Black men and women. Quality of life and effects of antihypertensive medications. *Arch Intern Med* 1990; **150**:1733–41.

11 Palmer AJ, Fletcher AE, Rudge P, Andrews C, Callaghan TS, Bulpitt CJ. Quality of life in hypertensives treated with atenolol or captopril: a double blind cross over trial. *J Hypertens* 1992; **10**:1409–16.

12 Fletcher AE, Bulpitt CJ, Chase D et al. Quality of life on three antihypertensive treatments: cilazapril, atenolol, nifedipine. *Hypertension* 1992; **19**:499–507.

13 Moeller JF, Poulsen DL, Kornerup HJ, Bech P. Quality of life, side effects and efficacy of lisinopril compared with metoprolol in patients with mild to moderate hypertension. *J Hum Hypertens* 1991; **5**:215–21.

14 The Treatment of Mild Hypertension Research Group. The Treatment of Mild Hypertension Study. A randomised placebo-controlled trial of a nutritional hygienic regimen along with various drug monotherapies. *Arch Intern Med* 1991; **151**:1413–23.

15 Os I, Bratland B, Dahlof B, Gisholt K, Syvertson JO, Tretli S. Lisinopril or nifedipine in essential hypertension? A Norwegian multicenter study on efficacy, tolerability and quality of life in 828 patients. *J Hypertens* 1991; **9**:1097–104.

16 Zubenko GS, Nixon RA. Mood-elevating effect of captopril in depressed patients. *Am J Psychiatry* 1984; **141**:110–11.

17 Testa MA, Anderson RB, Nackley JF, Hollenberg NK. Quality of life and antihypertensive therapy in men. *N Engl J Med* 1993; **328**:907–13.

18 Fletcher AE, Palmer AJ, Bulpitt CJ. ACE inhibitor cough – how much of a problem. *J Hypertens* 1994.

19 Testa MA, Hollenberg NK, Anderson RB, Williams GH. Assessment of quality of life by patient and spouse during antihypertensive therapy with atenolol and nifedipine gastrointestinal therapeutic system. *Am J Hypertens* 1991; **4**:363–73.

20 Fletcher AE, Chester PC, Hawkins CMA, Latham AN, Pike LA, Bulpitt CJ. The effects of verapamil and propranolol on quality of life in hypertension. *J Hum Hypertens* 1989; 3:125–30.

21 Bulpitt CJ, Fletcher AE. Measurement of quality of life in hypertension: a practical approach. *Br J Clin Pharmac* 1990; 30:353–64.

22 Fletcher AE, Battersby C, Bulpitt CJ on behalf of the European Pinacidil Study Group. Quality of life on hypertensive treatment: results from a randomised double blind trial of pinacidil and nifedipine. *J Cardiovasc Pharmacol* 1992; 20:108–14.

23 Palmer A, Fletcher A, Hamilton G, Muriss S, Bulpitt C. A comparison of verapamil and nifedipine on quality of life. *Br J Clin Pharmacol* 1990; 30:365–70.

24 Fletcher A, Amery A, Birkenhager W et al. Risks and benefits in the trial of the European Working Party on High Blood Pressure in the Elderly. *J Hypertens* 1991; 9:225–30.

25 SHEP Cooperative Research Group. Prevention of stroke by antihypertensive drug treatment in older persons with isolated systolic hypertension: final results of the Systolic Hypertension in the Elderly Program (SHEP). *JAMA* 1991; 265:3255–64.

26 Gurland BJ, Teresi J, McFate Smith W, Black D, Hughes G, Edlavitch S. Effects of treatment for isolated systolic hypertension on cognitive status and depression in the elderly. *J Am Geriatr Soc* 1988; 36:1015–22.

27 Wassertheil-Smoller S, Blaufox D, Oberman A et al for the TAIM Research Group. Effect of antihypertensives on sexual function and quality of life: The TAIM Study. *Ann Intern Med* 1991; 114:613–20.

28 Slovick D, Fletcher AE, Daymond M, Mackay E, Vandenburg MJ, Bulpitt CJ. Quality of life and cognitive function on a diuretic compared with a beta blocker: a randomised controlled trial of bendrofluazide versus dilevalol in elderly hypertensive patients. Presentation at British Geriatrics Society Autumn Meeting 1990, Age and Ageing 1992.

29 Bird AS, Blizard RA, Mann AH. Treating hypertension in the older person: an evaluation of the association of blood pressure level and its reduction with cognitive performance. *J Hypertens* 1990; 8:147–52.

30 Medical Research Council Working Party on Mild to Moderate Hypertension. Adverse reactions to bendrofluazide and propranolol for the treatment of mild hypertension. *Lancet* 1981; 2:539.

31 Curb JD, Borhani NO, Blaszkanski RP, Simbaldi F, Williams W. Long-term surveillance for adverse effects of antihypertensive drugs. *JAMA* 1985; 253:3263.

32 Grimm R. Treating mild hypertension. Report from Hypertension Update II, Scotland, December 1990.

33 Croog SH, Levine S, Sudilovsky A, Baume RM, Clive J. Sexual symptoms in hypertensive patients. A clinical trial of antihypertensive medications. *Arch Intern Med* 1988; 148:788–94.

34 Lipson LG. Treatment of hypertension in diabetic men: problems with sexual dysfunction. *Am J Cardiol* 1984; 53:46A–50A.

35 Veterans Administration Co-operative Study Group on Antihypertensive Agents. Comparison of prazosin with hydralazine in patients receiving hydrochlorothiazide; a randomised double blind clinical trial. *Circulation* 1981; 64:722–9.

16

Assessing the published results

Richard C Horton

'Difficult' hypertension has several possible meanings. It might refer to hypertension that is difficult to control; to raised blood pressure among groups for whom treatment is either urgent or potentially dangerous; or to hypertension among those who have an underlying condition that is driving blood pressure upwards. 'Difficult' might also relate to a more abstract concept, i.e. the difficulties that face clinicians when making treatment decisions for which there are few or conflicting data to guide their practice. How can physicians navigate their way through a voluminous and, at times, misleading literature? Analysis of evidence is central to decision making in all areas of clinical practice. Yet these skills are frequently neglected.

There are 3 broad themes that will be developed in this chapter.

1. Every clinician can – indeed must – learn the techniques necessary to evaluate research evidence. To rely on the judgement of journal editors and their system of peer review alone is to put too much faith in a process that has yet to be independently validated.
2. These techniques form part of an emerging discipline that is likely to transform medical practice: evidence-based medicine. Multispecialty and cross-disciplinary, this approach is likely to become *the* method of teaching postgraduate medicine in the future. Physicians, epidemiologists, and biostatisticians at the McMaster University Health Sciences Center have been at the forefront of advancing this approach.[1-4]
3. A critical (but as yet unacknowledged) part of this method is the practice of uncertainty analysis. Clinical decision making is inherently uncertain, especially with patients who have 'difficult' conditions. Neither the interplay of causal factors that we believe underlie disease processes nor the targets that we select for therapeutic intervention interact in a linear fashion. For instance, there is no easy way to summarize 'risk factors', such as those for hypertension, in a way that will produce a single point–risk estimate for an individual patient; there is no simple relation in a given individual between the use of an antihypertensive agent and subsequent prevention of myocardial infarction. Biological systems, the development of disease states and their modification by drug therapy are unpredictable.

When we evaluate clinical evidence, we should not give each part of that evidence equal positive value. Rather, we should begin by analyzing systematically the sources, nature, and implications of the uncertainties that these data possess. This approach to data analysis will provide us with a far more muscular grasp of how to translate research evidence into practice. This chapter focuses on 4 sources of evidence relating to the evaluation of drugs in the management of hypertension: the research paper, the review, the consensus guideline, and the meta-analysis.

The McMaster group advocate a twofold approach to patient management: first, when faced with a clinical scenario, physicians should apply the available research data in as precise a way as is reasonable; and second, to achieve this end, a method of critically appraising research literature is essential. David Sackett and his colleagues[2] have developed rules of evidence for reading medical literature which satisfy this second requirement.

I shall draw on McMaster methodology, and add some thoughts of my own, to the problems of interpreting and understanding uncertainty in research evidence.

The research paper

There are 3 broad categories of research study (Table 16.1). In clinical practice, we rely on intervention trials to determine our day-to-day treatment decisions, but we also draw intuitive conclusions that are clinically relevant from pathophysiological and observational data. For example, if laboratory animal data suggest that an antihypertensive agent has few effects on glycemic control, we are likely to choose that agent on the basis of the 'best available evidence' in the absence of clinical data. These intuitive generalizations are potentially misleading. To draw inferences that directly affect clinical practice from animal-based data is wholly unreliable. Animal work can do no more than provide signals to researchers about promising or unpromising avenues of study in human beings.

Observational data – case reports, descriptive studies, cross-sectional studies (analyzing

1. Pathophysiological studies (basic science)
2. Observational studies
   - case reports
   - descriptive studies
   - cohort studies
   - case-control studies
3. Intervention studies
   - preventive trials (primary prevention)
   - therapeutic trials (secondary prevention)

Table 16.1
Classification of primary research.

exposure and disease at the same time point in the same individual), and correlational analyses (relating potential risk factors to disease in a population) – all serve the same function as animal studies. That is, they raise hypotheses that require further testing in controlled conditions. As evidence that has any bearing on clinical practice, they too are unreliable unless several studies point independently to the same conclusion. The uncertainty inherent in these designs is so great that it dwarfs any explanatory power that they might seem to have. In essence, the uncertainty lies in the weakness with which cause and effect can be established.

Only when we come to studies that have attempted to include controlled data do we arrive at anything that is clinically meaningful. These are, in epidemiological terms, analytic as opposed to descriptive studies. It is here that skills to evaluate the meaning of these data in the context of clinical practice are needed. Clinical trials come in different forms. Again, the reader must discriminate between these and rely on multicenter, randomized, controlled study designs. The multicenter nature of such trials is critical, since it eliminates biases that might accrue from a single institution's or a single researcher's practice, though it may introduce greater variability in the application of inclusion and exclusion criteria and in the determination of endpoints. Phase I studies of maximum tolerated dose, phase II studies of toxicity and indications of efficacy, and phase IV studies devoted solely to postmarketing surveillance (outcomes research) may be unreliable sources of clinically meaningful information.

The importance of this critical approach has been summarized by Altman, who virtually equates poor quality research with scientific misconduct.[5]

HELP

There are many complex lists of variables that readers of research papers are encouraged to

consider when evaluating data.[6] For a physician who is overloaded with information, this idealized view of how the literature should be read is merely an epidemiologist's dream and a practicing clinician's nightmare. Yet a simple glance at the bottom line of an abstract, structured or otherwise, is inadequate. The users of medical literature need to have the skills to make their own judgements about the value of research data. The method of critical appraisal summarized in Table 16.2 can be applied to all newly presented primary research data.

The hypothesis
The hypothesis should be clearly stated and should provide a convincing argument about the clinical importance of the study.

The experimental method
The experimental method must be evaluated according to its design, end point, statistical method, summary measures, and validity. As a critical reader you are not attempting to design the experiment yourself; rather, you are attempting to evaluate the article in front of you. You need signposts for criticism rather than a complete map and road index. Such an evaluation gives a methodological estimate of the scientific strength of the study. Randomized controlled trials are the most secure means of judging the efficacy of a particular treatment. When assessing end points (the primary outcome measures) in a trial of the primary preventive efficacy of a new antihypertensive agent, we must judge whether they are hard (e.g. death from myocardial infarction), soft (e.g. reduction in blood pressure), or surrogate (e.g. changes in the electrocardiogram).

A statistical assessment is also necessary; this may prove the most difficult aspect of the evaluation, but the correct choice of statistic can be easily judged (Fig. 16.1).[7] Statistics sets out only to provide rules for drawing inference,

---

H : Hypothesis
E : Experimental method
    • Design (see Table 16.1)
    • End-point
    • Statistical method
        power
        confidence intervals
        errors (see Table 16.4)
    • Summary measures
    • Validity (see Table 16.5)
L : Language
P : Practical implications
    • Clinical importance
    • Toxicity
    • Quality of life
    • Cost

Table 16.2
HELP in reading a primary research paper.

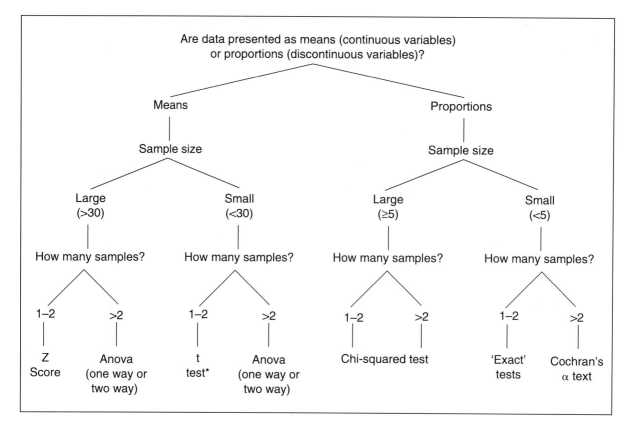

Figure 16.1
Is the statistical test appropriate?

Data can be measured according to three categories, each of which has its own measure of central tendency:
- *nominal (non-ranked categories) – mode*
- *ordinal (ranked categories) – median (best used for summarizing data with extreme values)*
- *interval (ordinal with equal distance between measurements) – mean*

Interval observations are distributed continuously and can be evaluated by tests of parametric data (t, anova). Ordinal observations are distributed discontinuously and must be evaluated by non-parametric methods (e.g., chi-squared). (Adapted from Hennekens and Buring.[7])

*The non-parametric analogue of the t test is the Mann–Whitney rank sum test.

and an excellent (non-mathematical) summary of these rules is provided by Bailar and Mosteller.[8] In statistics, one places most trust in authors, editors, and statistical reviewers for accurate assessment of an article's analysis.

However, for correct interpretation, the reader also needs pointers (Table 16.3).

In addition, one must judge the degree of uncertainty present in a trial. Uncertainty is measured in 3 ways; the power of the study,

Look for:
- A description of how the sample size was calculated (power)
- A clear indication that there were no baseline differences between groups
- Measurements of intra- and inter-observer variability
- Intention-to-treat analysis rather than calculations based on actual treatment received.
- SD not SE when referring to means[1]
- Correct use of the t test[2]
- Exact p values[3]
- A description of the parent statistic in association with the p value
- p values calculated by two-sided tests
- The elimination of inferences drawn from post-hoc subset analyses (these can only be hypothesis generating)

[1]For normally distributed data, within 1 SD lie 68% of observations; within 2 SD lie 95% of observations. SE is a measure of the SDs of all possible sample means, i.e. the precision with which a sample mean estimates a true population mean. The SE measures the certainty with which one can estimate the population mean from a sample. SE is almost always less than SD.
[2]There should be adjustment (Bonferroni) for multiple comparisons (true p = p × number of tests) or at least an estimation of the chance that a comparison may demonstrate false significance. Ideally, for multiple comparisons, use ANOVA, not t.
[3]p indicates whether the observation is compatible with a given hypothesis, i.e. it is the probability of being wrong when a true difference exists.

Table 16.3
Pointers to statistical precision.

the width of confidence intervals, and the inherent errors that are present.

The ability of a statistical test to discover a difference between groups is called its power; power depends on sample size and how large a difference we wish to detect. A difference alone is not sufficient; the difference must be clinically meaningful. For example, as of 1987 the median number of patients enrolled into one group of trials was 96,[9] far too few to detect even moderate differences between treatments. The danger of small trials is twofold: first, there is a risk of producing false-positive results (type I errors), and these are more likely to contribute to publication bias; second, there is a risk of producing false-negative results

(type II errors) because of their lack of power. Without a measure of the sensitivity of the study – e.g. the confidence interval – interpretation is impossible.

Error is a central component in our uncertainty analysis of the primary research study. The classification of error is shown in Table 16.4. Random errors can be largely eliminated by increasing the size and hence the power of the study. Systematic bias is equivalent to systematic errors in research methodology. Selection and observation biases are particularly important in case-control and cohort studies. Careful study design can go a long way to diminishing their importance – e.g. in randomized double blind trials, the randomization

1. Random error
   - Type I
   - Type II
2. Systematic error (bias)
   - Selection bias
   - Observation/information bias
      interviewer
      recall
      loss to follow-up
      misclassification

Table 16.4
Classification of error.

process eliminates selection bias and the double blind nature of the trial eliminates interviewer and recall bias.

The reader should also ensure that the investigators who have planned an intervention trial have adhered to the right protocol for ending the trial (stopping rules). An independent data and safety monitoring committee should have been established (with up to 5 members, including an epidemiologist or statistician and excluding the sponsor), and predetermined times for interim analysis should have been set. The investigators should define an (extreme) level of statistical significance beyond which they should be alerted to the possibility of ending the trial. The decision to terminate the trial should only be made in the light of all of the evidence – i.e. whether the observed difference is plausible at this stage in the study.

There are 3 key summary measures that the reader should be looking for: the relative risk, the absolute risk, and the number needed to treat (NNT) to prevent 1 adverse outcome. Each of these should be presented with a 95% confidence interval. In addition, one must be wary of the authors' attempts to persuade by

their biased reporting of data.[10,11] In analyzing treatment studies of patients with hypertension, the NNT summary measure is especially valuable. This variable measures the treatment burden that needs to be invoked to obtain 1 unit of treatment benefit: that is, the effort-to-benefit ratio.

The reader's interpretation of a study will depend on the way summary measures are presented. For instance, the estimate of relative risk tends to produce a more positive evaluation of data than the absolute risk, and both of these tend to lead to optimistic conclusions when set beside NNT. For example, the Medical Research Council trial of treatment of mild hypertension (diastolic 90–109 mmHg in men and women aged 35–64 years) found that treatment with bendrofluazide or propranolol significantly reduced the stroke rate: 60 strokes took place in the treatment group and 109 in the placebo group.[12] This difference was statistically significant (p< 0.01) and was the main finding reported in the abstract. Yet, in their conclusion, the authors admit that, according to the NNT, one would have to treat 850 mildly hypertensive patients for 1 year to prevent 1 stroke, though the patients had very mild hypertension. The effort-to-benefit ratio is the only ethically sound measure of treatment efficacy.

By contrast, one can compare this interpretation of the MRC trial with that of the Treatment of Mild Hypertension Study.[13] The TOMHS investigators compared placebo (advice to increase exercise and to reduce weight, dietary sodium intake, and alcohol intake; this advice was given to all trial participants) with chlorthalidone, acebutolol, doxazosin, amlodipine, and enalapril. In reporting their results, they failed to use NNT measures and concluded that, although there was no significant difference in deaths or major non-fatal cardiovascular events (a mix of 7

- Study design, e.g. randomized, double-blind.
- Implementation of that design, e.g. method of randomization, success of blinding.
- Analysis
  - intention-to-treat
  - use of correct summary measures
- Inference
  - confining generalizations to the study population

Table 16.5
How to measure the validity of a clinical trial.

other outcomes, such as hospitalization for unstable angina, congestive heart failure, and aortic aneurysm surgery), the reduction in total clinical events (including angina, intermittent claudication, transient ischemic attacks, and diminished peripheral pulses) was significant enough (11.1% in total drug treatment group compared with 16.2% in placebo group; p = 0.03) to justify treatment. This interpretation probably stretches the bounds of believable probability too far.

The validity of the study rests largely with components of the study methodology or with elements depending on this methodology (Table 16.5).[14]

The next two variables in our HELP scheme make up the science of interpretation.

Language

Language may seem an unusual analytic variable, but the way in which implications are made and arguments are set out may completely invalidate an excellent investigative protocol. Language is an instrument of power and, although the investigative protocol may

have been objective, language can never be. Linguistic bias is not uncommon.[15] The application of rhetorical language to manipulate results to a predetermined end is a crucial but often neglected part of criticism. For instance, when a study finds no beneficial effects of a particular treatment, the (statistically) accurate conclusion is that no significant difference has been found. Often, authors go further and conclude that *no* difference exists. Moreover, in any discussion of results, the authors should include their own calculation of their study's limitations. Also, they should recognize and discuss the 4 possible interpretations of any study: that the result may be due to chance; that the result may depend on an unrecognized confounding variable; that the result may be due to systematic or random errors; and, only lastly, that the result may actually be true.

Practical implications

Finally, the practical implications of the research must be considered. What is the clinical importance of the result as opposed to the statistical significance? What is the degree of certainty with which such an inference can be made? Is the initial hypothesis strengthened or weakened? Is the result applicable to a particular patient population?[16] Additionally, other clinically important measures may not have been included in the analysis, e.g. toxicity, cost, and estimates of quality of life. These all need to be taken into account when evaluating the efficacy of a particular intervention.

The review

The review article is, for most physicians in training or in specialty practice, the main means by which they keep up to date with the current literature and, most importantly, with the interpretation of that literature. Yet the review article is potentially one of the more misleading elements in the entire range of scientific communication. The review represents the literary equivalent of clinical instruction by a respected professor. Indeed, editors of medical journals are constantly seeking such high-profile figures to write in their pages. The chosen expert may well provide extremely valuable guidance; however, the reader should be aware that the views of the expert may be biased and not reflect the best possible interpretation of the available literature.

When reading reviews, one should take them for what they are: a series of personal interpretations of selected data, which are put together to persuade the reader of a particular point of view. They are for the most part non-systematic: that is, they make no claim to be impartial or comprehensive.

However, reviews represent original research in themselves. Their authors aim to collect primary data and synthesize these findings into some sort of narrative overview. Such secondary research must have a defined methodology before one can begin to accept it as a legitimate means of communication. Iain Chalmers, Director of the UK Cochrane Collaboration, has done much to provide a framework for judging whether the methodology adopted by the reviewer is satisfactory.[17] As in any scientific investigation, the main difficulty is bias. Oxman and Guyatt[18] have proposed guidelines that the reader should follow when confronted with a review article. These can be summarized in four simple rules (Table 16.6). The most important of these is to provide the reader with an explicit methodology about how articles were retrieved (sources of articles, search terms, limits of search by date); how articles were selected (number of studies reviewed and criteria for selection); and how data were extracted (guidelines according to which data were chosen for discussion). This information is important since

Rules of methodology
1. Are the methods of article retrieval and selection, together with data extraction, clearly stated?
Rules of interpretation
2. How were conflicting results in the primary research literature analyzed?
3. How were data from the primary research literature synthesized?
4. Are the specific conclusions individually supported by cited data?

Table 16.6
How to evaluate a review article.

it allows the reader to assess the possible influence of author bias.

The three remaining rules – analysis of heterogeneity, data synthesis, and drawing correct inferences – are rules of interpretation, as opposed to rules of methodology. The key point is that systematic rules of evidence will go far in removing systematic biases.

A further framework that authors and editors should place on reviews is that of the structured abstract.[19] The structured abstract not only forces authors to adopt rules of methodology, but also enables readers to judge whether reviews are reliable or not. The elements of the structured abstract for review articles are shown in Table 16.7. Readers must work hard when reading a review that adopts neither the structured abstract nor explicit rules of methodology. In such a case, the reviewer cannot be trusted to have eliminated bias.[20] An excellent example of how to construct a structured narrative review on isolated systolic hypertension in the elderly has been published by Howard.[21]

Objective	– a clear statement of the aim of the review
Data sources	– a description of where articles were drawn from
Study selection	– criteria for article selection
Data extraction	– a description of which data were used and why
Data synthesis	– the bulk of the narrative overview should explain how data were used to reach the conclusions drawn
Conclusion	– cite and reference the key evidence for each conclusion and comment on clinical relevance

Table 16.7
Structured abstracts for review articles.

The clinical practice guideline

If readers cannot trust review articles, then perhaps they should look to consensus statements or clinical practice guidelines generated from groups of opinion leaders in a particular field. Unfortunately, as is so often the case, the products of committees are no less free from criticism than the ideas of a single individual. Even when the same extensive world literature is available to them, different committees can and often do come to different conclusions.

Let us take as our example the treatment of mild hypertension and the recommendations of 3 committees: the British Hypertension Society,[22] the World Health Organization/International Society for Hypertension,[23] and the US Joint National Committee on Detection, Evaluation, and Treatment of high blood pressure.[24]

The British Hypertension Society[27] defines mild hypertension as a diastolic blood pressure of 90–99 mmHg. Sever et al[22] recommend treatment in older patients (over 60 years) or if target-organ damage is present, e.g. left ventricular hypertrophy, renal impairment, or if the patient has diabetes. If none of these conditions is present, one should look for additional risk factors, such as higher pressures within the range, advanced age, male sex, smoking, dyslipidaemia, and family history of heart disease.

In recommending drug treatment, the guidelines become more murky. The committee agreed that calcium entry blockers, converting enzyme inhibitors, and alpha-blockers should be considered as alternative agents in an individualized care program provided that diuretics and/or beta-blockers were contraindicated or ineffective. However, the committee disagreed about whether these newer classes of drug could be prescribed as first-line agents. The main difficulty is the lack of long-term data with these latest agents. In patients with mild hypertension who subsequently have consistently normal blood pressures without any evidence of target-organ damage, treatment can be gradually withdrawn, though continued monitoring of blood pressure is recommended.

The WHO/ISH guidelines[23] were reported 5 months later. Their definition of mild hypertension – diastolic 90–105 mmHg (borderline hypertension at 90–95 mmHg accounting for about half of these cases) – differed from the British Hypertension Society. The guidelines committee recommends that 4 weeks from the initial measurement, if the diastolic pressure remains between 90 and 105 mmHg, non-drug treatment should be initiated and the patient followed closely over 3 months. After 3 months, if the diastolic pressure is over 100 mmHg, drug treatment should begin. If the blood pressure is 95–100 mmHg, drug treatment should be considered and other cardio-vascular risk factors should be sought. If the blood pressure is 90–95 mmHg, the patient should be closely monitored. After a subsequent 3-month interval, drugs should be started if the blood pressure is 95 mmHg or above, irrespective of other risk factors.

In addition, the WHO/ISH group tackle the issue of mild hypertension as defined by systolic pressure of 140–180 mmHg. They recommend that after 3 months of monitoring, drug treatment should begin if the pressure is 160–180 mmHg, provided the diastolic pressure is over 95 mmHg or additional risk factors are present. After a subsequent 3-month interval, systolic pressures of 160–180 mmHg should be treated, irrespective of concomitant risk factors.

The WHO/ISH committee rank treatments in order of proven benefit: diuretics are superior to beta-blockers, both of which are superior to converting enzyme inhibitors, calcium antagonists, and alpha-blockers. They conclude that 'the choice of initial drug therapy . . . should not be restricted, on theoretical or economic grounds, to any one or two of the various classes of drugs that have been tested so far'.

The fifth report of the US Joint National Committee provides yet another view.[24] They drop the term 'mild hypertension' entirely in favour of high blood pressure stage 1. This category includes those with systolic pressure of 140–159 mmHg and diastolic pressure of 90–99 mmHg. Any statement about blood pressure should be accompanied by a comment on the presence or absence of target-organ disease and additional risk factors.

JNC-V is definite in its treatment recommendation: 'if blood pressure remains at or above 140/90 mmHg during a 3–6-month period, despite vigorous encouragement of life-style modifications, then antihypertensive medications should be started.' They recommend single agent therapy only for stage 1 hypertension and suggest that one should begin with either diuretics or beta-blockers. Alternatives should only be selected 'when diuretics and beta-blockers have proved unacceptable or ineffective'.

There are clearly subtle differences of definition, varying recommendations about when to intervene, and even different emphases on selection of drugs. There is no consensus about any of these matters. These differences are summarized in Table 16.8.

Similar discrepancies appear in those guidelines for other areas in addition to those on treatment of mild hypertension. For instance, hypertension in ethnic minorities is not mentioned in the guidelines produced by the British Hypertension Society and the WHO/ISH. Only JNC-V alludes to the facts that African Americans develop hypertension earlier in life, that hypertension is more severe at any age, and that African Americans have a greater risk of stroke and renal disease.

Nowhere in these 3 guidelines is there any attempt to evaluate efficacy by summary measures (e.g. NNT) that I have discussed earlier, and there are many generalizations

	British Society of Hypertension	WHO/ISH	JNC-V
Definition of hypertension	diastolic = 90–99 mmHg	diastolic = 90–105 mmHg	diastolic = 90–105 mmHg systolic = 140–159 mmHg
Indications for drug treatment	Older or target-organ damage or risk factors after 3–6 months	diastolic >100 mmHg after 3 months; diastolic 95–100 mmHg after 3 months plus additional risk factors; diastolic 95–100 mmHg after 6 months, irrespective of risk factors; systolic > 160 mmHg after 3 months (if diastolic > 95 mmHg or risk factors); systolic > 160 mmHg after 6 months, irrespective of risk factors	> 140/90 mmHg for 3–6 months
Drugs	First line: diuretics, beta-blockers Second line: calcium channel blockers, ACE inhibitors, beta-blockers	Ranked: 1. diuretics 2. beta-blockers 3. calcium channel blockers, ACE inhibitors, beta-blockers	First line: diuretics beta-blockers Second line: calcium channel blockers, ACE inhibitors, beta-blockers

Numbers indicate preferential use

Table 16.8
Lack of consistency between three sets of 1993 guidelines on mild hypertension.

unsupported by any data. In the WHO/ISH guidelines, the authors state that 'it is well established that lowering of even mildly elevated pressures reduces cardiovascular morbidity and mortality'. When one reviews the NNT data from the MRC trial of mild hypertension, one shrinks from agreeing with such a conclusion.

The idea that consensus statements and practice guidelines offer an unbiased and agreed interpretation of research data is another myth that needs to be quashed. They often seriously confuse or ignore important aspects of their subject.

The best example of dissonance between guidelines from experts and the true nature of the data comes from Antman et al.[25] This group compared data on the treatments for myocardial infarction, as compiled in meta-analyses, with the recommendations of experts. They found that the experts consistently 'failed to mention important advances or exhibited delays in recommending effective preventive measures'.

The difficulty with consensus statements is that they are often written without the involvement of an epidemiologist trained in evaluating research data. If the process of analyzing evidence is left to medical specialists, who may be natural enthusiasts for their subject, critical appraisal of evidence may be severely lacking. The same principles that apply for presenting evidence in research articles should also apply when writing guidelines; i.e. summary measures should be used appropriately. When you read a consensus statement or clinical practice guideline, look at the authorship. If you cannot discover the involvement of an epidemiologist, you should read on with a heavy measure of scepticism.

The meta-analysis

Meta-analyses[26] are quantitative reviews. This simple statement hides a controversy that still remains unresolved. Chalmers, for instance, believes that meta-analyses 'epitomize the . . . methodologically sound review article;[17] and Haynes has described them as 'advanced clinical research'.[27] However, Bailar, who was the principal statistical advisor to the *New England Journal of Medicine* throughout the 1980s, remains sceptical of their value and believes that their potential for bias is a lethal criticism.

Nevertheless, meta-analyses are increasingly being reported in medical journals and the reader needs a means of evaluating their worth (Table 16.9). In hypertension, meta-analyses are now a common means of linking many disparate clinical studies.[28-35] Meta-analyses will continue to gain ground in the medical literature since they aim to draw conclusions on important issues of clinical relevance. Critical skills are especially necessary given the definitive claims that authors sometimes make of such analyses.

While systematic error can be eliminated from review articles by insisting on explicit descriptions of article retrieval and selection, random errors can only be diminished by combining results according to certain statistical rules. Although randomized trials of a particular intervention are never going to be exactly the same in terms of their size, the characteristics of their study groups, and the duration of follow-up, provided that the selected studies have focused on closely related questions, they will produce results that have their own measure of central tendency. The meta-analysis is an attempt to quantify this central tendency.

Data are conventionally displayed graphically as odds ratios, represented as point estimates whose area indicates sample size, together with 95% confidence intervals (the usual measure of statistical uncertainty). They can be listed according to chronology, quality, or treatment effect.

Search	– Have the authors searched for, obtained, and included unpublished (abstracts and data submitted to journals or in press), as well as published, primary research data?
Quality	– Are explicit criteria given about the quality of research articles selected?
Similarity	– Are the studies selected for combination similar with respect to treatment, patients, and end points?
Sensitivity	– If unpublished data are included, have the authors conducted a sensitivity analysis?
Bias	– Is there evidence of publication bias?
Heterogeneity	– Are tests of heterogeneity included in the analysis?

Table 16.9
Rules for judging a meta-analysis.

The advantages of meta-analysis are clear. They are able to answer objectively a hypothesis that has led to conflicting results from randomized trials. Such an answer may be definitive and prevent the conduct of what may be unethical trials to investigate the so-called unresolved question further. New hypotheses may be raised by the meta-analysis, which require testing in subsequent randomized trials. Type I and type II errors can be largely eliminated. Overall, the degree of uncertainty that is frequently attached even to randomized controlled trials can be substantially diminished.

Concerns remain. These focus around Bailar's suspicion of bias. The meta-analysis is an observational study, not an experiment, and so it is prone to a particular form of bias: the tendency for authors to submit, and journal editors to accept, articles according to the result of the study rather than the quality of the study. Dickersin and colleagues[36] and Easterbrook et al[37] found that positive results were 2.5 times more likely to be published than results showing no differences between study groups. Reliance by meta-analysts on data reported in peer-reviewed journals is unsound. The first question that readers should ask of a meta-analysis is: have the authors sought unpublished as well as published primary research data (Table 16.9)?

The risk of this approach is that some unpublished data may be of inferior quality compared with those appearing in peer-reviewed journals. To avoid this possibility, sensitivity analyses should be performed in which results are presented with and without unpublished studies.[38] If the result is substantially the same, one can trust the validity of the unpublished data; if the results are divergent, one must question the quality of the data set. In truth, the only way publication bias can be eliminated is by the construction of clinical trials registries.[39]

One way to elicit evidence of publication bias is to draw up a funnel plot, first described by Light and Pillemar[40] (Fig. 16.2). The idea is that if bias exists against negative studies, this can be shown graphically by a relative absence of studies in that part of the funnel indicated by the odds ratio 1.0 (no effect). One would expect

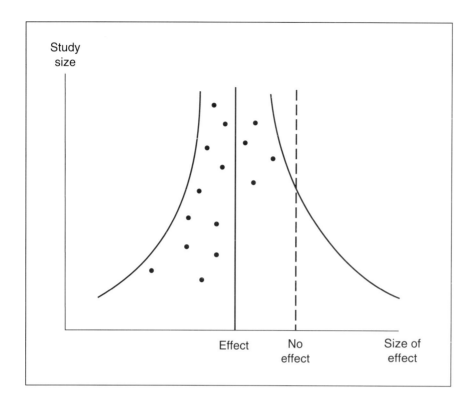

Figure 16.2
The funnel plot for discovering publication bias.

scatter fairly evenly about the truth; this scatter will be largest for the smallest studies, and is indicated by the funnel in Fig. 16.2. If publication bias exists, one would expect a relative absence of these smallest studies, since they are the ones least likely to be submitted to, or accepted by, journal editors. A good example of this approach – in a non-hypertension field – has been provided by Vandenbroucke.[41]

The reader should also determine whether the studies selected for inclusion in the meta-analysis have sufficient similarity to be combined. Three tests judge this criterion: treatment; patient group; and end points. Moreover, readers should ask themselves whether rigorous criteria have been applied in the selection of the types of research studies –

e.g. only randomized, controlled, double-blind clinical trials? This last point is critical since no amount of statistical manipulation will overcome poor study design.

The similarity of the results from selected studies can be measured by tests of heterogeneity. A simple method of assessing heterogeneity is to look at the degree of overlap of the confidence intervals of individual studies. If overlap is substantial, heterogeneity is unlikely. However, the authors should also attempt to calculate a value for the statistical heterogeneity of their meta-analysis. This value indicates whether individual point estimates vary around the pooled estimate to a greater extent than would have been expected by chance. If statistical heterogeneity is present (although the statistical tests are somewhat insensitive), a different statistical model (a random-effects model as opposed to a fixed-effects model) is necessary to combine the data. The fixed-effects model assumes the existence of a single effect that is common to all studies, while the random-effects model treats 'among-study variability' as an essential component in the analysis. Random-effects assumptions can lead to alteration in the level of significance and produce wider confidence intervals, thereby introducing the necessary caution that heterogeneity implies.

Interpretation is a vital component of any meta-analysis. Often the apparent hubris of the statistical community leaves physicians wondering how they can effectively challenge a meta-analysis that carries with it a mathematical seal of approval. By applying the tests outlined here – search, quality, similarity, sensitivity, bias, and heterogeneity – the reader can decide whether the meta-analysis is methodologically sound or insecure. In addition, if heterogeneity is present, the reader should spend time trying to understand why such heterogeneity is present, rather than simply reading a re-analysis by a different method to obscure perhaps real and important differences in study selection. Most importantly, the results of any meta-analysis cannot be generalized beyond the populations studied in the individual trials.

For more detailed discussion, the reader is referred to excellent reviews by Dickersin and Berlin[42] and others[43–46] on the role of meta-analysis in medical research and clinical practice.

Finally, the inclusion of a structured abstract (as shown in Table 16.7) will help readers to navigate their way through what can be complex and lengthy statistical territory. Again, few journal editors insist on such a format, much to their discredit.

An example: meta-analysis of outcome trials in elderly hypertensives

Let us apply these rules – search, quality, similarity, sensitivity, bias, and heterogeneity – to a specific example.[34] In 1992, Thijs et al reported a meta-analysis of 6 randomized controlled trials in elderly hypertensives. Their published paper serves as a useful model to test our powers of critical appraisal. The paper was published without a structured abstract, so readers must work a little harder to discover if any flaws are present.

Search

The authors searched for trials by 'personal contacts'; they indicate that they had already selected some papers. Clearly, this search strategy is poor. They neither report the use of a literature database nor give the reader any indication of whether they sought published data from peer-reviewed journals only.

Quality

The authors set out explicit criteria for inclusion of studies in their meta-analysis. These criteria were: publication of data; randomization; and reporting of all-cause and cause-specific mortality. Of 11 published randomized studies, only 6 were included in their meta-analysis because the remainder failed to adhere to their inclusion criteria. The authors did not search out unpublished data – this should immediately signal to the reader that there is a risk of publication bias.

Similarity

The end-points that were prerequisites for inclusion were all-cause and cause-specific mortality. However, end-points are only one element in assessing similarity. What about treatment and patient groups? The treatment category is simply antihypertensive therapy. As for patient groups, the authors considered that isolated systolic hypertension should be a separate category, and so the SHEP study[47] was not included in the meta-analysis. The authors indicate that they thought carefully about which studies to include.

Sensitivity

The results of the meta-analysis were that coronary and cerebrovascular mortality were significantly reduced by antihypertensive therapy in elderly patients. There was a non-significant decrease in all-cause mortality. The authors then performed a sensitivity analysis and found that the treatment effect was greater in the double-blind studies than in the single-blind and open studies, but the differences were not statistically significant. Moreover, no single study led to the observed significant reductions in coronary and cerebrovascular mortality.

Bias

The authors' failure to search for unpublished data (e.g. by searching for relevant abstracts or by seeking information from colleagues) should warn the reader to be a little sceptical of the positive outcome of the study, especially since there was no benefit in all-cause mortality.

Heterogeneity

A test for heterogeneity was performed, which did not reach statistical significance. The authors note that this result did 'not contradict the hypothesis of a common underlying treatment effect in all studies'. A fixed-effects model was therefore used.

This meta-analysis was well conducted apart from the authors' lax search strategies. It incorporates most of the critical points – quality, similarity, sensitivity, and heterogeneity – that the reader should look for.

Meta-analyses involve complex statistical methods, but they are amenable to criticism and interpretation by the non-statistician providing that the reader applies the 6 tests described above. Given the increasing importance that meta-analyses will assume in medical decision making, this knowledge must become widely known if correct interpretations of these studies are to take place.

Conclusion

I hope to have drawn attention to the locus of uncertainty that can be uncovered by the literate clinician in each form of communication. This approach to reading the literature can be called clinical hermeneutics (the clinical application of the theory of interpretation).[48] Others[2] call it critical appraisal, which is, perhaps, a little too narrow a definition, since this description tends to focus on methodology alone, rather than the context of the whole piece of research. By targeting these wider uncertainties — e.g. in language — the reader is able to reach a pragmatic evaluation of the worth of a scientific article, be it research paper, review, consensus statement, or meta-analysis. I have summarized these uncertainties in Table 16.10.

These identifiable uncertainties reflect our lack of precise knowledge as to the truth of the evidence presented. Uncertainty exists in two forms, one of which – parameter uncertainty – has been dealt with in detail in this chapter (Table 16.11). But our focus on methodology, though in part correct, must not overwhelm our appraisal of evidence. This is where the hermeneutic approach adds to – perhaps even improves upon – the McMaster paradigm. We must also ask: are we applying the correct model when discussing any collection of complex data? For instance, is our assumption that lowering blood pressure is beneficial,

Research article	Review	Consensus statement	Meta-analysis
Hypothesis	Rules of methodology	Is there an epidemiologist	Search
Experimental method	Rules of Interpretation	involved?	Quality
• design	• conflicting data	Rules of interpretation	Similarity
• end-point	• data synthesis	• conflicting data	Sensitivity
• method	• correct conclusions	• data synthesis	Bias
• summary measures		• correct conclusions	Heterogeneity
• validity			
Language			
Practical implications			

Table 16.10
Discovering uncertainty in your reading.

1. Parameter uncertainty
    (i)   Non-representative sample
    (ii)   Measurement error
    (iii) Incorrect surrogate measures
    (iv)   Systematic bias
    (v)   Random error
2. Model uncertainty

Table 16.11
The elements of uncertainty.

irrespective of the agent used, correct? These model uncertainties frequently arise because of gaps in our theories which require us to make assumptions. Such assumptions are frequently made by invoking linear and causal relationships that may not exist. Part of one's critical armamentarium must be a willingness to question all assumptions made in any piece of research.

How should the clinician approach the medical literature on the management of common and important conditions like hypertension in order to keep up to date? Medical journals serve several functions: certainly, to inform, by publishing original research, but also to comment on wider issues in medicine, to review recent research in other journals, to report news, and to provide a forum for lively debate between readers. However, to find the best journals – that is, those that consistently report research of the highest quality (as defined in this chapter) – then one needs some measure of a journal's quality. This measure has been provided by Haynes, editor of the *ACP Journal Club*.[49] This supplement to the *Annals of Internal Medicine* publishes abstracts and commentaries on articles selected, according to strict methodological criteria, from a wide range of journals. Their top 5 journals are: *New England Journal of Medicine, Journal of the American Medical Association, Annals of Internal Medicine, The Lancet*, and *Archives of Internal Medicine*.

The traditional IMRAD – introduction, methods, results and discussion – structure of the research article is now in a precarious state. With the advent of meta-analyses, several observers believe that a research article should begin and end with a meta-analysis.[17] This approach would establish the value of the study at the onset by explicitly identifying gaps in our knowledge. An expanded discussion that includes a meta-analysis of existing data plus the results of the new trial also seems not only logical but also of most value for the reader. I suspect that we will gradually move towards both MAMRAD – meta-analysis, methods, results, and discussion – and MAMRADS – meta-analysis, methods, results, and data synthesis).

The future

What other sources of evidence that are relevant to clinical practice should the reader be looking for in the future? There are several possibilities and I shall briefly review four that I believe are especially important: electronic dissemination of information, decision analysis, n = 1 clinical trials, and Bayesian thinking.

Electronic dissemination of information
The *Online Journal of Current Clinical Trials* is the first truly electronic journal, though physicians have been slow to embrace its possibilities. A more likely means of obtaining information electronically is (until we become more accustomed to the information cyberspace) by fax on demand or CD-ROM.

However, as the Cochrane Collaboration completes its task of creating cumulative overviews in disciplines spanning all areas of medical practice, paper journals are unlikely to be able to cope with the enormous amount of data that these meta-analyses will inevitably contain.[17] Electronic databases will then become an essential archival source of material. The vision of the McMaster group is to have such on-line databases available on the ward as close to the patient as possible, so that evidence-based medicine becomes everyday medical practice. Only then will we be truly able to get research into practice. The likelihood is that the traditional scientific paper will mutate to enable the user to access data not horizontally, by reading a paper from start to finish, but vertically through problem-oriented data retrieval by means of hypertext (text behind the text).

Decision analysis
The method of decision analysis is an attempt to resolve the conflict in a decision between apparently similar treatments. This method has received increasing attention over recent years.[2,50] The elements of decision analysis are fairly straightforward.

1. One draws up a decision tree. This diagram (e.g. Figure 16.3) illustrates all of the potential diagnostic or treatment strategies, together with their outcomes.
2. Assign probability (p) to each branch that arises from a point of uncertainty (chance 'node'; circles)
3. Assign utility (u) to each outcome. Utility reflects the product of quality of life and quantity of life. This can best be done by ranking the outcomes from best to worst.
4. Combine probabilities and utilities for each branch in the decision tree and add these products at each node. This process involves multiplying probabilities by outcome utilities, and continues backwards to the final chance node.
5. Select the decision that has the highest projected utility.
6. Set your choice in the context of the individual patient – e.g. is the patient particularly reluctant to undergo a procedure?

This approach is helpful when one has a toss-up between different treatments. In

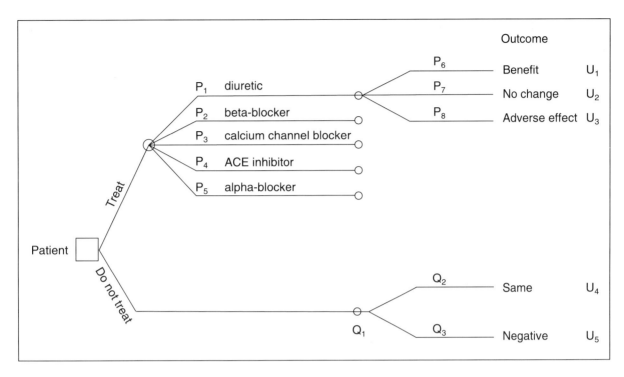

Figure 16.3
Hypothetical decision analysis for the treatment of a patient with mild hypertension.

addition, it takes account of quality-of-life issues by assigning a clinical value to the outcomes of treatment. Such quality-of-life estimates are increasingly important in determining treatment decisions[51] and are partly accounted for in NNT calculations. These issues are relevant to treatment decisions in hypertension. Those who set about drawing up practice guidelines might do well to adopt such analyses. They offer an explicit means of seeing how decisions and recommendations have come to be made.

n=1 clinical trials

If evidence about a particular treatment is lacking, then it might be appropriate to apply the principles of the n=1 trial.[52,53] There are 3 criteria that should be satisfied before performing an n=1 trial: the efficacy of treatment should be uncertain, the condition should be chronic, and the treatment should have a reasonably rapid onset.

The idea is a simple one. The patient receives pairs of treatment intervals, one for the treatment, one for the placebo or alternative treatment. These are given blind to both the patient and physician. The decision about which one takes place first is made by randomization. Moreover, the outcome measures are carefully monitored, together with the use of a patient diary. This process can be repeated until a clear difference emerges. This approach should replace the uncontrolled trial of treatment that is frequently applied on the ward and would bring clinical trial methodology directly to the bedside.

Guyatt and colleagues[52] reported on 73 double-blind, randomized, multiple crossover n=1 trials. Seventy were initiated and 57 were successfully completed. Of these 57, 50 provided clinically useful information, and the results of 15 led to a change in planned management. Larson et al[53] have described their 2-year experience of providing a single-patient trial referral service. Thirty-four trials were completed and 17 gave definitive results. They concluded that this method was not only feasible but also produced greater confidence among clinicians about their treatment decisions. When faced with various options for individualized antihypertensive therapy, n=1 trials might prove an extremely powerful means of assessing benefit.

Bayesian thinking

When we make a clinical decision in the real world of the patient we begin not with a null hypothesis that states that a particular treatment will have no effect but with a belief that the treatment will have a beneficial effect. Any other approach to patient management would be ridiculous. The question the clinician asks is: what certainty is there that the treatment will have this effect? This question is one of probability: the degree (probability) of belief that one has in a particular course of action. The statistical correlate of this qualitative uncertainty analysis is reflected in Bayesian thinking, after the eighteenth-century English clergyman, Thomas Bayes.

The essential notion seems obvious. One begins with a hypothesis that an intervention has a certain effect and then seeks evidence to increase or diminish the probability that this belief (hypothesis) is true. In an individual

patient, we do this by close follow-up using defined outcome measures: e.g. blood pressure, microalbuminuria. For instance, if we believe the hypothesis that one beta-blocker has greater efficacy than another in preventing myocardial infarction, one can assign a probability to that belief (or a range of probabilities) and then seek to modify it in the light of further experience.

In more abstract form, the probability that a hypothesis is true in the light of evidence (the posterior probability or our updated belief) is a function of the probability of the data and the probability of the hypothesis (the prior probability or our preconceived bias). In other words, the researcher assigns a prior probability to the hypothesis, collects evidence, and adjusts the prior probability accordingly (now called the posterior probability).[54]

It seems like common sense, but such a view is fiercely contested by those who adhere to classical significance testing, which attempts to remove the subjective element of belief by creating the more objective, but less realistic, null hypothesis.

One must ask why the vast number of research papers reporting 'significant' results for one form of treatment over another have not resulted in the eradication of most human disease? Because, perhaps, the methodology of research does not accord with the methodology of practice, and so research evidence never can be effectively translated into the clinical setting.

For instance, if we know that a drug reduces blood pressure effectively and if we believe that blood pressure reduction will prevent myocardial infarction, then we would have a high degree of belief that the drug would prevent infarction. If we conducted a trial according to classical statistics, we would begin with a null hypothesis and judge efficacy on the basis of both blood pressure reduction and the reduction in clinical events (as seen in Neaton et al.[13]). The result might be an optimistic one, since we know that blood pressure will be reduced and this positive result is already built into the trial. However, if we assign a probability to our original belief – e.g. 80% – and then, in the light of the trial's evidence, found that clinical events were not reduced by 80%, our hypothesis would not only be weakened but the result would also give a more practical answer to the question we began with: was our belief that lowering blood pressure is beneficial a sound one?

In hypertension, Bayesian approaches have been applied to diagnosis.[55,56] The application of Bayesian thinking to clinical trial methodology has been superbly summarized elsewhere.[57–59]

Bayesian reasoning approximates closely to the way we make clinical decisions and the statistical theory that goes along with it is a powerful method that deserves wider use. Decision analysis – assigning probabilities to interventions and modifying them according to expected utilities – is one form of Bayesian reasoning.

Despite my emphasis on uncertainty analysis, a technique that has conceptual (critical) as well as methodological value, let me end on a more optimistic note. Charles Sanders Peirce (1839–1914) was an American physicist and philosopher of science who passionately believed in the self-correctiveness of the scientific enterprise. His philosophical point of view has a precise parallel with our own modern notions of accumulating data into self-correcting meta-analyses. In 1902 he wrote:

> Science does not advance by revolutions, warfare, and cataclysms, but by cooperation by each researcher's taking advantage of his predecessors' achievements, and by joining his own work in one continuous piece to that already done.[60]

References

1   Evidence-based medicine working group. Evidence-based medicine: a new approach to teach the practice of medicine. *JAMA* 1992; **208**:2420–25.

2   Sackett DL, Haynes RB, Guyatt GH, Tugwell P. *Clinical Epidemiology: A Basic Science for Clinical Medicine*. Boston: Little, Brown, 1991.

3   Guyatt GH, Rennie D. Users' guides to the medical literature. *JAMA* 1992; **270**:2906–7.

4   Oxman AD, Sackett DL, Guyatt GH. Users' guides to the medical literature. I. How to get started. *JAMA* 1993; **270**:2093–5.

5   Altman DG. The scandal of poor medical research. *Br Med J* 1994; **308**:283–4.

6   Greenberg RS. Medical epidemiology. Norwalk: Lang, 1993: 119–30.

7   Hennekens CH, Buring JE. Epidemiology in medicine. Boston: Little, Brown, 1987.

8   Bailar JC, Mosteller F. Guidelines for statistical reporting in articles for medical journals: amplifications and explanations. *Ann Intern Med* 1988; **108**:266–73.

9   Begg CB, Pocock SJ, Freedman L, Zelen M. State of the art in comparative cancer clinical trials. *Cancer* 1987; **60**:2811.

10 Naylor CD, Chen E, Strauss B. Measured enthusiasm: does the method of reporting trial results alter perceptions of therapeutic effectiveness. *Ann Intern Med* 1992; **117**:916–21.

11 Bobbio M, Demichelis B, Giusetto G. Completeness of reporting trial results: effect on physicians willingness to prescribe. *Lancet* 1994; **43**:1209–11.

12 Medical Research Council working party. MRC trial of treatment of mild hypertension: principal results. *Br Med J* 1985; **291**:97–104.

13 Neaton JD, Guimm RH, Prineas RJ et al. Treatment of Mild Hypertension Study: final results. *JAMA* 1993; **270**:713–24.

14 Guyatt GH, Sackett DL, Cook DJ. Users' guides to the medical literature. II. How to use an article about therapy or prevention. A. Are the results of the study valid? *JAMA* 1993; **270**:2598–601.

15 Gore SM, Jones G, Thompson SG. The Lancet's statistical review process: areas for improvement by authors. *Lancet* 1992; **340**:100–2.

16 Guyatt GH, Sackett DL, Cook DJ. Users' guides to the medical literature. II. How to use an article about therapy or prevention. B. What were the results and will they help me in caring for my patients? *JAMA* 1994; **271**:59–63.

17 Chalmers I. Improving the quality and dissemination of reviews of clinical research. In: Lock S, ed. *The Future of Medical Journals: In Commemoration of 150 Years of the British Medical Journal*. London: BMJ, 1991; 127–46.

18 Oxman AD, Guyatt GH. Guidelines for reading literature reviews. *Can Med Assoc J* 1988; **138**:697–703.

19 Haynes RB, Mulrow CD, Huth EJ, Altman DG, Gardner MJ. More informative abstracts revisited. *Ann Intern Med* 1990; **113**:69–76.

20 Bulpitt CJ. A risk–benefit analysis for the treatment of hypertension. *Postgrad Med J* 1993; **69**:764–74.

21 Howard PA. Treating isolated systolic hypertension in the elderly. *Ann Pharmacother* 1994; **28**:367–73.

22 Sever P, Beevers G, Bulpitt C et al. Management guidelines in essential hypertension: report of the second working party of the British Hypertension Society. *Br Med J* 1993; **306**:983–7.

23 Guidelines subcommittee. 1993 guidelines for the management of mild hypertension. *Hypertension* 1993; **22**:392–403.

24 Joint National Committee of Detection, Evaluation, and Treatment of high blood pressure: the fifth report. *Ann Intern Med* 1993; **153**:154–208.

25 Antman EM, Lau J, Kupelnick B, Mosteller F, Chalmers TC. A comparison of results of meta-analyses of randomized controlled trials and recommendations of clinical experts. *JAMA* 1992; **268**:240–8.

26 Glass GV. Primary, secondary and meta-analysis of research. *Educat Res* 1976; **5**:3–8.

27 Haynes RB. Loose connections between peer-reviewed clinical journals and clinical practice. *Ann Intern Med* 1990; **113**:724–8.

28 Ramsay LE, Waller PC. Blood pressure response to percutaneous transluminal angioplasty for renovascular hypertension: an overview of published series. *Br Med J* 1990; **300**:569–72.

29 Dahlof B, Pennert K, Hansson L. Reversal of left ventricular hypertrophy in hypertensive patients: a meta-analysis of 109 treatment studies. *Am J Hypertens* 1992; **5**:95–110.

30 Weidmann P, Boehlen LM, de Courten M. Pathogenesis and treatment of hypertension associated with diabetes mellitus. *Am Heart J* 1993; **125**:1498–513.

31 Beto JA, Bansal VK. Quality of life in treatment of hypertension: a meta-analysis of clinical trials. *Am J Hypertens* 1992; **5**:125–33.

32 Cappuccio FP, Siant A, Strazzullo P. Oral calcium supplementation and blood pressure: an overview of randomized controlled trials. *J Hypertens* 1989; **7**:941–6.

33 Cappuccio FP, McGregor GA. Does potassium supplementation lower blood pressure? A meta-analysis of published trials. *J Hypertens* 1991; **9**:465–73.

34 Thijs L, Fagard R, Lignen P et al. A meta-analysis of outcome trials in elderly hypertensives. *J Hypertens* 1992; **10**:1103–9.

35 Collins R, Peto R, MacMahon S et al. Blood pressure, stroke, and coronary heart disease. *Lancet* 1990; **325**:827–38.

36 Dickersin K, Min Y, Meinert CL. Factors influencing publication of research results. *JAMA* 1992; **267**:374–8.

37 Easterbrook PJ, Berlin JA, Gopalan R, Matthews DR. Publication bias in clinical research. *Lancet* 1991; **337**:867–72.

38 Cook DJ, Guyatt GH, Ryan G et al. Should unpublished data be included in meta-analyses? *JAMA* 1993; **269**:2749–53.

39 Horton R. Data-proof practice. *Lancet* 1993; **342**:1499.

40 Light RJ, Pillemar DB. *Summing Up: the Science of Reviewing Research*. Cambridge, Massachusetts: Harvard University Press, 1984.

41 Vandenbroucke JP. Passive smoking and lung cancer: a publication bias? *Br Med J* 1988; **296**:391–2.

42 Dickersin K, Berlin JA. Meta-analysis: state-of-the science. *Epidemiol Rev* 1992; **14**:154–76.

43 Berlin JA, Laird NM, Sacks MS et al. A comparison of statistical methods for combining event rates from clinical trials. *Stat Med* 1989; **8**:141–51.

44 L'Abbe KA, Detsky AS, O'Rourke K. Meta-analysis in clinical research. *Ann Intern Med* 1987; **107**:224–33.

45 Gelber RD, Coates AS, Goldhirsch A. Meta-analysis: the fashion for summing up evidence. *Ann Oncol* 1991; **2**:461–8.

46 Gelber RD, Coates AS, Goldhirsch A. Meta-analysis: the fashion for summing up evidence. *Ann Oncol* 1991; **3**:683–91.

47 SHEP Cooperative Research Group. Prevention of stroke by anti-hypertensive drug treatment in older persons with isolated systolic hypertension. Final results of the Systolic Hypertension in the Elderly Program. *JAMA* 1991; **266**:3255–64.

48 Gadamer HG. *Reason in the Age of Science*. Cambridge, Massachusetts: MIT Press, 1992.

49 Haynes RB. Where's the meat in clinical journals. *ACP Journal Club* 1993; November/December: A22–A23.

50 Kassirer JP, Kopelman RI. *Learning Clinical Reasoning*. Baltimore: Williams and Wilkins, 1991.

51 Slevin ML. Quality of life: philosophical question or clinical reality? *Br Med J* 1992; **305**:466–9.

52 Guyatt GH, Kellner JL, Jaeschke R, Rosenbloom D, Adachi JD. The n-of-1 randomized controlled trial: clinical usefulness. *Ann Intern Med* 1990; **293**:99.

53 Larson EB, Ellsworth AJ, Oas J. Randomized clinical trials in single patients during a 2-year period. *JAMA* 1993; **270**:2708–12.

54 Howson C, Urbach P. *Scientific Reasoning: the Bayesian Approach*. Chicago: Open Court, 1993.

55 Elijovich F, Laffer CL. Bayesian analysis supports use of ambulatory blood pressure monitors for screening. *Hypertension* 1992; **19**(suppl 2):268–72.

56 Blinowska A, Chatellier G, Wojtasik A, Bernier J. Diagnostica – a Bayesian decision – aid system – applied to hypertension diagnosis. *IEEE Trans Biomed Engin* 1993; **40**:230–5.

57 Freedman LS, Spiegelhalter DJ. Application of Bayesian statistics to decision making during a clinical trial. *Stat Med* 1992; **11**:23–35.

58 Greenhouse JB. On some applications of Bayesian methods in cancer clinical trials. *Stat Med* 1992; **11**:37–53.

59 Lewis RJ, Wears RL. An introduction to the Bayesian analysis of clinical trials. *Ann Emerg Med* 1993; **22**:115–23.

60 Rescher N. *Peirce's Philosophy of Science.* Notre Dame: University of Notre Dame Press, 1978.

Index